Treating Eczema and Neurodermatitis with Chinese Herbal Medicine

by the same author

Treating Acne and Rosacea with Chinese Herbal Medicine
Sabine Schmitz
Foreword by Dan Bensky
ISBN 978 1 78775 227 6
eISBN 978 1 78775 228 3

Treating Psoriasis with Chinese Herbal Medicine
Sabine Schmitz
Foreword by Steve Clavey
ISBN 978 1 78775 349 5
eISBN 978 1 78775 350 1

of related interest

Treating Insomnia with Chinese Medicine
A Synthesis of Clinical Experience
Yoann Birling
Foreword by Jane Lyttleton
ISBN 978 1 83997 230 0
eISBN 978 1 83997 231 7

**Chinese Medicine and the Management of
Hypermobile Ehlers-Danlos Syndrome**
A Guide for Practitioners
Paula Bruno Ph.D., L.Ac.
ISBN 978 1 83997 498 4
eISBN 978 1 83997 499 1

Treating Eczema and Neurodermatitis with Chinese Herbal Medicine

Sabine Schmitz

Foreword by Z'ev Rosenberg

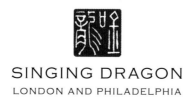

SINGING DRAGON

LONDON AND PHILADELPHIA

First published in Great Britain in 2025 by Singing Dragon,
an imprint of Jessica Kingsley Publishers
Part of John Murray Press

1

Disclaimer: The information contained in this book is not intended to replace
the services of trained medical professionals or to be a substitute for medical
advice. The complementary therapy described in this book may not be suitable for
everyone to follow. You are advised to consult a doctor before embarking on any
complementary therapy programme and on any matters relating to your health, and
in particular on any matters that may require diagnosis or medical attention.

A CIP catalogue record for this title is available from the
British Library and the Library of Congress

ISBN 978 1 78775 230 6
eISBN 978 1 78775 231 3

Printed and bound in China by Leo Paper Products

Jessica Kingsley Publishers' policy is to use papers that are natural, renewable and recyclable
products and made from wood grown in sustainable forests. The logging and manufacturing
processes are expected to conform to the environmental regulations of the country of origin.

Singing Dragon
Carmelite House
50 Victoria Embankment
London EC4Y 0DZ

www.singingdragon.com

John Murray Press
Part of Hodder & Stoughton Limited
An Hachette UK Company

For my husband. I thought it was time to dedicate one of my books to you.

In Buddhism, the First Noble Truth is the idea that everyone suffers and that suffering is part of the world. Now that I have been working with patients for more than 30 years, I can say that I have seen diverse manifestations of suffering in life. Interestingly, I have only fully understood–not to say felt–the importance and truth of this over the past few years. I feel very fortunate to have a job with meaning and purpose, a profession with which I can alleviate the suffering of many. This makes me incredibly thankful.

I hope that you will bring the knowledge in this book to life and use it for the benefit of your patients, because that is exactly what it is for: to use TCM to relieve the suffering of others for a better and healthier life!

Yours, Sabine

Contents

Foreword

FROM THE BEGINNINGS of humankind, dermatological disorders have afflicted our ancestors. The Han Dynasty medical classics such as the *Sùwèn* 素問, *Língshū* 靈樞 and *Shāng Hán Lùn* 傷寒論 all mention specific skin ailments such as boils, ulcers, rashes, flaking, itching and deep-rooted sores. Later generations developed new formulas and treatment strategies, establishing a vast pharmacopeia of herbal medicines and formulas for treating these conditions.

There has been a noticeable lack of definitive information on the Chinese medical treatment of dermatological disorders in English language textbooks. As a recognized specialty in Chinese medicine, rectifying this issues is of extreme importance, because dermatological disorders (a subdivision of *wàikē* 外科/external medicine) affects a significant percentage of our patient population. Sabine Schmitz has already published two textbooks, *Treating Psoriasis with Chinese Medicine* (2020) and *Treating Acne and Rosacea with Chinese Herbal Medicine* (2022), and continues her excellent work here in this new text *Treating Eczema and Neurodermatitis with Chinese Herbal Medicine* (2024). This is clearly the most comprehensive manual for the treatment of eczema and neurodermatitis, with voluminous information heretofore unavailable to Western practitioners in a Western language. This text contains sections on terminology (both Chinese and Western), case histories with tongue photos, and pattern differentiation by *zàngfǔ* 臟腑/viscera/bowel diagnosis. I found the section on historical sources and the evolution over time of different approaches to skin disorders to be in depth and fascinating. It is rare to find a practitioner/author like Sabine who has done the hard study in a Chinese university of Chinese medicine, and is devoted to a specialty. Her hard study and years of clinical practice have paid dividends not only in clinical success, but also in the development of a high-quality line of external applications for skin disorders, such as creams, lotions and other delivery systems for herbal medicine. This textbook also deals with the common clinical conundrum of patients on multiple medications, and how to handle herbal treatment in such cases.

And with that, I will say no more. Sabine has provided a veritable ency-clopedia on skin disorders in Chinese medicine, as deep as it is vast. This book deserves a place in the clinical library of every Chinese medical prac-titioner who treats patients with skin issues, specifically the overly common occurrence in the modern world of eczema and neurodermatitis.

Z'ev Rosenberg, L. Ac.
Xiǎoxuě 小雪
Tenth Lunar Month, 2023
San Diego, CA

Acknowledgments

P UBLISHING A BOOK without the help of other people is basically unthinkable. Yáng Zǐ, faithful friend, you deserve special recognition for your outstanding, generous, and continuous support in the translations from Chinese to English (and vice versa). My gratitude goes to you; you were always there for me. I cannot express this enough! And Fāng Yīmiào, my friend, I thank you as well for always being at my side and helping me in the collecting of pictures of the skin. Thank you both for being my "back-up" in China and always being there for me when I needed help! I would like to thank my dear colleague, Mary-Jo Bevin, for conscientiously editing and proofreading my manuscript. I appreciate your knowledge and I like it when you are strict, because this is the only way a book can get better. I love working with you! And further thanks to Vera Sugar for polishing up my adventurous English, formatting and arranging my text neatly. I would also like to thank Claire Wilson and the whole team at Singing Dragon, you are not just a wonderful and friendly team, but also incredibly professional. I really appreciate this way of working. Finally, I offer my gratitude to my beloved dermatology teacher in China, my former tutor, Professor Mǎ Lìlì. Without her guidance, my work in Chinese dermatology would certainly not be the same. But most of all, I would like to thank my husband, Hans. You are a very patient man! I'm grateful you exist.

Disclaimer

THE INFORMATION in this book is given to the best of the author's knowledge. However, the author cannot be held responsible for any error or omission. The author disclaims any responsibility for any injury and/or damage to persons or property in connection with the use of the material contained in this book. Chinese medicine is professional medicine and this is a specialist book. The author does not advocate or endorse self-medication by laypersons. Laypersons interested in availing themselves of the treatment described in this book are advised to seek out a qualified professional practitioner of Chinese medicine. It is the responsibility of the treating physician to determine the method, the dosages of each therapeutic drug, and duration of treatment for the patient.

About the Author

SABINE SCHMITZ (M. Med. TCM) is an award-winning Traditional Chinese Medicine (TCM) practitioner, author and a graduate of the Zhèjiāng Chinese Medical University in Hángzhōu, China. One of very few Western students majoring in Chinese medical dermatology, she has developed unique expertise on the subject. She runs a successful TCM practice specializing in skin diseases, gynaecological disorders, and infertility treatment in Cologne, Germany, where she works mainly with Chinese herbal medicine and acupuncture. Sabine has also authored the best-selling TCM handbook series on the most common skin diseases–the first handbook series dedicated specifically to TCM dermatology outside of China–and numerous articles on skin health and Chinese herbal medicine.

Dedicating her entire career to the treatment of patients, before completing her studies in Chinese medicine and setting up her own practice over 20 years ago, Sabine worked in hospitals, laboratories, universities, and national and international clinical research.

Sabine is also the founder and owner of CHINAMED COSMETICS®, an exciting new range of natural facial skincare products. Based on the principles of TCM and using Sabine's unique herbal formula, these natural TCM skincare products are created using only the best quality TCM herbs, carefully selected for their efficacy and nourishing properties for dry, sensitive and normal skin. Find out more at www.chinamed-cosmetics.com.

Preface

TREATING ECZEMA *and Neurodermatitis with Chinese Herbal Medicine* is the third volume in my series of Traditional Chinese Medicine (TCM) handbooks on the most common skin diseases seen in clinical practice. My TCM Dermatology series–the first of its kind published outside China, and in English–launched in 2020 with *Treating Psoriasis with Chinese Herbal Medicine*, and the second volume, *Treating Acne and Rosacea with Chinese Herbal Medicine*, was published in 2022. My aim with the series is to provide a comprehensive overview of skin diseases, as well as practical information on how to treat them with Chinese herbal medicine, to TCM practitioners across the globe.

This book details how to treat eczema and neurodermatitis (atopic eczema or atopic dermatitis) with Chinese herbal medicine, internally and externally. The initial idea for this book was to write solely about eczema from the TCM perspective. It is a skin condition that TCM practitioners, me included, see very often in our practice. There were two reasons why I decided to expand this topic: completeness and practical usability as a handbook. In TCM, eczema and neurodermatitis belong to the same category–TCM eczema–despite displaying different characteristics on the skin. Even in Western dermatology, neurodermatitis is categorized as a sub-type of eczema (I discuss sub-types in Western medicine in detail in Chapter 2). So, it seemed illogical to leave neurodermatitis out of the picture, and I have decided to include both topics. Readers can learn about their similarities and differences in internal and external treatment with Chinese herbs.

There are many reasons why I felt the need to write about individual skin diseases in such detail. During my studies in China, majoring in Chinese medical dermatology, I struggled to find any literature in English that dealt with individual topics from a TCM perspective–including dermatology. This meant that, as a Westerner, I had to spend hours searching for books and reading literature that wasn't specific or detailed enough, and often repetitive in its superficiality. It seemed obvious to me that TCM practitioners needed specific publications in English for specific subjects.

In Western medicine there are a variety of resources that deal with a certain area or specialty. In my opinion, a medicine with more than 2500 years of expertise should also be reflected in proper publications on these subject matters. There should be books that introduce TCM practitioners to a specific topic and provide real guidance on treating patients. And the feedback I have received from readers, colleagues and even patients from all over the world seems to also corroborate this view. My handbook series therefore aims to close this gap in knowledge sharing for those that cannot read Chinese.

This is a handbook, rather than merely a textbook. This difference is crucial to my work as an author. The approach is broader and more comprehensive with regards to a particular topic. Despite the handy format of the text, the subject at hand (in this case eczema and neurodermatitis) is systematically explored, contextualized and treated in its entirety. This way, readers can access the subject in a holistic, in-depth manner. For experts, it can serve as a reference book in everyday practice.

The topics covered in this book include:

- an overview of the skin and its functions

- theoretical knowledge on the Western perception and treatment of eczema and its sub-types

- in-depth background information on the TCM perspective on eczema over the past 2000 years

- prescriptions and treatment options for all types of eczema, including neurodermatitis, and TCM syndromes

- pharmacological properties of the 15 most commonly used Chinese herbs in the treatment of eczema

- advice on diet, lifestyle, skincare and patient communication, including detailed information on relevant psychological factors that may be affecting the skin

- a complete section on how to make external applications such as washes, wet compresses or ointments

- high-quality color images of the skin and tongue for precise diagnosis

- numerous case studies for better practical understanding.

With some background knowledge of TCM and Chinese herbal medicine

assumed, this handbook helps develop diagnostic and therapeutic competence in TCM treatments of eczema and neurodermatitis. It provides up-to-
date information on these skin diseases, and guides readers through their
treatment with Chinese herbal medicine, both internally and externally. It
also helps to develop the confidence to write prescriptions and to modify
basic TCM formulas to suit individual patients.

The text is designed as a practical, easy-to-understand manual that can
be used immediately in everyday practice. It is neither a dry, standard text,
nor a listing of existing literature. In this book, I pass on the knowledge I
have gained in China and through my own experience treating complex skin
conditions with Chinese medicine for many years. And not only that, I also
provide extra practical tips, because I strongly believe that the extras that are
not necessarily part of the so-called "standard" therapy are an essential part
of successful treatment. It is the ultimate resource for practitioners to use in
clinical practice.

Introduction

S KIN DISEASES are the fourth most common of all human diseases.[1] It is estimated that they affect between 30% and 70% of individuals[2] at any given time.[3,4] A recent study found that 5.5% of the European population suffers from atopic dermatitis or eczema, making it the second most prevalent skin condition in Europe.

This data is relatively fresh. However, I dare say these trends of complex skin diseases are on the rise–at least this is what I observe daily in my own dermatological TCM practice. Without a doubt, we are living in fast-paced times; the world has changed so much during the last few years. Take the pandemic or the rising cost of living, for example. There is more strain on our health, both physical and mental. In practice, I see patients becoming increasingly tense, stressed or anxious depending on their personality type. They either develop new skin symptoms or, quite often, old processes flare up and worsen. Not only are these chronic skin conditions often difficult to treat but they also seriously affect patients' quality of life on multiple levels. Their burden is often underestimated, despite the visibility of their condition. Skin diseases that are rarely life-threatening or physically handicapping are thought not to pose much of a problem for those who experience them. For those who have lived with the consequences of skin disease, however, it is obvious that the effects are more than skin deep. Eczema is a very good example of this.

Stop for a minute and imagine: you have had eczema since early childhood. Ever since you've been conscious of it, you have been mourning for your "normal" appearance. Your skin feels painful, your whole body is itching and on top of that you often feel stigmatized because of your skin condition. All your life you have had the experience that Western dermatologists are sometimes unhelpful or dismissive. You are told, "It's only a cosmetic disorder," "It has no debilitating effects," or "You just have to live with it." Unfortunately, these utterances capture neither the severity nor the complexity of your experience. In a society where there is so much emphasis on looks and appearance, there seems to be little attention paid to feelings and the challenges you face day by day. And the same thing happens each time. The standard treatment will be given, a pure symptom-related treatment without targeting the root cause: corticosteroids (cortisone). In the best case, it will be given only externally, in the worst case as an internal medication, which of course can bring considerable side effects.[5]

That's exactly the story I keep hearing over and over again. And after a certain point, many patients become frustrated, perhaps because of the way they are being treated and/or the treatment results from conventional medicine, which are either unsatisfying or just not long-lasting. This is what causes them to look for alternative treatment options for their disease, which are gentler and most of all effective.

My aim is to break this vicious cycle: I really think that our wonderful medicine is needed more than ever! TCM, with all its possibilities, can help many, if not most patients with complex skin conditions, eczema in particular. And this is exactly what my series of TCM handbooks on the most common skin diseases is for: helping colleagues in their daily practice to deal with these diseases, and most of all, to help patients to have a better life!

About This Book

In this book I set out to address how to treat eczema with Chinese herbal medicine. Before starting to write, I considered how to structure the book for a very long time. It was not as easy as I had first thought because, during many conversations with colleagues, I discovered how different the understanding in definitions and classification of eczema are. In this book, I share my views and understanding of "TCM eczema," explained in a clear, in-depth, structured, and easy-to-understand manner.

First, I want to briefly clarify the differences between general terminology and the terminology I use in this book. The term "eczema" is widely used as an umbrella term to describe inflammatory skin diseases, and many colleagues use the terms "eczema" and "dermatitis" interchangeably. Theoretically, there is a difference: "eczema" refers to chronic disease, while "dermatitis" describes an acute process—in general, inflammatory skin reactions that are accompanied by certain symptoms, such as itching, erythema, vesicles, papules, and/or papulovesicles. In the chronic stage, dry skin, scaling, and lichenification are predominant. However, as most of these types of diseases are traditionally called eczema, I use this term throughout the book.

That brings me directly to the term "TCM eczema," which can be seen as a kind of superordinate category within Chinese medicine. According to

Western medicine, eczema and neurodermatitis both belong to the TCM category of "eczema," also called "TCM eczema." In my opinion, although they belong to the same TCM category, these are two completely different skin conditions with different visibilities and appearances of the skin. Both have unique characteristics: in Chinese, eczema is called "*shī chuāng*" (湿疮),[6] which means "wet boils" or "damp boils." What you usually see is a skin condition marked by inflammation, rash, itching, exudation and crusts. In contrast, neurodermatitis, in Chinese most commonly called "*sì wān fēng*" (四弯风), is a chronic inflammatory skin condition where severe itching, dry skin, scaling, and lichenification is predominant. It typically starts at birth or during childhood and persists in many cases into adulthood. At least this is what I see in my practice, as I mainly treat adults. Neurodermatitis[7] is synonymous with "atopic eczema" and "atopic dermatitis." I will generally use the term "neurodermatitis" throughout this book. As I've already mentioned, these conditions present different appearances of the skin and so they have different needs and ways of treatment in TCM. Figuratively: when standing at a crossing, it makes a huge difference if you go right or left. As a result, I divided the book into an *eczema* part and a *neurodermatitis* part. This book will help you differentiate the type and determine the appropriate treatment strategy.

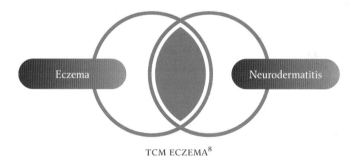

TCM ECZEMA[8]

How This Book Is Structured

In Chapter 1, I begin with background knowledge and key information on the anatomical structure and physiological functions of the skin–crucial awareness to have before treating any skin disease. This way, we can better understand how dysfunction develops, the role individual components play, and finally, how to treat chronic skin diseases successfully.

In Chapter 2, I turn your attention to the Western view of eczema, investigating causes, the most common types and current treatment options.

Chapter 3, on the other hand, is dedicated to the basics of Chinese medical dermatology, providing you with an overview of the history, developmental changes and important aspects in the correct Chinese diagnostic process of skin diseases, and presenting the available Chinese herbal treatment options for acute and chronic skin conditions in detail.

In Chapter 4, I look at the TCM perspective of eczema, giving an overview of the definition, history and treatment of eczema over the last 2000 years. It is surprising how far the wealth of experience in TCM goes back! I also describe the differentiation according to the affected areas, providing you with the different terms for eczema per appearance as well as location in TCM, and explain the classification of eczema according to the clinical presentation of the lesions. This is assisted by high-quality color images of the skin to make the differences clear—because a picture is worth a thousand words.

Chapter 5 examines the most common causes for the development of eczema. I describe the *zàng fŭ* organs that play the greatest role in the process, elaborating on the possible internal and external pathogenic factors in detail, and stress the importance of diet and food for keeping the skin healthy.

In Chapter 6, I focus specifically on the syndrome differentiation and treatment of *eczema* according to TCM, highlighting the characteristics of the skin, and explaining the prescriptions and treatment options with Chinese herbal medicine—both internally and externally—of the most common TCM syndromes seen in practice. All this is accompanied by photographs of the tongue and skin, helping you to develop the confidence to write prescriptions, and modify basic TCM formulas to suit individual patients.

Please note that I will not differentiate between the various subtypes of eczema seen in conventional medicine. In TCM, we treat what we see and it makes no difference whether it is, for example, nummular eczema, seborrheic eczema or dyshidrotic eczema. TCM is an independent field with its own framework and understanding. The TCM syndrome/pattern patients present with is more important than the subtype of eczema they have. For me, it is just not plausible to divide eczema types as conventional medicine does. What sense does it make when, ultimately, we treat the TCM syndrome? What is more important for you in this context are the modifications of the basic formulas for each pattern, enabling you to treat patients regardless of their eczema subtype. However, I make an exception and include extra information on contact eczema in Chapter 6, because the two TCM syndromes I am describing in this context are predominantly found in this type of eczema. I have also added an extra paragraph about the four main TCM syndromes of infantile eczema, because I describe a special TCM syndrome that mainly occurs in children, as well as how the treatment of children differs to adults.

The next big section, Chapters 7 and 8, are solely dedicated to *neuro-dermatitis (ND)*. In Chapter 7, I describe the decisive characteristics of this skin condition, its origin according to conventional medicine, and give an overview of the definition according to TCM and the different stages. Following that, I will discuss the most common causes for the development of ND according to TCM in detail, wherein I will be elaborating the aspect of "fetal toxicity" in particular in great detail. Finally, I also include a complete section on emotions and other psychological factors that can affect ND patients to keep in mind, because often this is neglected in training and education.

In Chapter 8, I focus specifically on the syndrome differentiation according to TCM and treatment of ND with Chinese herbal medicine, both internally and externally. The structure is the same as that of the section on eczema: I describe very precisely the characteristics of the skin, and the representative formulas of the most common TCM syndromes seen in my practice, accompanied by high-quality color images of the tongue and skin. I discuss patient education, skincare, dietary, and lifestyle advice, as well as the course and prognosis of the treatment of ND, to conclude this chapter.

Chapter 9, I call "Modern Pharmacological Research," in which I explore the pharmacological properties of the 15 most commonly-used Chinese herbs in the treatment of eczema and neurodermatitis. This background knowledge on the chemical constituents and quality of Chinese herbs is very beneficial when talking to your patients, explaining the mechanisms of action in a language they understand.

In Chapter 10, "Preventive Healthcare: Dietary, Lifestyle and Skincare Advice; Patient Communication," I talk about foods that should be avoided, and provide preferable alternatives. In addition, I share information on healthy eating habits and other practical tips on lifestyle, skin care, patient communication and the use of herbs during pregnancy. In Chapter 11, "Useful Advice on the Practical Application of Chinese Herbs," I answer the most frequently asked questions on taking Chinese herbal decoctions.

And finally, following the tradition of my previous books, you will also find a whole chapter with numerous case studies of eczema and neuro-dermatitis for better practical understanding in Chapter 12, and detailed information on how to make external applications such as washes, wet compresses or ointments at the end of this book in Appendix 1.

My hope is that this book will provide you with ideas and profound knowledge about understanding and treating *eczema* and *neurodermatitis* with Chinese herbal medicine, and better prepare you to deal with patients who have often had these complex skin conditions their whole lives. I am convinced that with TCM we can make many people's lives healthier and happier by improving and keeping their skin condition stable. Eczema and neurodermatitis are complex skin diseases, but they are definitely treatable with TCM in a gentle, effective and safe way. Never forget that and be confident!

This book is easy to understand and just as easy to navigate in day-to-day practice. You may wish to use it as a source of information in your clinical practice or to expand on existing knowledge. However, the one thing my book should do is bring you joy and self-confidence in our wonderful medicine, TCM!

Endnotes

1 Flohr, C. and Hay, R. (2015) "Putting the burden of skin diseases on the global map." *British Journal of Dermatology 184*, 189–190.

2 Hay, R.J. et al. (2014) "The global burden of skin disease in 2010: An analysis of the prevalence and impact of skin conditions." *The Journal of Investigative Dermatology 134*, 6, 1527–1534.

3 Richard, M., Paul, C., Nijsten, T., Gisondi, P. et al. (2022) "Prevalence of most common skin diseases in Europe: A population-based study." *Journal of the European Academy of Dermatology and Venereology 36*, 1088–1096.

4 Other prevalent conditions include fungal skin infections (8.9%) and acne (5.4%).

5 Yasir, M., Goyal, A., and Sonthalia, S. (2022) *Corticosteroid Adverse Effects.* Treasure Island, FL: StatPearls Publishing. Available from: www.ncbi.nlm.nih.gov/books/NBK531462.

6 *Pīnyīn* will be named first for all Chinese terms throughout the book, then Chinese. This should make it more accessible for all those who do not speak Chinese.

7 In German: Neurodermitis.

8 Source: Sabine Schmitz.

1

The Skin

THIS CHAPTER PROVIDES vital background knowledge and key information for those specializing in skin diseases, or regularly treating skin conditions. Before treating any skin disease, it is crucial to know the anatomical structure and functions of the skin. This way, we can better understand how dysfunction develops, the role individual components play and, finally, how to treat chronic skin diseases successfully. This knowledge is also an advantage for explaining processes and mechanisms to patients. All this information not only serves us, but ultimately our patients.

This overview may contain new information for you, it may give you a better understanding of the skin, or perhaps simply reinforce and complete existing knowledge.

The Anatomical Structure of the Skin

Did you know that, with a surface area of 1.5–2 m², the skin is our largest organ? It is also the heaviest, with its weight ranging from 3.5 to 10 kg, depending on the size of the person. When fatty tissue is included, it can weigh as much as 20 kg.

It is also the most vulnerable organ—and its vulnerability is clearly visible. This is one of the reasons why patients are often frustrated or even depressed when they experience changes to their skin. Many patients feel uncomfortable and ashamed, particularly if a skin disease is located on the face, as is very often the case.

The skin is the boundary between the individual and the outside world. It is our first line of defense, the body's primary barrier against microbial pathogens—it protects us every day. It also contains adnexal structures such as hair, nails, and sweat glands, as well as vessels, nerves, melanocytes, and the skin-associated immune system.

The skin has three layers: the epidermis, the dermis, and the subcutaneous fatty region. Each layer performs specific tasks, as described below.

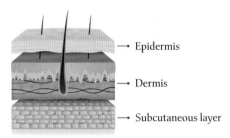

Epidermis

Dermis

Subcutaneous layer

THE THREE LAYERS OF THE SKIN[1]

Epidermis

The epidermis, relatively thin and tough, is the outermost of the three layers that make up the skin. It acts as the shield for the body. The epidermis is composed of multi-layered keratinized, stratified squamous epithelium which, as proliferation tissue, is subject to constant renewal. The epidermis has many nerves, but no blood vessels of its own. It is entirely nourished by the underlying dermis.

From the inside to the outside, the five layers of the epidermis include:[2]

- Stratum basale, also known as stratum germinativum: A layer with cuboidal to columnar mitotically active stem cells that are constantly producing keratinocytes. This layer also contains melanocytes, which synthesize the pigment melanin, the main photo-protective factor, which also gives our skin its color.

- Stratum spinosum, also called prickle cell layer: Keratinocytes are connected by spiky intercellular bridges (desmosomes).

- Stratum granulosum, or granular layer: A thin cell layer of diamond shaped keratinocytes (granule cell) containing fine granules.

- Stratum lucidum: The undermost cell layer of the stratum corneum. Cells appear visually denser, palmoplantar particularly pronounced.

- Stratum corneum: The outermost layer of the epidermis, also known as corneocytes, is the final outcome of keratinocyte maturation. This layer consists of flattened dead cells, relatively densely packed, with no nuclei or cell organelle.

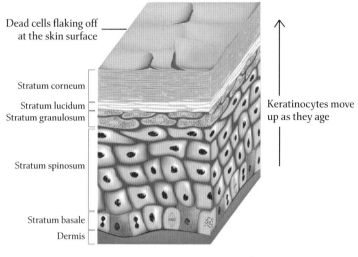

Dead cells flaking off at the skin surface

Stratum corneum
Stratum lucidum
Stratum granulosum

Stratum spinosum

Stratum basale
Dermis

Keratinocytes move up as they age

THE ANATOMY OF THE EPIDERMIS[3]

Keratinocytes are the predominant cell type of the epidermis and originate in the basal layer. The turnover time from the stratum basale to the stratum granulosum is usually about two to three weeks. From the stratum granulosum to the stratum corneum it usually takes another two weeks. The epidermis varies most in thickness, and within this layer, the dead keratinocytes are our first immune defence. So, what we actually see on the surface of our body are dead horn cells. One could also say that this makes the concept of beauty relative.

Other cell types contained in the epidermis include Langerhans[4] cells, the skin's first-line defenders. They play a significant role in antigen presentation by uptaking the antigens from the skin via phagocytosis and transporting them to the lymph nodes. The epidermis also contains Merkel cells. These neuroendocrine cells serve a sensory function as mechanoreceptors for light touch and are mainly found in sensitive skin regions—for example, in fingertips, the tip of the nose, and also in the palms, soles, and oral and genital mucosa.

When talking about the epidermis one must also mention the natural skin surface potential of hydrogen (pH). But what is it exactly? The pH is a protective acid mantle (protective skin mantle) of the stratum corneum, which forms a resistant layer against any damaging influences. The pH on the surface of the skin is below 5 on average, which is beneficial for its resident flora. An acidic pH (4–4.5) keeps our skin healthy: it prevents the growth of bacteria and fungi, and thus protects the outer layers of the skin. In contrast, with an alkaline pH (8–9), important skin fats required for the protective acid mantle can no longer accumulate. The skin loses water, dries out, and is no longer able to offer sufficient protection.

Dermis

The dermis is the layer beneath the epidermis and, as a dense connective tissue, it is the major structural component of the skin. In the dermis, the predominant cells are fibroblasts. They secrete elastin and collagen fibers that form a dense extracellular matrix, giving the skin its flexibility and strength. The dermis houses nerve endings, sweat glands and sebaceous glands, hair follicles, blood and lymph vessels, as well as mast cells. Blood vessels nourish the dermis, while lymphatic fluid is drained through the lymph vessels to the lymph nodes. Blood vessels also help regulate temperature by dilating or contracting, which is why the skin pales when a person feels cold and reddens when he or she flushes.

In summary, the dermis provides elasticity and firmness of the skin; its vessels supply the epidermis with nutrients; and it is responsible for temperature regulation and protection against pressure, pain and cold.

Subcutis (Hypodermis)

Between the dermis and the muscle fascia lies the subcutaneous tissue, a layer of loose connective tissue and fat tissue, that serves as a shifting layer between the skin itself and the connective tissue sheath (adventitia), which delineates the muscles of the musculoskeletal system.

The subcutis helps insulate the body from heat and cold, provides protective padding for shock absorption, and allows the storage of fat for energy reserves. The fat remains in adipose (fat) cells, held together by fibrous tissue. It is surrounded by connective tissue and some skin appendages like hair follicles, sensory neurons, and blood vessels. The fatty layer varies in thickness, from very thin on the eyelids to several centimeters on the abdomen and gluteal region in some people.

The Physiological Functions of the Skin

The skin carries great responsibility for our well-being. It protects us every single day. It literally holds us together. This is why it is essential to treat it well. A big problem is excessive personal hygiene, such as showering too often or with water that is too hot, using excessive amounts of shower gel, or, even worse, shower gel which contains chemicals, irritating substances, and perfumes. Visits to a solarium or using chemicals to make the skin look tanned, which might have a positive visual effect at first, are not a good way to take care of our skin in the long term. These habits harm our skin, which then is no longer able to sustain its natural function as a barrier: the skin becomes irritated, inflamed, or so dry that it can no longer be nourished. Therefore, patients often need to reconsider their skin routines. It can be helpful to advise them to use mild and pH-neutral shower gels without perfume—the best choice for sensitive skin anyway. Most of all, however, we need to create awareness that not only is the skin highly sensitive to internal and external factors, but its functions as an organ are crucial for our well-being.

As the interface between the body and the environment, the skin protects the body by performing several vital physiological functions:

Protection
Due to the keratinization of the epithelium and glandular secretions, the skin forms a stable barrier to water, invasion by microorganisms, mechanical, chemical, and thermal trauma, and damage from UV light.

Immune Response
The skin is the first site of immunological defense via the action of the Langerhans cells in the epidermis, which are part of the adaptive (acquired) immune system and are activated when the tissue is under attack by invading pathogens. Memory T cells patrol the skin and are capable of responding to repeated attack from the outside by supporting the reaction of the monocytes and mast cells. Memory T cells are T cells that remain long after an infection has been eliminated. They have learned how to fight off an invader by "remembering" the strategy used to defeat previous infections. This mechanism is particularly important in gaining life-long immunity to infections such as scarlet fever, rubella, mumps, or chickenpox.

Temperature Control
Temperature control is the process of keeping the body at a constant of 37°C. Sweat regulation and skin blood flow are both essential for maintaining the body's core temperature. Sweating begins almost precisely at a skin temperature of 37°C and increases rapidly as it rises above this value, regulated

by neural feedback mechanisms which operate primarily through the hypo-thalamus.[5] If skin temperature drops below 37°C, a variety of responses are initiated to conserve heat within the body and to increase heat production. These include vasoconstriction to decrease the flow of heat to the skin and the cessation of sweating.

Water Resistance

The skin also acts as a barrier to water–an essential function as it prevents the body from losing essential nutrients and minerals. Skin barrier function depends on the lipid-enriched stratum corneum cell membrane in the epidermis.

Sensation

Another important role of the skin is detecting the different sensations of heat, cold, touch, pressure, vibration, tissue injury, and pain. Sensation is felt through a rich network of nerve endings with a variety of sensory receptors in the dermis.

Synthesis of Vitamin D

Vitamin D occupies a special position among vitamins, since it is both supplied through the diet[6] (endogenous) and formed by humans themselves through UVB light exposure (exogenous sunlight). That's why some call it the "sunlight vitamin." It is crucial for building and maintaining strong bones and teeth.

When human skin is exposed to sunlight, the solar UVB light penetrates through the epidermis, where pre-vitamin D3 (cholecalciferol) is formed. Further metabolic processes in the liver and kidney result in production of the biologically active form of vitamin D, called calcitriol. Calcitriol increases the blood calcium level by promoting the absorption of dietary calcium from the gastrointestinal tract into the blood. It also stimulates the release of calcium from the bones, therefore affecting the human bone's mineral density and bone turnover. In addition, the body can convert vitamin D3 into a storage form called calcifediol, primarily located in muscle and fatty tissue. This is particularly important when, in winter, the solar radiation in our latitudes is too weak for sufficient vitamin D production in the skin, and the body can utilize the vitamin D3 stored in the form of calcifediol, if available.

Vitamin D deficiency can cause osteomalacia, called rickets when it occurs in children, or other musculoskeletal symptoms, such as bone pain, myalgias, and generalized weakness in adults. Optimal nutrition and outdoor activities for sufficient sunlight exposure are both important for adequate vitamin levels and to prevent chronic illness.

Absorption and Excretion

Although the skin is a waterproof barrier, certain drugs and remedies can be administered through the skin by means of ointments, adhesive patches or essential oils. The process by which these substances can penetrate through the skin's layers, the hair follicles and sweat glands is called "percutaneous" absorption: per = via, cutaneous = relating to the skin. The extent of penetration is limited by the skin's health and condition, of course.

The skin also serves as an excretory organ, disposing of waste material and toxins. Waste substances are expelled from the body through the skin via the sweat glands and normally take the form of salts, carbon dioxide, urea, and ammonia.

Communication

Finally, a word about the function of communication, as the skin also communicates, albeit unconsciously and perhaps often unintentionally. Just think of paling in fear or fright or blushing in shame as an expression of unconscious (vegetative) reactions. This is also the reason why the skin is often called "the mirror of the soul."

If all these tasks are performed properly, our skin will be healthy and resilient. We are warm and protected. The complexion looks bright and there are no pathological changes. We simply look good. However, these functions are all affected by the structural changes in the skin with ageing and, after middle age, most functions are reduced, some by as much as 50–60%.[7]

Endnotes

1   Source: Adobe Stock.

2   You will find that, if you know Latin terms, many of the names of the layers and/or the cells are self-explanatory.

3   Source: Adobe Stock.

4   Please don't confuse the Langerhans cells with the so-called islets of Langerhans located within the pancreas. These are two completely different types of cells with different functions.

5   The hypothalamus is an important "control centre" of our body. It is an area of the brain in the interbrain (diencephalon) and it is located below (= hypo) the thalamus. It contains not only control mechanisms for water, salt balance, and blood pressure, for instance, but also the key temperature sensors. It is also an important inceptor within the endocrine system because it regulates the timing and quantity of hormonal formation.

6   Such as oily fish, variably fortified foods (milk, juices, margarines, yogurts, cereals, and soy), and oral supplements. Source: Kennel, K.A., Drake, M.T., and Hurley, D.L. (2010) "Vitamin D deficiency in adults: When to test and how to treat." *Mayo Clinic Proceedings 85*, 8, 752–758.

7   Cerimele, D., Celleno, L., and Serri, F. (1990) "Physiological changes in ageing skin." *British Journal of Dermatology 122*, 13–20.

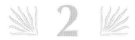

The Western View of Eczema

B EFORE GOING INTO more detail, a short reminder of the use of terms in this book: As already mentioned, the term "eczema" is widely used synonymously with the term "dermatitis." I will generally use the term "eczema" throughout this book.

The Definition and Etiology of Eczema According to Western Medicine

Eczema is an inflammatory, non-infectious disease of the skin. It has three stages: acute, subacute, and chronic. During the acute stage, it is clinically characterized by itching, erythema (abnormal reddening of the skin), vesicles (small fluid-filled blisters on the skin), papules (small raised solid lesions of the skin) and/or papulovesicles (presence of both papules and vesicles). In this stage, the skin lesions easily can become infected when left untreated. Subacute stage of eczema is marked by mild to moderate inflammation that may come and go. In the chronic stage, dry skin, scaling and lichenification are predominant. The term lichenification refers to the process by which the skin becomes hardened and leathery, usually the result of constant irritation due to scratching and rubbing. The epidermis becomes hypertrophied (overgrown), resulting in thickened skin with a leathery bark-like appearance, and characteristic features of thickening, hyperpigmentation, and exaggerated skin lines.

Microscopic examination (histology) reveals the following features:

- Acanthosis: an enlargement of the epidermis in the stratum spinosum

- Spongiotic tissue reaction: intracellular oedema within the epidermis

- Hyperkeratosis: thickening of the stratum corneum

- Parakeratosis: abnormal retention of nuclei in the stratum corneum due to incomplete maturation of epidermal keratinocytes

- The dermis shows a lymphocyte dominated infiltration.

The Most Common Types of Eczema

Eczema is very common in our modern fast-paced society. The most common types of eczema are the irritant-toxic contact eczema, allergic contact eczema, neurodermatitis (also known by the terms: atopic eczema, atopic dermatitis) and seborrheic eczema. Let's take a closer look at these different forms.

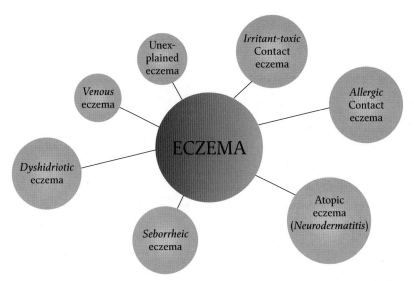

THE MOST COMMON TYPES OF ECZEMA ACCORDING TO WESTERN MEDICINE[1]

Irritant-Toxic Contact Eczema

This type of eczema is also called "irritant-toxic contact dermatitis." It results when the epidermal protective mechanisms are overwhelmed. This nonallergic skin reaction is provoked by contact with potential irritants like water, detergents, soaps, alkalis, acids, oils, and other chemicals, and most commonly occurs on the hands. Of course, the extent of the reaction depends on the dose and the exposure time. This type of eczema is very common in the household and also plays a major role in certain workplaces as well.

Different Types of Irritant-Toxic Contact Eczema

- Acute toxic contact eczema: provoked by highly toxic substances, such as alkalis and acids.

- Cumulative toxic contact eczema: the continuous exposure to substances that are intrinsically low in toxicity, such as water, surfactants or body secretions.

- Napkin dermatitis: occurs in infants but also in incontinent patients, due to the permanent exposure to urine and/or stool.

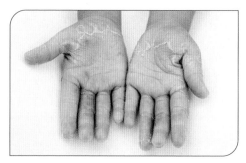

WORK-RELATED CONTACT ECZEMA ON THE HANDS (LATEX ALLERGY)[2]

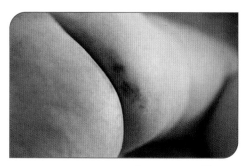

NAPKIN DERMATITIS (DIAPER RASH)[3]

Allergic Contact Eczema

Allergic contact eczema, also called allergic contact dermatitis, occurs when an allergen triggers a T-cell[4] mediated immune reaction in the skin. It usually affects only the area that came into contact with the allergen, such as contact with nickel, fragrances, hair dyes, or preservatives, for instance. It may also be triggered by substances that are taken internally, including foods, spices, medicine, or medical or dental procedures, just to name a few. In this case it is called "systemic contact dermatitis." However, contact allergies occur predominantly from an allergen on the skin surface rather than from internal sources or food. It is also not uncommon that, prior to the reaction, patients may have been in contact with the allergen for years without it causing any dermatitis. As soon as the allergic substance has been identified, general prevention usually includes avoiding the irritants and allergens.

Two Types of Allergic Contact Eczema

- Acute allergic contact eczema: a relatively rapid development of erythema, followed by formation of itchy vesicles and papulovesicles, which can burst. Erosions then develop, which are covered by drying secretions (crusts). Healing occurs after allergen abstinence.

- Chronic allergic contact eczema: if exposure to the contact allergen continues, the eczema becomes chronic. Vesicles will regress, erythema and hyperkeratoses dominate, rhagades (cracks or fissures in the skin) and lichenifications develop.

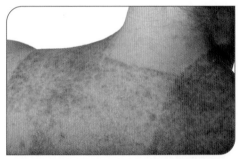

ALLERGIC SKIN REACTION TO PLASTER (PLASTER ALLERGY)[5]

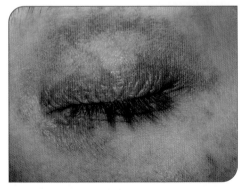

ALLERGIC CONTACT ECZEMA CAUSED BY COSMETICS[6]

Atopic Eczema

Atopic[7] eczema, also called atopic dermatitis, neurodermatitis atopica or colloquial neurodermatitis (ND) is classified as the most common inflammatory skin disease affecting up to 20% of children and adolescents worldwide, and can significantly decrease the patient's quality of life.[8] It is speculated that the prevalence has consistently increased over the last four decades in Europe.[9] I would like to delve into this type in more detail, as I see it very often in practice and if you treat skin conditions, you will too. While this condition is known by several names as mentioned above, I will generally refer to it as neurodermatitis or ND in this text.[10]

Similar to hay fever and allergic asthma, ND is an atopic disorder characterized by the production of allergen-specific immunoglobulin E antibodies (IgE). Briefly explained, if a person has an allergy, their immune system overreacts to an allergen by producing IgE antibodies. IgE stimulates mast cells and basophils to release biologically active chemicals, causing an allergic reaction. Within seconds or minutes, the chemicals give rise to symptoms in the nose, lungs, throat, or on the skin.

Four pathogenic factors appear to be relevant in the pathogenesis in conventional medicine:

- Impaired epidermal barrier, which seems to be the leading cause
- Impaired innate immunity[11]
- Infection with Staphylococcus aureus[12]
- Altered immunity with elevated skin and serum levels of IgE.

We all know patients with ND. They usually come with a long list of allergies and react to literally everything. As a rough guide, the main diagnostic features of this skin disease are: [13]

- severe itching (pruritus)
- very dry and scaly skin
- lichenification
- chronic relapsing dermatitis.

A short note on lichenification: ND can also be called *lichen simplex chronicus*. This term describes nothing other than thickening of the skin with variable scaling, arising secondary to repetitive scratching. It is definitely not a primary process. While the use of this term is extremely rare, it is always good to know these fine details.

ND usually appears for the first time between ages zero to two, progresses in episodes, and can vary in appearance depending on the age of the affected person. Due to itching and visible skin rashes, ND can severely affect the psyche and quality of life of those affected. The disease is both aggravated by stress and is itself a major source of stress, for children and adults alike. Anyone who sees these patients in their practice knows this. The emotional component is discussed in detail in Chapter 7.

Typical Locations of Neurodermatitis (Predilection Sites)
Experience shows that there are age-dependant differences in the location of the lesions, which I would like to summarize below.

- Infants/small children: skin eruptions usually initially develop on the cheeks, forehead, arms and legs.

- Adolescents: after puberty, eruptions are more likely to develop on the neck, backs of hands and feet, elbow creases and backs of knees.

- Adults: primarily involvement of trunk including chest and arms, but also backs of hands and feet, and neck.

The Occurrence and Risk Factors of Neurodermatitis
European trends remain in line with those reported from global studies, including the following:[14]

- ND is more prevalent in overcrowded urban areas.

- Symptoms are worsened in cold or temperate climate.

- Significantly more frequent occurrence of ND is reported in children compared to adults.[15]

A higher prevalence of ND is associated with the following risk factors:[16]

- urban environment

- higher socioeconomic status

- higher level of family education

- family history of ND

- females six years and older

- smaller family size.[17]

We will explore neurodermatitis in detail in Chapter 7, since many patients seek other treatment options to help their skin and TCM can help very well here. Their path of suffering is often long, characterized by cortisone creams, psychotherapy and setbacks.

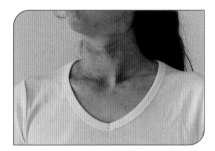 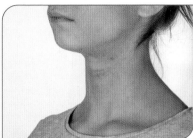

NEURODERMATITIS ON THE NECK AND DÉCOLLETÉ[18]

Seborrheic Eczema

Seborrheic eczema, or seborrheic dermatitis, is a chronic inflammation of the skin that occurs in episodes and is accompanied by greasy scaling. Where does the name come from? Seborrhea means hyperfunction of the sebaceous glands; eczema is an inflammation of the skin. Once we understand the name, it makes sense that the foci of inflammation occur in the areas of the skin rich in sebaceous glands. Microbial factors such as yeast fungi are often involved.[19] The composition of the skin lipids and the skin flora is thought to play a crucial role in the pathogenesis of the disease, but this has not been fully clarified to date. It is a non-contagious skin disease that is harmless in most cases.

Clinically, seborrheic eczema manifests as plaques associated with reddening of the skin, covered by greasy, yellowish and symmetrically arranged scales. In addition, seborrheic skin may also be accompanied by itching. In my practice, patients mainly show up with lesions on the scalp and face. It is important for me to mention here that patients frequently report that they use dandruff shampoos. I have observed that this does not improve the condition on the head but actually worsens it. Many chemical substances really do not contribute to an improvement. Talk to your patients about this!

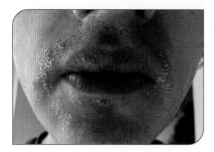
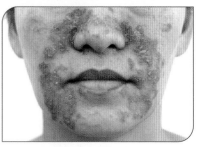

SEBORRHEIC ECZEMA ON THE FACE   20

Vesicular Hand Dermatitis, or Dyshidrotic Eczema

This is a less common type of eczema, but one which I often see in my practice. That is why I would like to mention it here. In China, I have often seen it classified as "sweat acne."

Vesicular hand dermatitis is also known as dyshidrotic eczema, palmoplantar eczema, or pompholyx from the Greek word meaning bubble or blister.[21] It involves the fingers, hands, and, although named "hand dermatitis," sometimes also the feet. In this case, it is called palmoplantar eczema. It is an acute type of eczema, characterized by tiny vesicles or blisters. The blisters cause itching or a burning sensation. Blisters usually peel away and the skin then appears red, like raw skin (especially immediately after the peeling); dry with painful fissures (cracks). Aggravating factors include emotional stress, hyperhidrosis, weather changes, atopy, mycosis, irritants, contact allergens, and systemic exposure to metals, drugs, and food.[22] The cause is often unknown, making the condition challenging to treat. Patients need to be aware of secondary bacterial infections, which will cause pain, swelling, and pustules on the affected areas of the skin, on the hands and/or feet.

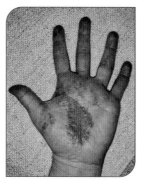
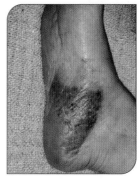

DYSHIDROTIC ECZEMA ON THE HANDS AND FEET

Other Types of Eczema
Nummular Eczema

Nummular eczema, also known as *discoid eczema* and *nummular dermatitis*, is characterized by round or oval-shaped lesions, often itchy and sometimes oozing patches. The name originates from the Latin word *nummus*, which means "coin."[23]

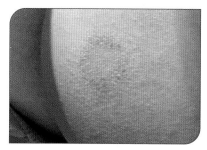
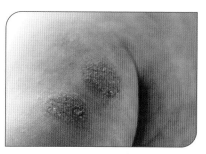

NUMMULAR ECZEMA ON BUTTOCKS   NUMMULAR ECZEMA ON ARMS [24]

Venous Eczema

Venous eczema, also called stasis dermatitis, gravitational dermatitis, or venous stasis dermatitis, happens when there is venous insufficiency, or poor circulation in the lower legs. Venous insufficiency happens when the valves in leg veins that help push blood back to the heart weaken and leak fluid. As a consequence, water and blood cells pool in the lower legs and put pressure on the skin.

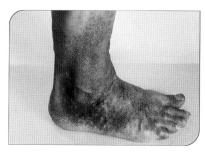
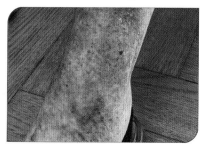

25   VENOUS ECZEMA ON THE LOWER LEG

Unexplained Eczema

In these cases, the cause of eczema remains unknown. Note: It is advised that such patients should be tested, questioned, and re-examined to hopefully find out the possible cause of the eczema.

CLINICAL NOTE: Please keep in mind that in conventional medicine it is often difficult to diagnose the type of eczema clinically. There are so many triggers, such as atopy, irritation, sensitization or dryness which all produce quite similar changes on the skin. This makes a fundamental difference from TCM, in which the aim is to precisely target the pattern according to Chinese medicine and not the clinical type of eczema.

Psycho-Social Aspects

The skin is the mirror of the soul–this statement is probably familiar to everyone. If the skin is healthy, its function as a protective organ goes almost unnoticed. However, when problems begin to appear this has a gradual detrimental effect on the general sense of well-being. Experience proves that dermatological diseases are often associated with a troubled soul, and studies consistently confirm that the psyche has an enormous influence on skin health. We all know the popular saying "it gets under your skin." As previously mentioned, as the interface between body and soul, the skin is a crucial organ of communication. If the skin is smooth and clean, it is considered attractive and a sign of health and well-being. A visibly diseased skin, on the other hand, is often met with social rejection. Especially for sensitive patients, skin condition definitely has an impact on many interpersonal relationships.

Essentially, psychologically caused skin problems can be said to be stress-related, and we all know how much pressure and stress exists in today's society. This means that many skin diseases have important psychosocial implications for those affected, in addition to the medical ones. Neurodermatitis is a very good example of this. However, it is not only the psyche that triggers skin diseases. Conversely, changes in the skin can also have a significant influence on the personality and self-confidence of those affected. Experts call this "coping."

Although conventional medicine recognizes these mechanisms, they are often neglected in daily routine. Patients are nonchalantly prescribed medication and advised to undergo psychotherapy. They are being told that they should just relax! Whether it is due to lack of time or for the simple reason that conventional medicine works in a fundamentally different way, the consequence is that many patients feel abandoned. I hear this reported in my practice again and again. Ideally therapy starts with a conversation, and with understanding and empathy for the patient. Especially with chronic skin diseases, this is crucial. No matter which skin disease, no matter whether the psyche is the trigger or an exacerbating factor in an already existing skin disease, the emotional causes must be addressed. We as practitioners have to take time for the patient and also discuss emotions. Anything else will not lead to a satisfactory and lasting result.

Current Treatment Options in Western Medicine
Topical Treatment

In conventional dermatology, the most important pillar of therapy for eczema, irrespective of the type, are glucocorticoids, which are used topically as ointments or creams in varying strengths depending on the localization and severity. This is due to their (conventionally seen) potency in treating inflammatory skin disease. Unfortunately, with chronic use of topical glucocorticoids, patients develop side effects including cutaneous atrophy, which affects all skin compartments and compromises the barrier function of the skin. Skin atrophy following long-term use of steroids may be irreversible.[26] Hence, substances with an increased benefit–risk ratio are urgently needed and it is high time that research on new drugs focuses on safer ones.

If a fungus is detected in seborrheic eczema, for example, topical antifungal agents are used including creams, shampoos, and oral formulations. These antifungals can reduce the number of yeasts on the skin.[27] Apart from that, in my opinion, these remedies are not very effective because once again the root cause is not addressed.

Oral Treatment

Systemic glucocorticoids are very rarely used in the treatment of eczema. This is because they can cause serious side effects which can be musculoskeletal, endocrine, gastrointestinal, neuropsychiatric, cardiovascular, dermatologic, ocular or immunologic in nature.

In the case of severe itching, antihistamines may also be used. The use of traditional antihistamines has, until recently, been associated with a number of undesirable side-effects, the most troublesome being sedation.[28] Patients very often tell me that antihistamines make them feel very tired, and they struggle to maintain focus at work or when driving.

Light Therapy

If topical therapies in moderate to severe eczema do not lead to improvement, UV light therapy can be used. There are different kinds of light with different wavelengths, known as UVA (broadband) and UVB (narrowband). The major difference between broadband and narrowband is that narrow band UVB light units release a more specific, or smaller (narrow), range of ultraviolet light. Treatment of eczema nowadays mostly uses narrowband UVB phototherapy. Here the skin is only exposed to UVB rays with a wavelength of 311 to 313 nanometers.[29] However, this therapy is used mostly for adults. It is used less for children, and should be avoided in patients who have UV-sensitive dermatitis or a photo allergy. Patients should also be aware of an increased risk of developing skin cancer. Therefore, the benefit must be carefully weighed against potential risks.

Prevention

If eczema is allergic in nature, avoidance of any identified triggering factors is essential to prevent re-exposure. It must be said, however, that this is not always possible. If, for example, the irritating substance is present in the workplace, it can be difficult to just change jobs. Patients should, however, be educated regarding the presence of identified allergens. This makes them easier to avoid.

Conclusion

It seems quite clear that conventional therapy can only alleviate the symptoms of eczema for a time, without any impact on the underlying cause of the disease (proved when the symptoms of the disease reoccur after drug cessation). One might also question at what price, in terms of the side effects of many medications. And, apart from that, if emotional factors are not taken into account and the disease is not approached holistically, there will be no target-oriented, long-lasting solution.

Endnotes

1   Source: Sabine Schmitz.

2   Source: Adobe Stock.

3   Source: Adobe Stock.

4   T cell, also called T lymphocyte, is a type of leukocyte (white blood cell) that is an essential part of the immune system. They help protect the body from infection.

5   Source: Adobe Stock.

6   Source: Adobe Stock.

7   Atopic originated from the Greek term atopos, which means "unusual" and

indicates that the condition has no clear cause.

8 Kowalska-Olędzka, E., Czarnecka, M., and Baran, A. (2019) "Epidemiology of atopic dermatitis in Europe." *Journal of Drug Assessment 8*, 1, 126–128.

9 Williams, H., Stewart, A., von Mutius, E., Cookson, W., and Anderson, H.R. (2008) "International Study of Asthma and Allergies in Childhood (ISAAC) Phase One and Three Study Groups." *Journal of Allergy and Clinical Immunology 121*, 4, 947–954.

10 In Germany, we typically use the term "neurodermatitis" (in German: Neurodermitis).

11 Immunity that is present at birth and lasts a person's entire life. Innate immunity is the first response of the body's immune system to a harmful foreign substance.

12 Staphylococcus aureus is a gram-positive bacteria that causes a wide variety of clinical diseases.

13 Hanifin-Rajka criteria (HRC), 1980.

14 Kowalska-Olędzka, E., Czarnecka, M., and Baran, A. (2019). "Epidemiology of atopic dermatitis in Europe." *Journal of Drug Assessment 8*, 1, 126–128.

15 Nutten, S. (2015) "Atopic dermatitis: Global epidemiology and risk factors." *Annals of Nutrition and Metabolism 66*, Suppl 1, 8–16.

16 Kowalska-Olędzka, E., Czarnecka, M., and Baran, A. (2019). "Epidemiology of atopic dermatitis in Europe." *Journal of Drug Assessment 8*, 1, 126–128.

17 DaVeiga, S.P. (2012) "Epidemiology of atopic dermatitis: A review." *Allergy and Asthma Proceedings 33*, 3, 227–234.

18 Source: Adobe Stock.

19 Adalsteinsson, J.A., Kaushik, S., Muzumdar, S., Guttman-Yassky, E., and Ungar J. (2020) "An update on the microbiology, immunology and genetics of seborrheic dermatitis." *Experimental Dermatology 29*, 481–489.

20 Source: Adobe Stock.

21 Sobering, G. and Dika, C. (2018) "Vesicular hand dermatitis." *The Nurse Practitioner 43*, 11, 33–37.

22 Thyssen, J.P. and Menné, T. (2012) "Acute and Recurrent Vesicular Hand Dermatitis." In T. Rustemeyer, P. Elsner, S.M. John, and I.H. Maibach (eds) *Kanerva's Occupational Dermatology*. Berlin, Heidelberg: Springer.

23 Greek: noummos.

24 Source: Adobe Stock.

25 Source: Adobe Stock.

26 Baida, G., Bhalla, P., Kirsanov, K., Lesovaya, E., et al. (2015) "REDD1 functions at the crossroads between the therapeutic and adverse effects of topical glucocorticoids." *EMBO Molecular Medicine 7*, 42–58.

27 Gupta, A.K., Nicol, K., and Batra, R. (2004) "Role of antifungal agents in the treatment of seborrheic dermatitis." *American Journal of Clinical Dermatology 5*, 417–422.

28 Hindmarch, I., and Shamsi, Z. (1999) "Antihistamines: Models to assess sedative properties, assessment of sedation, safety and other side-effects." *Clinical and Experimental Allergy 29*, 133–142.

29 InformedHealth.org [Internet] (2017) Eczema: Light therapy and oral medications. Cologne, Germany: Institute for Quality and Efficiency in Health Care (IQWiG) [Updated 2019 Mar 20].

3

Overview and Basics of Chinese Dermatology

I T IS ASSUMED that the reader of this book is familiar with the foundations of Traditional Chinese Medicine (TCM). This section on the basics of TCM dermatology is primarily aimed at TCM students and beginners, or those interested in TCM medical history. Experts can, of course, skip this section. Nonetheless, the information here can be a valuable resource and refresher for everyone—TCM dermatologists, general TCM doctors, and students of TCM.

An Overview of the History of Chinese Medical Dermatology (*pí fū kē* 皮肤科)

Chinese medical dermatology draws on many centuries of experience, with detailed records of the effects of Chinese herbs and acupuncture on the condition of the skin. Comprehensive descriptions of the treatment of specific skin diseases were put down in writing by ancient scholars, and their clinical histories and treatment notes provide a depth of experience that we still utilize in our practice today. Early Chinese medical literature contains references to Chinese medical dermatology within the text. Later texts focus solely on dermatology, such as the *Wài Kē Jīng Yào* (Essence of Diagnosis and Treatment of External Diseases), written by Chén Zì-Míng in 1263. Please see below for more details of the development and documentation of Chinese dermatology.

Yet time does not stand still. A great deal of research into Chinese medicine has been conducted both inside and outside of China. In addition to clinical studies, official monographs on almost every Chinese medicinal plant are available at the European Medicines Agency (EMEA) and the

World Health Organization (WHO). These monographs provide a detailed introduction and scientific overview of the safety, efficacy, and quality control of commonly used medicinal plants in Chinese dermatology. Moreover, gathered information about chemical composition, pharmacological effects, toxicology, clinical studies, and research has been incorporated into many *Materia Medica*, the herbal textbooks used by TCM doctors worldwide.[1]

The result of this combination of rich history and modern developments is an independent and sophisticated specialty in Chinese medicine, which can be effectively employed in the treatment of many, if not most, skin diseases. This is particularly true for the most common skin problems presenting in our clinics, where the effectiveness of conventional medicine therapy is often very poor.

Developmental Changes in Chinese Dermatology

In ancient China, Chinese dermatology was a part of the general category *wài kē* 外科. Medical fields such as traumatology and surgery were also classified as a part of *wài kē* at that time. *Wài* refers to the outside of the body and comprises the skin, hair, muscles, flesh, sinews, and bones. The term *kē* means subject, branch, or field. *Wài kē*, or "external medicine," refers to the diagnosis and treatment of conditions on the exterior of the body. This includes skin conditions such as sores and abscesses, and diseases of the eye, ear, nose, and mouth. In contrast, *nèi kē* 内科 (internal medicine) refers to diseases occurring inside the body and the *nèi*, or the inside, comprising the viscera and bowels. Chinese dermatology was recognized much later in history as a separate specialty in TCM.

The following presents a short overview on the development and documentation of Chinese dermatology.

Early classical literature	Small sections dedicated to Chinese dermatology (*pí fū kē*)	• Many important doctors devoted to the study and practice of external medicine • References to external medicine scattered in medical textbooks • No independent section of medical literature
Sòng Dynasty[2] 1263	*Wài Kē Jīng Yào* (Essence of Diagnosis and Treatment of External Diseases) by Chén Zì-Míng	• First book solely focused on *wài kē* • Establishment of external medicine and traumatic surgery as independent branches of Chinese medicine

Yuán Dynasty[3] 1335	*Wài Kē Jīng Yì* (Treatment of Surgical Diseases) by Qí Dé-Zhī	▪ Compilation of the medical knowledge of external diseases prior to the Yuán dynasty ▪ Treatment of external diseases should start with regulating body's internal system considering pathogenic factors ▪ External disease arises from disharmony between yīn 阴 and yáng 阳, or stagnating qì 气 and xuè 血 ▪ Creation of new therapies, e.g., wet compresses and methods for draining pus
Míng Dynasty[4]	*Wāng Jī* (1463-1539)[5]	▪ Medical writer and clinical practitioner from Ānhuī Province south of Nánjīng
1531	*Wài Kē Lǐ Lì* (Exemplars for Applying the Principles of External Medicine)	▪ Preface: "external medicine [i.e., surgery] deals with ulcers, abscesses, sores and boils…seen on the exterior" ▪ Wāng Jī's views on *wài kē*: "surgical" doctors (TCM dermatologists). (While the term surgical doctors has been used, TCM dermatologists do not undertake surgical procedures in the sense of what modern medicine would now classify as "surgical") ▪ All external manifestations of illness have internal roots ▪ Emphasized the combination of internal treatments, i.e., herbal decoctions, and external treatments, i.e., ointments, washes, acupuncture, or moxibustion ▪ Vast number of case histories
1522-1633	*Wāng Shí-Shān Yī Shū Bā Zhǒng* (Wāng Shí-Shān's Eight Medical Books) One book of this compilation is *Shí Shān Yī Àn* (Medical Cases of Wāng Jī)	▪ Numerous cases of *wài kē* categories, e.g., itchy body, foot sores, and breast lumps[6] ▪ More than one hundred of Wāng Jī's medical cases (collected by his students and published in 1531 by Chéng Zēng, one of his disciples)
Míng and Qīng[7] Dynasties		▪ Chinese dermatology flourished with the publication of several works that presented treatment of external diseases
1604, late Míng Dynasty	Wài Kē Qǐ Xuán (Profound Insights on External Diseases) by Shēn Dǒu-Yuán	▪ Consisting of 12 volumes ▪ Considered China's first atlas of skin diseases ▪ Contains about 200 different diseases and treatments

1617	Wài Kē Zhèng Zōng (Orthodox Lineage of External Medicine) by Chén Shí-Gōng	• New therapeutic recommendations for skin diseases, including ointments • Summary of medical achievements before the Míng Dynasty • Diagnoses, therapies, medical records and prescriptions • Precise surgical procedures, e.g., removal of nasal polyps,[8] trachelorrhaphy, and cancer therapies
1665	Wài Kē Dà Chéng (Great Compendium of External Medicine) by Qí Kūn	• Chinese dermatology became increasingly sophisticated and numerous specialist books were published, such as the Wài Kē Dà Chéng for example
1740	Wài Kē Zhèng Zhì Quán Shēng Jí (Complete Compendium of Patterns and Treatments in External Medicine) by Wáng Wéi-Dé	• A summary of 40 years clinical experience • In the treatment of sores: division into yáng-type (red, excessive) and yīn-type (white, cold, qì and blood stagnation) pattern • Treating yīn-type patterns by activating the yáng and supplementing qì and blood • Many warming and blood stasis dispelling formulas
1831	Wài Kē Zhèng Zhì Quán Shū (Complete Book of Patterns and Treatments in External Medicine) by Xǔ Kè-Chāng	• Based on the former book, similar academic thoughts • Division of syndromes into two categories, namely those with definite location and those without a definite location • Pointed out the importance of Stomach qì and opposed the abuse of cold and attacking medicines • One volume includes different treatments on poisoning, e.g. food poisoning, animal poisoning etc.
		• Most classics about treating external diseases have been republished in modern times • New dermatological textbooks • Some available in English

The Daily Routine in Chinese Medical Dermatology

Chinese medical dermatology is said to be one of the most difficult areas of TCM. The disease patterns are complex, and many skin diseases are deep-rooted and most of them resistant to treatment. The challenge of diagnosing and treating skin diseases requires patience and a highly skilled ability to observe and analyze. Every student of Chinese medicine soon finds that the knowledge one acquires from one's teachers cannot simply be copied in clinic: imitation will not work; you must use your teacher's knowledge as a basis to build your own expertise over the years. There are some factors that cannot be adapted, such as environmental circumstances or emotional and cultural factors.

No matter how much experience you have gained throughout the years, the continuing process of learning enables you to deepen both theoretical and practical understanding, learning refinements that improve your practice and prevent mistakes in application. This is the only way to deepen expertise and refine knowledge–an experience that will serve your patients as well. Thus, the goal of every Dermatology course or textbook should be to empower practitioners to confidently and independently prescribe and modify classical formulas after identifying the disease pattern.

A constant challenge in daily practice is that disease patterns often overlap. It is also important to note that most patients who come into a TCM practice have a long history of visiting allopathic skin specialists and have already tried multiple therapies. This is particularly true for patients with neurodermatitis. Don't forget, they've had this condition since they were very young and have usually tried everything before coming to see us. Again, most cases present not only with a skin disorder but also with other factors such as digestive or emotional issues. This is why patience is required from both the doctor and the patient over the course of the treatment. Patients need to be made aware of the fact that long-term conditions will take much longer to treat than conditions with a more recent onset. As a rule of thumb, you can always give the advice: It generally takes one month of treatment for one year of illness. This allows the patient to estimate how long their treatment might take.

Chinese dermatology deals with profound processes that manifest on the body's surface–the skin. Skin diseases must be understood in the context of the entire body, a perspective that is fundamentally different from conventional medicine. Diseases are considered through complex patterns of signs and symptoms that define each individual clinical presentation. I always say: We treat what we see. This means, in TCM, the goal is always to treat the pattern, which is regarded as the root cause. A purely symptom-based treatment, as is frequently employed in conventional Western dermatology, will not reach a long-lasting resolution.

The initial diagnosis of the skin disease leaves us with multiple options for internal and external treatments. The following presents a step-by-step description of this process.

For a correct diagnosis of skin diseases according to TCM, it is essential to consider the following factors:

- an examination of the skin lesion (its onset, duration, location, appearance, and temperature)

- the exacerbating or relieving factors such as stress, certain foods, climate etc.

- all associated symptoms such as itching,[9] pain, burning sensation, scaling, bleeding, or pus and discharge.

The focus in Chinese dermatology is always the skin lesion with all its presenting characteristics. Besides the presenting skin disease, factors such as emotions, sleep, diet, digestion, lifestyle (potential stress, overwork, night shifts), and environment, and the menstrual cycle in female patients, are all important aspects of the Chinese diagnostic process. Moreover, by taking pulse and tongue diagnosis into consideration, the therapist gathers information on how the body works as a whole.

Please note that there are some factors which can distort the pulse condition, such as certain Western drugs, emotions and foods:

- antibiotics might slow the pulse and make it slippery (cold and damp)

- cortisone can generate internal heat and accelerate the pulse

- beta-blockers can produce internal cold and decelerate the pulse

- caffeine, restlessness, arguments, exertion can all lead to internal heat which accelerates the pulse

- after larger meals and during pregnancy: a slippery pulse can occur

- dislocated pulse due to atypical pulse location: this is very rare but makes it sometimes nearly impossible to take the pulse.

Moreover, please remember that it is also very helpful to tell your patients not to eat or drink anything that could stain their tongue about two to three hours before their appointment, in particular before the first consultation. They should also avoid scraping their tongue for about 2–3 days before the appointment–all this is important for accurate tongue diagnosis according to Chinese medicine.

Once all this information has been gathered and the Chinese medicine diagnosis established, an individual treatment plan is created.

In severe or long-lasting skin diseases, Chinese herbs can be prescribed for both internal treatment and external application. Especially for conditions like eczema, the list of potential external combinations is nearly endless.[10]

One important but often overlooked issue in stubborn cases: it is particularly important to enquire in detail about diet, living circumstances, and lifestyle habits. This is especially true for those patients with a chronic skin disease who expect instant results, or patients who state that they have already tried every method available. Practitioners might be surprised by what they will learn about bad eating habits, excessive alcohol consumption, or a constant lack of sleep. For those patients, it is essential to provide dietary advice and to explain what role their own behavior plays in maintaining their disease. Telling them to go to bed early or to reduce their workload to lessen stress may seem to be simple and obvious advice, but patients often find it hard to break long-standing habits. One approach is to help the patient understand that they are doing it for themselves and their health. How many times have you heard from patients, "I can't do it!" It actually means nothing other than "I don't want to." Thus, if you can help a patient realize that they are an integral part of the therapeutic process, substantial progress can be made.

Chinese Herbal Treatment Options in Chinese Medical Dermatology

The wide variety of treatment options developed over the centuries and the extensive range of internal and external applications that Chinese herbal medicine offers are a direct response to the flexibility required in curing complex disease patterns.

This section offers a general overview of commonly used internal and external treatment options in Chinese medical dermatology. Advantages and disadvantages of each application will be explained, and examples are listed by way of illustration. All of this is part of basic Chinese medicine education, but it can be helpful for explaining the process to your patient and can serve as an overview for students and beginners. A brief outline of specific external treatment options for eczema can be found in Appendix I.

Decoctions (*Jiān Jì* 煎剂)

Decoctions, or teas, of raw herbs are the most effective form of treatment. Herbal decoctions are prepared in three steps: firstly soaking, which allows the cell walls of the medicinal substances to expand for better extraction during boiling; then boiling in a ceramic pot (a ceramic pot is usually the best choice, because some herbs such as *ē jiāo*, *hé shǒu wū*, or *shú dì huáng* are not suitable for cooking in a metal pot); and lastly straining. The patient then drinks the strained liquid. To obtain the highest efficacy of the herbs when brewing, the herbs are usually boiled twice. Some herbs are added early, some later; some herbs are bagged, and others are dissolved in water and taken directly without boiling.

To provide a guide for colleagues lacking experience with raw herbs, I am sharing the standard cooking times and doses I give to my patients:

- Standard soaking time: 20–30 minutes

- Standard boiling time: 30 minutes, twice, using fresh water each time, and then mixing the decoctions before drinking

- Standard intake of decoction: 100–150 ml, twice a day. The dose depends on the severity of the (skin) disease, and in acute or severe cases, herbs can be taken three times a day. It is a flexible process.

Each prescription combines individual medicinal herbs selected to fulfil the individual's needs. Decoctions are very flexible in their application and allow easy adaptation of the prescription to the condition as it presents on a particular day. Thus, the patient will obtain an individually tailored prescription fitting his or her medical condition and current situation. One single pill can never be effective for thousands of patients, as seen in conventional medicine, when every one of these people has their own individual symptoms and different situation in life.

The substances extracted from a freshly brewed herbal decoction are more potent than from any other form of prepared Chinese herbal medicine. Raw herbs can also be modified through processing techniques, known as *páo zhì* 炮制. This traditional preparation process enhances the therapeutic effect of medicinal plants. *Páo zhì* reduces toxicity and unwanted side effects, for instance, changing pharmacological properties, enhancing the precision of therapeutic effects, and changing the smell and taste of the plants. There are many different preparation methods, such as roasting, frying, steaming, baking, calcining, germinating, fermenting, or cooking individually or in special combinations. Applied in daily practice, this means that if you want to change the action—for example, strengthen a certain effect of a herb—or you want to make it more tolerable for patients with a weak digestion, then you can use *páo zhì*—depending on your needs. Any qualified TCM pharmacist is able to prepare it.

Another advantage of herbal decoctions is that the ingredients can be cooked for different lengths of time. Flowers, for example, are very light in nature and should only be cooked for a few minutes. Heavy substances such as minerals should be cooked for a longer time, at least 60 minutes, and they are often pre-cooked for this reason. In general, a fresh herbal decoction with a long cooking time is best for deep-rooted processes, because it can reach the deep layers of the body and quickly attack the disease. This means that the correct location of the disease must be taken into account in order to cure illness. For external applications, the opposite applies–herbs are only boiled very briefly because the effects must address the surface.

In summary, within a complex and individual tailored herbal formula, many chemical reactions occur between the active ingredients of every single herb. The dosages of decoctions can be used with precision. A decoction can be modified in many ways and works quickly. Additionally, in the West, raw herbs are considerably cheaper than other application forms such as herbal granules. Considering all this, when treating a serious case, raw herbs are always recommended. Although herbal decoctions do not taste good, patients usually tolerate them once the benefits are explained. Herbal decoctions are usually the best choice to treat difficult skin conditions, such as eczema and neurodermatitis, which almost always have been present for a very long time.

Granules (*Kē Lì Jì* 颗粒剂) and Pills (*Piàn Jì* 片剂)

Granules are Chinese medicinal herbs extracted and concentrated into granules, using modern extraction and concentration technologies to replicate the traditional method of preparing medicinal decoctions. Please do not confuse granules with powdered herbs, which are raw herbs, uncooked and ground or pulverized into a powder. In pills, the extracts are further processed and pressed into pill form for ease of consumption.

As granules and pills are not given in a fresh form, fillers such as cellulose and carrier substances such as lactose, cornflour or maltodextrin are added. Although there are no significant pharmacological, toxicological, and clinical studies to demonstrate equivalence with decoctions,[11] it can be seen in clinical practice that granules are less effective as symptoms return and conditions worsen when patients switch from raw herbs to granules. Moreover, it can be quite difficult to determine the exact ratio of herb available in the granules. The industry mentions several yield ratios–that is, the amount of product yielded from the extraction process. The standard yield ratio seems to be 5:1,[12] but the industry often does not publish the exact ratio because yields can differ. This is because so many other factors can further affect the yield ratio, such as whether the herbs (especially roots and fruits/seeds) are ground coarse or fine, the length of extraction time, the solubility of the herb's ingredients in water, whether organic solvents are used or not, the pH of the extract solution, and so on. The size of the measuring spoon[13] used by patients and whether it is a level or heaped spoonful must also be taken into account. As a consequence of all these factors, determining how to properly dose granules can be a very difficult process. Furthermore, for granules often neither *páo zhì* nor different cooking time options are available. Other simple practical disadvantages of granules are that they often clump together, they do not taste any better than herbal decoctions, and they are usually more expensive than raw herbs.

However, granules are convenient and helpful in some situations, and better than no remedy–for instance, during travel, in circumstances where refrigeration is not available, or in situations where the patient does not want to or cannot drink decoctions. I find that many patients return after taking granules during travel and ask for herbal decoctions once more. Most agree that granules don't taste significantly better than decoctions and they notice the difference in their efficacy.

Tinctures (*Dīng Jì* 酊剂)

Tinctures are herbal preparations made in alcoholic bases. Tinctures are called medicinal liquor in Chinese, and they can be used internally or applied topically. Taken internally, the use of herbal tinctures is not that common, but it can be a good interim solution when the patient is not drinking herbal tea. For example, patients are commonly advised to drink one bag of Chinese herbal tea per week in less severe conditions. One bag of tea does not usually last the whole week, and so for the remaining days of the week the patient can take the tincture to support the effect of the raw herbs. However, the use of tinctures for eczema in general–externally and internally–is extremely rare.

Washes (*Xǐ Dí* 洗涤) and Wet Compresses (*Shī Fū* 湿敷)

Herbal washes, which are applied topically directly to the skin lesion, can help with various types of skin problems such as itching, heat, inflammation, pustules, swellings, and ulcerations, and can promote healing of the skin. Herbal washes can be used externally as a wash or locally as a wet compress. For wet compresses, a folded piece of material, bandage, or small towel is immersed in herbal decoction and then placed over the affected area for a certain period of time. This is usually done once or twice a day for at least 15–30 minutes, depending on the severity of the skin lesions.

Again, I am sharing my standard cooking process for herbal washes and wet compresses, to help colleagues with less experience in raw herbs:

- Standard soaking time: 15–20 minutes

- Standard boiling time: max. 20 minutes, once only

- Standard application time: 15–30 minutes depending on severity of the skin lesions. This can be done once or twice a day, and in severe cases even three times a day.

- The liquid will stay fresh for up to seven days when refrigerated, but should be assessed for freshness in appearance and smell before use. When the liquid is no longer aromatic it should be discarded.

In general, herbal washes, wet compresses and baths are mainly used in skin conditions involving discharge. This method still allows the skin's secretion of pathogenic fluids and pus, while relieving heat, inflammation, pustules, or swellings. During acute stages of serious skin conditions, washes, compresses, but particularly baths, should be taken with caution because of the potential risk of secondary inflammation. This can happen to compromised skin very easily if there is any contamination, and so herbal liquid that comes in contact with the skin should only be used once. However, in skin conditions such as eczema and neurodermatitis, herbal washes and wet compresses are incredibly helpful and give very good results.

Special herbal combinations are known to have a disinfecting effect, such as the formula *Sān Huáng Xǐ Jì*, made of *huáng bǎi*, *huáng qín*, *dà huáng*, and *kǔ shēn*. Because "yellow" (*huáng* in Chinese) is part of three of these four herb names, the formula is called "Three Yellow Cleanser Formula." This ancient topical formula is known for its effects of clearing heat, stopping itching, and arresting secretion, and it is often used in skin conditions such as eczema. This topical formula is also useful in treating deep acne and furuncles (boils) and has shown very good effects for psoriasis. In eczema, you can work with single herbs or combinations for topical use. It doesn't require many herbs to be effective, just work precisely and cleanly, including instructing your patient in detail on how to properly use them at home. I will give many examples later in the book.

In summary, when using topical treatments for inflamed skin, herbal decoction is always the best choice because its light texture offers a non-occluding effect when applied externally, and this method is able to heal the skin on a deeper level. A cream, on the other hand, would enclose the discharge, and instead of pathogens exiting the body, they are trapped and move transversely back into the body. Interestingly, this is very often seen in conventional medicine. Although skin lesions are still discharging, patients are prescribed creams. The skin cannot breathe, the secretion or pus is trapped, and the healing process is thus impeded. Almost all my patients report feeling uncomfortable using creams while their skin lesions are still weeping, particularly those with oozing eczema. Similarly, patients with neurodermatitis are often advised by a conventional dermatologist to apply thick cream to nourish and soften their skin, but in most cases the opposite is achieved. Skin care must aim to actively support nourishing and moistening of the skin in the long term, rather than just providing a short-term improvement. Creams based on mineral oil (Paraffin) or with silicones do not help here. They just occlude the skin and block the pores, without any added benefit. A better treatment strategy is to first use Chinese herbs to reduce inflammation and allow wounds to heal, followed with a high-quality oil or thin lotion if the skin feels dry after application of herbs.

Pastes (*Hú Jì* 糊剂)

Pastes are prepared by combining finely powdered herbs with a carrier substance. One type of paste is prepared using a greasy medium such as oil. In Chinese dermatology, sesame oil is very frequently used. The other type of paste is prepared with water. The paste is then applied to the affected area of the skin in order to protect dry skin, serve as a barrier, protect the affected area from bacterial infection, and promote the healing process of the skin.

Pastes should not be applied topically if there is profuse discharge. They should also be avoided in case of damp-heat (*shī rè* 湿热), as damp-heat could move transversely back inside to the interior and the pathogenic process would be aggravated. Zōu Yuè pointed out in his *Wài Kē Zhēn Quán* (Personal Experience in Wài Kē, 1838) that "pastes are contraindicated when damp-heat toxins exist on the lower extremities. If misused, the confined heat will move transversely and spread even more extensively. Pastes are advisable in protected cases." Therefore, the application of pastes when the patient shows profuse pus or discharge will impede the drainage of the fluids.[14] However, pastes are rarely used externally to treat eczema.

Ointments (*Yóu Gāo* 油膏)

An ointment, also called a salve or balm, is a semi-solid preparation for external application on damaged skin. Oil-based ointments consist of finely powdered herbs heated in an oil base, such as almond oil, jojoba oil, olive oil or sesame oil. A note regarding the sesame oil: The oil of roasted sesame seeds is best because it is comparatively stable and does not turn rancid on contact with air due to the toasting process.

The texture of an oil-based ointment is thick (but not too thick) and often looks yellowish. Creams, by contrast, are water-soluble and usually have a white hue. An ointment can be smoothly applied on damaged skin, and it is absorbed easily and quickly. Ointments usually have good permeability and are therefore often used after herbal baths and washes as I have already mentioned. Oil-based ointments are often used to stop itching, clear heat, and dispel inflammation. Ointments are particularly suitable for chronic skin diseases or when the skin is very thick, such as in neurodermatitis. Ointments, like pastes, are not suitable if there is profuse discharge.

Cream (*Rǔ Gāo* 乳膏)

A cream is a semi-solid emulsion of either oil in water or water in oil for topical use. Creams are spreadable substances, they adhere well, and they are often more appropriate for application on exposed skin areas such as the face and hands.

For compound creams, either oil-based herbal extracts or water-based herbal extracts (decoctions) are carefully blended with the base cream and other substances such as essential oils, aloe vera, or dexpanthenol[15] to achieve a homogenous and consistent product. In Chinese dermatology, base creams often consist of high-quality and skin-friendly substances such as shea butter, cocoa butter, jojoba oil, or natural white beeswax. It should be emphasized that petroleum jelly (e.g., Vaseline®) should not be used, although it is still often mentioned in medical textbooks. Petroleum jelly, a petroleum by-product of the oil industry, is not a high-quality solution. It is thick and often poorly spreadable and has a very unpleasant smell. Cheap and low-quality substances such as petroleum jelly, paraffin, or propylene glycol usually leave a greasy film on the skin with increased sweating underneath. In sweating, salt crystals are produced, which can further worsen already existing itching, and therefore these substances should be avoided. The skin must be able to breathe in order to heal! For those who still prefer to use petroleum jelly, wool wax alcoholic cream (also called lanolin) can be used as an alternative.

Wool wax alcoholic cream is a cream base, consisting of white petroleum jelly, cetyl-stearyl alcohol, and wool wax alcohol. Due to its lighter texture, it spreads easily and feels more pleasant on the skin.

However, when making your own creams and ointments, it is important to know exactly what ingredients are being used. Only pure, natural, environmentally friendly options should be used, ensuring that the ingredients do not irritate the skin and are suitable for sensitive skincare. If there is an ingredient a patient is allergic to, one can simply leave it out or replace it with something else.

Neurodermatitis is a perfect example of a skin condition where creams are frequently used in practice. Due to lichenification, the skin is very thick and dry, with scaling and itching. The patient feels very uncomfortable: as well as the visual appearance and itching sensation, the skin feels very tight which can be quite painful. In this case, creams made from herbs such as *shēng dì huáng, dāng guī, gān cǎo, sāng shèn*, or *bǎi hé* are frequently prescribed. Two or three of these herbs can be used in combination, or as part of a larger formula, if needed. Herbs such as *gǒu qǐ zǐ* or *mài mén dōng* can also be used to moisten the skin. The choices here are endless. For my patients with dry skin and lesions located on the face, I usually recommend my specially formulated TCM skincare products, CHINAMED COSMETICS®. These products are non-irritating and contain highly potent Chinese herbs and no harmful substances. Through balanced formulations, these TCM skincare creams can moisturize the skin, reduce irritation and help maintain its balance in a very natural way. This allows even sensitive skin types, such as ND patients, to be nurtured and thus maintain and protect their skin health.

In summary, in order to treat the root cause of the disease, internal TCM herbal remedies must be the core of treatment. Nonetheless, external applications are often also prescribed. According to clinical experience, external treatments supplement and enhance the healing process, and the effect for the patient is more immediate. The psychological factor cannot be underestimated here. When applying external remedies, the patient is more of an active participant, which can be very important for some patients.

One more practical hint: patients are often very sensitive and can easily have an allergic reaction to various kinds of external influences. Some patients say that they are even sensitive to water. This is why it is always advisable to start with a mild approach when it comes to external treatments, and then slowly increase the strength. The same applies for internal treatment. If in the first consultation your patient mentions allergies to almost everything, I recommend starting with just one bag of herbs and waiting for the patient's feedback. If the prescription is well tolerated, more bags can be ordered. This saves the patient money and also builds trust, because these patients have often already experienced bad reactions to medicines in the past.

Endnotes

1 For example: Bensky, D., Clavey, S., and Stöger, E. (2004) *Materia Medica* (3rd edition). Seattle, WA: Eastland Press; or Chen, J.K. (2013) *Chinese Medical Herbology and Pharmacology*. City of Industry, CA: Art of Medicine Press.

2 Sòng Dynasty: Běi Sòng, Nán Sòng (Northern Sòng, Southern Sòng) (960–1279 AD).

3 Yuán Dynasty (1206–1368 AD).

4 Míng Dynasty (1368–1644 AD).

5 Aka Wāng Shí-Shān.

6 Grant, J. (2003) *A Chinese Physician: Wang Ji and the Stone Mountain Medical Case Histories*. Abingdon: Routledge.

7 Qīng Dynasty (Before the Opium Wars of 1840) (1644–1911 AD).

8 With a pair of copper wires and a loop at the end of each wire.

9 Important to differentiate here is whether the itching is worse during the day or at night. We will discuss the difference later in this book.

10 Examples will be given for each individual TCM pattern later in this book.

11 Luo, H., Li, Q., Flower, A., Lewith, G., and Liu J. (2012) "Comparison of effectiveness and safety between granules and decoction of Chinese herbal medicine: A systematic review of randomized clinical trials." *Journal of Ethnopharmacology 140*, 3, 555–567.

12 Sturgeon, S. (2012) *Powders and Granules RCHM*. Norwich: Register of Chinese Herbal Medicine.

13 Teaspoon, tablespoon etc.

14 Taken from my TCM Dermatology seminar notes.

15 Dexpanthenol, also known as panthenol, pantothenol, or provitamin B5, is often used as a moisturizer and to improve wound healing in creams, ointments, and lotions.

4

The Traditional Chinese Medicine Perspective on Eczema

BEFORE TAKING an in-depth look at the causes, levels, and stages of eczema, including the corresponding clinical features, TCM syndrome differentiation and treatment, let us first explore the long history of Chinese medicine and its perspective and development in naming, diagnosing, and treating eczema. Please note again, eczema and neurodermatitis in Western medicine both belong to the TCM category of "eczema," also called "TCM eczema." The following descriptions are primarily those of eczema, whether it is, for example, contact eczema, nummular eczema, seborrheic eczema or dyshidrotic eczema. Neurodermatitis is discussed in a separate part of this book (please see Chapter 7).

There is an extensive history of TCM being used to treat inflammatory skin diseases, like eczema. Eczema was first mentioned in the Warring States Period, although with a name we no longer use today. It is amazing that TCM knowledge about this skin condition dates back more than 2000 years, and as TCM practitioners we can be very proud of this wealth of medical experience. Nevertheless, the depth of understanding and corresponding treatment strategies of eczema in TCM has been constantly refined over the centuries and will continue to be. This rich traditional and experiential knowledge is ultimately the basis that we practitioners can use every day in our own practice.

The Definition and History of Eczema According to Traditional Chinese Medicine

According to TCM, eczema belongs to the category of "*shī chuāng*" (湿疮). Translated, this means "wet boils" or "damp boils," an inflammatory skin disease characterized by symmetrical distribution of multiform skin lesions, accompanied by itching (pruritus), skin redness and rash, watery discharge (exudation), and the development of scales, crusts, and skin infections due to repeated scratching. Scratching breaks the skin and can cause open sores and cracks, which understandably increase the risk of infection from bacteria and viruses. Eczema tends to be recurrent and chronic. Coming back to the classification, when "boil" is called "sore," then eczema is called "*shī yáng*" (湿疡), which means "wet sores." Colloquially, eczema can also be called "*shī zhěn*" (湿疹). *Zhěn* is the term for "rash," and again *shī* for "wet or damp." While there are differing names, you can already tell that the emphasis is always on "wet or damp" because that's exactly what is seen in eczema: "weeping" lesions caused by itching, which scab over and often become infected.

The possibilities of naming are manifold, so eczema is termed differently depending on where it occurs on the body and what characteristics it has. A detailed list can be found later in the text under the heading "Differentiation According to the Areas Affected with Eczema." Before we get to that, I would like to give you a historical overview of eczema, and how this skin condition is described in classical TCM books and sources.[1]

Warring States Period (475–221BC)	*Wǔ Shí Èr Bìng Fāng* (Formulas for Fifty-Two Diseases), author unknown	• Earliest name of eczema, "*lù bǐ*," which means "flaws outside" in literal translation.
Qín and Hàn Dynasties (221–206 BC) (206 BC–220 AD)[2]	*Huáng Dì Nèi Jīng*[3] (The Yellow Emperor's Classic of Internal Medicine), author unknown	• Mentions: "All kinds of pain, itchiness and sores belong to the Heart." It means that all the sores are related to Heart. • Further mentions: "All kinds of dampness and swelling belong to the Spleen." • Recognizes: There is a close relationship between the lesions of the viscera and the onset of skin lesions.
Eastern Hàn Dynasty (25–220)	*Jīn Guì Yào Lüè* (Essentials from the Golden Cabinet) by Zhāng Jī	• Earliest reference to the term "*jīn yín chuāng*," which means that the sores are spread over the body with much exudation.

Suí Dynasty (589–618)	*Zhū Bìng Yuán Hòu Lùn* (Treatize on the Origins and Manifestations of Various Diseases) by Cháo Yuán-Fāng	▪ Describes the cause of the term "*jīn yín chuāng*" in detail. ▪ Caused by wind-heat attacking the Heart, located on the skin. ▪ Very small at the beginning, starts with itching and sensation of pain, and finally becomes the lesion. ▪ Exudation comes out and the skin lesions will spread throughout the body. It equals eczema in its acute phase. ▪ Mentions: When eczema appears on the navel, it is called "*qí chuāng*." Cause: wind-dampness attacks the body, while body has internal heat and exterior deficiency; then eczema will occur. ▪ Another passage mentions the term "*shī xuǎn zhě*" (damp ringworm): It feels like worms (insects) are moving on the skin, spreading, itching and weeping (discharging) after scratching. Cause: wind and dampness dwell at the muscular interstices. Here, the dampness is predominant, not wind, so it is called "damp ringworm."
Eastern Jīn Dynasty (317–420)	*Zhǒu Hòu Bèi Jí Fāng* (Emergency Formulas to Keep Up One's Sleeve) by Gě Hóng	▪ Acute eczema accompanied with exudation is caused by Heart problems.
Sòng Dynasty (960–1279)	*Chuāng Yáng Jīng Yàn Quán Shū* (Complete Manual of Experience in the Treatment of Sores) by Dòu Hàn-Qīng & Dòu Mèng-Lín[4]	▪ First reference to "*xuè fēng chuāng*," which means that there is bleeding after scratching the sores.
Jīn Dynasty (1115–1234)	*Rú Mén Shì Qīn* (Confucians' Duties to Their Parents) by Zhāng Cóng-Zhèng	▪ Eczema is caused by water and dampness.
Yuán Dynasty (1271–1368)	*Wài Kē Jīng Yì* (Quintessence of External Medicine) by Qí Dé-Zhī	▪ Toxins in the Lung will be transported to the four limbs and can't be dispersed quickly.
Míng Dynasty (1368–1644)	*Wài Kē Zhèng Zōng* (Orthodox Lineage of External Medicine) by Chén Shí-Gōng	▪ Eczema is due to interaction of wind-heat, damp-heat and blood heat. ▪ Babies have eczema because their parents prefer spicy and grilled food before the conception.

Qīng Dynasty (1644–1911/12)	*Dòng Tiān Ào Zhǐ* (Collection of Secrets of External Medicine)[5] by Chén Shì-Duó	• The pathogens of eczema are described as water and dampness.
	Wài Kē Xīn Fǎ Yào Jué (Essential Teachings on External Medicine)[6] by Wú Qiān	• Eczema is caused by Heart fire and Spleen dampness in the body and attack from external wind.
	Yáng Kē Xīn Dé Jí (Collected Experience on Treating External Sores) by Gāo Bǐng-Jūn	• Dampness and heat are combined together, attacking the skin, so eczema will occur. • Storms, heavy raining, coldness, dampness, summer-heat or heat: all these factors can attack the skin, resulting in eczema. • "*Shī dú chuāng*," a name of eczema, which means that the lesions appear in a certain position in the body. • When the lesion is located at the extensor side, it pertains to the foot meridian of the Stomach (*zú yáng míng jīng* 足阳明经) and foot meridian of the Gallbladder (*zú shǎo yáng jīng* 足少阳经). • When the lesion manifests at the flexor side, it pertains to the foot meridian of the Liver (*zú jué yīn jīng* 足厥阴经) and the foot meridian of the Spleen (*zú tài yīn jīng* 足太阴经).
	Yī Zōng Jīn Jiàn (The Golden Mirror of Ancestral Medicine) by Wú Qiān	• *Jīn yín chuāng* is like scabies at the beginning. • It itches continuously and can spread all over the body. • There will be yellow secretion after scratching the skin lesion. • Caused by internal Heart fire and Spleen dampness and attack of external wind.
	Wài Kē Zhèng Zhì Quán Shū (Complete Treatise of Patterns and Treatment in External Medicine) by Xǔ Kè-Chāng	• Eczema caused by dryness-heat in the body combined with dampness, and wind attacking the exterior. • Wind and dampness combine to become pimples, with itching sensation. • Accompanying symptoms: irregular urination, vexation, and thirst, which will be worse at night.

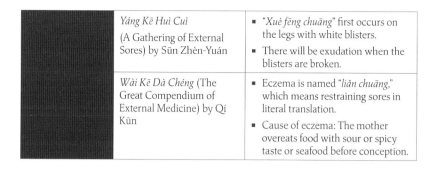

Yáng Kē Huì Cuì (A Gathering of External Sores) by Sūn Zhèn-Yuán	• "Xuè fēng chuāng" first occurs on the legs with white blisters. • There will be exudation when the blisters are broken.
Wài Kē Dà Chéng (The Great Compendium of External Medicine) by Qí Kūn	• Eczema is named "liǎn chuāng," which means restraining sores in literal translation. • Cause of eczema: The mother overeats food with sour or spicy taste or seafood before conception.

The History of Treatment of Eczema According to Traditional Chinese Medicine

Just as the definition of eczema has changed over time, so have treatment strategies. The following table explains the treatments applied at different time periods.[7] Interestingly, many of the herbs and formulas are still used today, which speaks for their effectiveness. Herbal prescriptions and individual herbs are described in detail for both internal and external applications, whereas acupuncture seems to play little role in the old texts. From my own clinical experience, I can only agree that in severe cases of eczema (like any other serious skin condition), Chinese herbal medicine always comes first, and acupuncture should always be considered a secondary treatment. At least that's my experience and that's how I work.

Eastern Hàn Dynasty (25–220)	Jīn Guì Yào Lüè (Essentials from the Golden Cabinet) by Zhāng Jī	Huáng Lián Sǎn (Coptis Rhizome Powder)	huáng lián	• "Jīn yín chuāng" could be treated externally with Huáng Lián Sǎn.
Sòng Dynasty (960–1279)	Shèng Jì Zōng Lù (Comprehensive Recording of Divine Assistance), anonymous, Song Imperial Court	Shēng Má Tāng (Cimicifuga Decoction)	shēng má, huáng qín, dà huáng, dāng guī, sháo yào, gān cǎo, zhī shí	• "Jīn yín chuāng" is mostly caused by wind-heat accumulation in the Heart meridian. • Treatment with Shēng Má Tāng.
Míng Dynasty (1368–1644)	Dān Xī Xīn Fǎ, (Teachings of [Zhu] Dan-Xi) by Zhū Zhèn-Hēng, aka Zhū Dān-Xī	Modified Sì Wù Tāng (Four Substances Decoction)	chuān xiōng, dāng guī, dì huáng,[8] sháo yào,[9] huáng lián, huáng qín, niú bàng zǐ, gān cǎo	• Modified Sì Wù Tāng can treat sores, which are mostly related to fire and heat.

Yī Zōng Jīn Jiàn (The Golden Mirror of Ancestral Medicine) by Wú Qiān	*Shēng Má Xiāo Dú Yǐn* (Cimicifuga Decoction to Eliminate Toxins)	*dāng guī, chì sháo, jīn yín huā, lián qiào, niú bàng zǐ, zhī zǐ, qiāng huó, bái zhǐ, hóng huā, fáng fēng, gān cǎo, shēng má, jié gěng*	▪ Eczema should be treated by firstly "clearing heat." ▪ *Shēng Má Xiāo Dú Yǐn* as first treatment used.
	Xiāo Fēng Sǎn (Wind-Dispersing Powder)	*jīng jiè, dāng guī, fáng fēng, shēng dì huáng, kǔ shēn, cāng zhú, chán tuì, hu má rén, niú bàng zǐ, zhī mǔ, shí gāo, gān cǎo, mù tōng*	▪ When the skin is broken and exudation occurs, wind dispersing method shall be used, i.e., by the use of *Xiāo Fēng Sǎn*.
	Shé Chuáng Zǐ Tāng (Cnidium Fruit Decoction)	*shé chuáng zǐ, dāng guī, wēi líng xiān, shā rén, dà huáng, kǔ shēn, cōng bái*	▪ Used as external application for scrotum eczema.
Wài Ke Dà Chéng (The Great Compendium of External Medicine) by Qí Kūn	Modified *Dāng Guī Yǐn Zǐ* (Chinese Angelica Drink)	*dāng guī, shú dì huáng, chì sháo, huáng qí, chuān xiōng, bái jí lí, hé shǒu wū, jīng jiè, fáng fēng, gān cǎo, chái hú, zhī zǐ*	▪ This formula can treat vulvar eczema.[10]

Differentiation According to the Areas Affected with Eczema

Eczema can occur anywhere on the body and its symptoms are different for everyone. However, ancient texts have classified different types and areas of eczema and, thus, gave further names depending on the appearance and the location. The following table lists the different terms for eczema per appearance as well as location:[11]

Pīnyīn Name	Chinese Name	Characteristics and Location
fēng shī yáng	风湿疡	An acute condition where rashes cover the whole body (rheumatic ulcer/sores)
guō chuāng	瘑疮	Eczema of the hand

jīn yín chuāng	浸淫疮	Generalized eczema with weeping blisters (soaking sores)
miàn yóu fēng	面游风	The rash mainly affects the face and scalp, Chinese term for: seborrheic dermatitis (face travelling wind)
nǎi xuǎn	奶癣	Eczema in infants (milk ringworm)
qí chuāng	脐疮	Eczema of the navel (navel sore)
rǔ tóu fēng	乳头风	Eczema of the mamilla (papilla mammae) (nipple wind)
shèn náng fēng	肾囊风	Scrotal eczema (renal capsule wind)
sì wān fēng	四弯风	Eczema affecting the knee bend and crook of the arm. Chinese term for: neurodermatitis (four bends of wind)
shī dú yáng	湿毒疡	When the lesions are infected (damp sores)
sù chuāng	粟疮	Eczema papulosum (miliary sore)
wán xuǎn	顽癣	When eczema is a chronic condition (stubborn or persistent ringworm)
xuán ěr chuāng	旋耳疮	Eczema of the ear (ear sore)
xuè fēng chuāng	血风疮	When the lesions bleed after scratching (blood sores)

I would like to mention that "*sì wān fēng*" (four bends of wind) is the most commonly used Chinese term for neurodermatitis at present. And it simply refers to the four commonly affected skin sites: the insides of the elbows and the backs of the knees. We will discuss this condition later in this book.

Example Pictures of the Skin According to the Affected Areas with Eczema

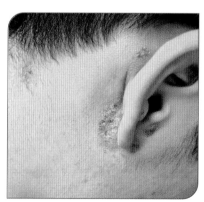

ECZEMA ON THE EAR

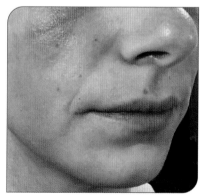

ECZEMA RASH MAINLY
AFFECTING THE FACE

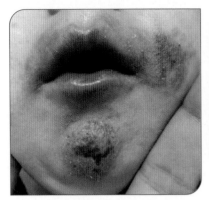

ECZEMA IN INFANTS

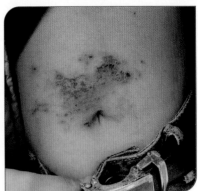

ECZEMA AROUND THE NAVEL

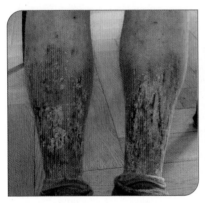

INFECTED ECZEMA LESIONS

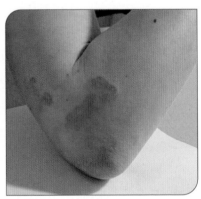

ECZEMA ON THE ARM

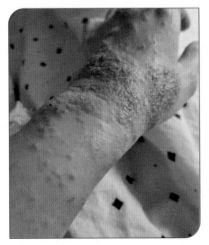

ECZEMA WITH WEEPING BLISTERS

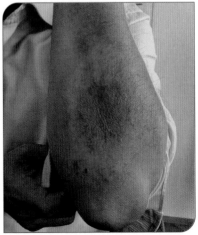

CHRONIC ECZEMA

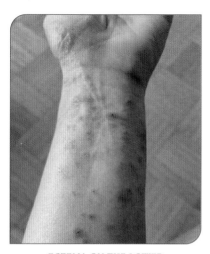

ECZEMA ON THE LOWER
ARM AND WRIST

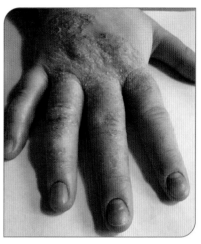

ECZEMA ON THE HAND

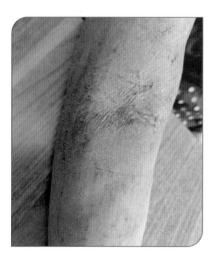

ECZEMA ON THE CROOK OF THE ARM

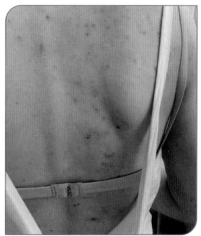

ECZEMA ON THE BACK

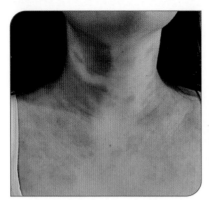

ECZEMA ON THE DÉCOLLETÉ

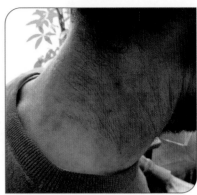

ECZEMA ON THE NECK

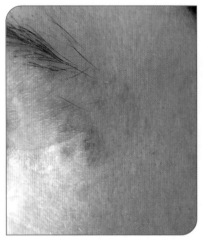

ECZEMA ON THE EYE

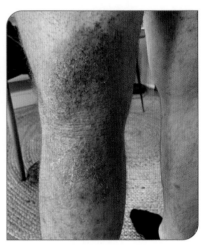

ECZEMA ON THE LEGS

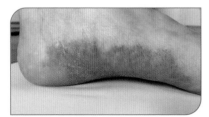

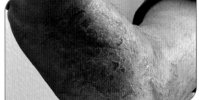

ECZEMA ON THE FOOT

Endnotes

1   The list makes no claim to be complete, but does provide a good overview of classical TCM texts.

2   The dates in brackets refer to the periods of Chinese dynasties.

3   In the *sù wèn* · 素问 (Basic questions).

4   This book is attributed to Dòu Hàn-Qīng (1196–1280) but it is said that it is actually written by his grandson, Dòu Mèng-Lín. The book appeared in 1569 but has been published/re-printed many times since (the publishing year differs depending on the source).

5   Other English names of this book: *Mysterious Teachings in a Cave* and *The Secret Meaning of a New World*.

6   Also known as Principles of External Medicine Treatments.

7   This summary does not claim to be complete but should provide a good idea of how treatment has changed throughout time—and the ways in which it has remained the same.

8   If caused by fire and heat, *shēng dì huáng* is more suitable than *shú dì huáng*. Please keep in mind, if the lesions are redder and a blood cooling aspect is needed, *shēng dì huáng* is always better.

9   If eczema is caused by fire and heat, *chì sháo* should be used instead of *bái sháo*. As well as invigorating the blood, *chì sháo* can also cool the blood and clear heat.

10   Affects the skin of the vulva and the surrounding area.

11   This list does not claim to be complete. For example, in my notes from China I found the terms *shen leng feng* = eczema of the anal region, *wo chuang* = eczema of the elbow and popliteal fossa, but I could not find these names mentioned in other Chinese texts.

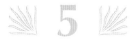

Classification of Eczema According to the Clinical Presentation of the Lesions

I T SHOULD NOW be clear that eczema can occur on different parts of the body and can have very different characteristics. However, eczema also progresses in three stages: acute, subacute, and chronic. There is no set timeline for the progression of eczema through the three stages; it is not always linear and the reason for the progression of eczema rashes is also not exactly understood. This chapter will outline the clinical features according to the different stages.

Acute Stage

This refers to the beginning phase of an eczema rash with a sudden onset. It can occur on any part of the body. The rash appears as symmetrical multiform skin lesions, erythema, papules, papulovesicles, blisters and pustules, followed by exudation, erosions, and formation of crusts. The skin rash is more severe in the center and has indistinct borders. In the acute stage eczema is usually accompanied by itching and burning sensations of the skin, and it is not uncommon that the skin becomes infected after scratching. Infection, of course, aggravates the skin lesion causing erosion, oozing, suppuration and further leading to boils and/or painful swelling. A high standard of hygiene is advisable here to avoid infections. Keep this in mind when reading Chapter 10 on preventative healthcare.

> CLINICAL TIP: When thinking about TCM syndrome differentiation, you should keep damp-heat in mind here as a main cause.

Subacute Stage

This stage refers to the transitional phase between acute and chronic stages. In this stage, the skin rash is less severe than in the acute stage. With milder skin lesions this stage mainly involves small papules, scales, crusts, and smaller numbers of blisters. Intense itching may occur, accompanied by a burning or stinging sensation.

> CLINICAL TIP: Here, it is very advisable to consider Spleen deficiency and lingering dampness as a main cause.

Chronic Stage

These eczema flares are long-lasting, and can be mild or severe. They can develop independently but can also be a result of inappropriate treatment of acute and subacute eczema. This stage tends to appear on tender skin areas, for example in the genital area, mammillae or wrists, and inside the elbows and behind the knees. The skin appears thick, coarse, and leathery, also known as lichenification. The skin may have dark red, brownish or purple colored discoloration with many cracks. Itching tends to be intense, again resulting in a vicious cycle of scaling, scratching, and bloody crusts. Papules, blisters, and oozing may be present.

> CLINICAL TIP: Considering the color of the skin lesions, it is very advisable to keep blood deficiency and blood stasis, resulting in insufficient nourishment of the skin, in mind at this stage. Always remember that when the disease course is long, yīn and blood will be exhausted, which leads to pathogenic wind or blood stasis. At the very end, qi and blood have stagnated, which results in skin mal-nourishment. Thus, the longer the disease lasts, the more the blood stagnates and wind-dryness symptoms appear. However, no matter the stage, the treatment in TCM is always based on the corresponding TCM syndrome.

CLINICAL TIP: In clinic, it can be observed that eczema is often found in places where there are varicose veins. If there are lesions which aren't healing well, check if varicose veins are present. Treatment will take a little longer in these cases.

Differentiating Eczema and Psoriasis

Eczema may not look the same in every patient. Different types of eczema may even affect different areas of the body at different times. However, care should be taken not to confuse eczema with other skin conditions. For example, some people mistake symptoms of psoriasis for eczema, although the two conditions are completely distinct and require completely different treatments. It is important to know the differences and characteristics of both diseases. If eczema is misdiagnosed, it becomes more difficult to treat and takes longer to respond.

The table below clearly highlights the differences between eczema and psoriasis:

	Eczema	Psoriasis
Symmetric	yes	no
Vesicle	yes	no
Fluid	yes	no
Crust	yes	no (only in pustular psoriasis type)
Scaling	+ (normal)	+++ (silvery white)
Itching	+++	+ / ++
Thickness of the skin	+	+++ (because of hyperproliferation and scaling)
Season	worse in winter	worse in winter
Main causes (TCM)	damp	heat
Inflammation	++	+++
Auspitz phenomena	no	yes
First onset	infancy	later in life, usually more common in adults
Trigger factors	seafood; dust mites; stress	hot food, hot spices, stress, alcohol, tobacco
Stress as trigger	+/++	+++
Edge of lesions	unclear	clear

	Eczema	Psoriasis
Types	acute, subacute, chronic; there are symptom free intervals	progressive and latent phases alternating; the patient is rarely without lesions. Lifelong.
Location	mostly in the yīn areas according to TCM	yáng areas (excluding inverse psoriasis type) according to TCM

+: mild, ++: moderate, +++: severe

Etiology and Pathogenesis of Eczema in Traditional Chinese Medicine

As I have already mentioned, when it comes to eczema the terminology can be as difficult as treating the disease itself. Eczema is the overall term for any type of "inflammation of the skin." This section will outline the etiology and pathogenesis of eczema "*shī chuāng.*"

Eczema, as is the case with all other skin conditions, has an etiology which is always multifactorial and very complex. As we see in our practices, there is usually never just one single cause as triggering factor. It is rather an interplay of various internal and external factors that ultimately lead to inflammation of the skin. Internal factors such as a weak constitution, overall state of health, chronic gastro-intestinal disorders, stress, overwork, insomnia, and also long-term emotional imbalances may lead to eczema. External factors including climate and environmental changes, extreme heat, damp or humid weather, often combined with profuse sweating or inappropriate diet, and also chemical exposure can play a role in the onset of eczema. It's all so complex that we as practitioners have to start by identifying the cause (or causes) in order to treat the disease successfully. However, let's go into more detail.

When we live in accordance with nature, we can achieve a harmonic and healthy lifestyle. Yet it must be said that in today's world, many people do not respect their own needs or boundaries, and do not treat their body and mind well. This literally means neglecting mental and physical health. Resisting the laws of human nature leads to imbalance, and the result can be illness and disease. In modern society, it is challenging to perceive what ourselves and our bodies need, and people often live rather disconnected from themselves. They have lost the ability to determine their needs, and even act in conflict with them. Wealth, status symbols, professional achievements—these are only necessary on the surface. Yet people tend to confuse basic needs with wants. In fast-paced societies, where "time is money," the idea of doing nothing, resting, and recharging is not valued enough. Time for mental and physical healthcare is not usually integrated into people's schedules, and if it is, it becomes another item on the to-do list, with clear targets and often a competitive aspect. Constant time-pressure and perceiving life as a series of scheduled events can have devastating effects on people's health. The great paradox here is that our societies not only fail in promoting health and taking precautions against becoming sick, but they also do not handle illness very well. Many cases confirm this in my own practice, particularly with skin diseases. Patients do not receive anything beyond a superficial treatment of symptoms; neither extensive consultation nor investigation of the root causes is provided by traditional Western medicine. Rethinking health and disease management is overdue. TCM's central philosophy tells us that living in balance is key to a healthy and long life. And even in today's society, this is possible. It is high time to understand that our health comes first!

TCM never just treats isolated symptoms in isolated parts of the body. Its holistic approach assesses each individual aspect of the patient's situation: physical condition, but also their living situation, psycho-emotional factors, and lifestyle habits. The following details these individual aspects in the context of eczema.

Zàng Fǔ

As TCM practitioners are well aware, according to the theory of Chinese medicine, all internal organs are divided into two major categories, namely the five *zàng* (脏) organs and the six *fǔ* (腑) organs. The five *zàng* organs comprise the Heart (*xīn* 心), the Liver (*gān* 肝), the Spleen (*pí* 脾), the Lung (*fèi* 肺) and the Kidney (*shèn* 肾). The six *fǔ* organs include the Gallbladder (*dǎn* 胆), the Stomach (*wèi* 胃), the Small Intestine (*xiǎo cháng* 小肠), the Large Intestine (*dà cháng* 大肠), the Urinary Bladder (*páng guāng* 膀胱), and the Triple Burner (*sān jiāo* 三焦). They differ not only in their functions but also in their characteristics. The main function of the five *zàng* organs is "to store" and the main function of the six *fǔ* organs is "to transport and transform." The individual organs serve different energetic functions. It can be very beneficial to inform patients that TCM practitioners are familiar with the organs as they are seen in Western medicine's anatomy. Yet, though they are named similarly, TCM's perspective is different. TCM views the organs as physical-anatomical structures, obviously with similar functions as in Western medicine, but with much broader energetic functions and purposes. The following section discusses the most important organs in this context, namely the ones that play the greatest role in the development of eczema: the Spleen and Stomach, Liver, and Heart.

Spleen and Stomach

In TCM, the primary cause of eczema is defined as a weak Spleen and Stomach. This can be caused by a constitutional weakness itself and/or an improper diet, amongst other factors. Spleen and Stomach can be damaged by an over-consumption of hot, spicy, or greasy food but also by fish, seafood, and excessive alcohol intake. Irregular eating habits over a long time can have a similar effect. The Stomach and the Spleen are also adversely affected by overwork, which can cause deficiency through both mental taxation and long hours of work. When the Spleen's ability to transform, transport, and eliminate dampness is thus impaired, foods and fluids will accumulate in the middle *jiāo* (*zhōng jiāo* 中焦). This leads to generation of internal dampness, which then–at a later stage–transforms into heat. The longer dampness accumulates in the body, the more easily it transforms into heat. This damp-heat then travels and often accumulates in the skin. Consequently, red, burning, and oozing skin rashes can occur. If heat is prevalent, we usually see erythema, papules, blisters, pustules, erosions, and crusts. This is often complicated by infection, which is very painful. If dampness is the predominant factor, meaning there is little or no heat involved, the trapped fluids present in papules. Multiple blisters with exudation and crusts can be seen. In this case, the onset is relatively slow. A reminder: everything related to dampness is characterized by slowness, sluggishness, and heaviness.

> CLINICAL TIP: It is not uncommon that the skin gets worse following tiredness or overthinking.

Liver

According to TCM, all diseases arise from an upset of qì. Regarding the Liver, the *Huáng Dì Nèi Jīng* (The Inner Canon of the Yellow Emperor, *sù wèn* chapter 39), which was written over 2500 years ago, states: "When there is anger, the qì rises up." Thus, anger always has the tendency to harm the Liver, which should be explored in more detail.

The Liver prefers a smooth flow of qì within the body, and therefore ensures balanced emotions and that all blood vessels remain open and unobstructed. If qì no longer flows smoothly, the psychological and physiological functioning of the organs is disrupted. Liver qì stagnation can easily arise from several causes. One of these–very commonly seen in contemporary societies–is emotional problems or excessive emotions. This means that a person is either experiencing their emotions too intensely, or on the contrary, repressing them. However, root causes can be very diverse. When talking about "emotional problems," it is essential to understand that, regarding the Liver, we mean specific emotions: anger and rage, but also frustration. Anger and rage are obvious and easily perceivable, and so frustration is often overlooked in this context. Yet frustration is directed inward and constrains the qì. It's an example of how internal workings and emotions can be just as important for and detrimental to our health as what we see on the outside.

On a physical level, the TCM mechanism behind this is as follows. Once blocked, Liver qì cannot move freely, and if it stagnates for a longer period the body starts to produce heat, which then builds up and eventually turns into fire if there is no intervention. In this case, skin lesions will appear red. If the fire lasts too long, blood stagnation might appear, because fire tends to consume yīn and/or blood. When blood becomes deficient, it stagnates. There is quite a simple analogy: when a river dries out, nothing remaining in the riverbed can move, because there is no more water. Like the riverbed, the blood is parched and no longer supplies the skin with moisture. The skin usually becomes dry and taut. So, if a patient presents with eczema that looks red-purple, TCM practitioners need to remember to also move blood in order to resolve blood stasis. The analogy of the dry riverbed and its relation to blood within the body according to TCM is also very easy for patients to understand.

It is obvious, but nonetheless practitioners need to be aware that this can easily turn into a vicious cycle. Once the Liver is impeded—no matter what the initial trigger is—the person will be more prone to feel anger. This increased anger or rage will further harm the Liver, which results in more anger or rage, which then further damages the Liver, and so on. The same applies, of course, to frustration. Thus, the aim is to break this vicious cycle and lead everything back to balance, namely to a free flow of qì. In my practice, I often observe that skin conditions worsen in times of stress or after episodes of frustration, anger, rage, or even arguments. This is anything but uncommon, and eczema is a very good example. This emotional turmoil, in combination with a large quantity of alcohol, red meat, and coffee, is a sure way to flare up a patient's eczema. The saying "the Liver is on fire" is meant literally in TCM. Patients need to become aware of how important balanced emotions are for the health of their body and skin. Prolonged emotional turmoil and being constantly upset should be avoided in any case. Everyone gets upset or annoyed from time to time. This is normal. But patients need to deal with their emotions and long-lasting situations or circumstances that cause emotional upset, because these make people ill!

CLINICAL TIP: Whenever the skin gets worse after feeling angry, you should keep the Liver in mind.

Heart

Heart fire is another possible cause of eczema, but of the three organs mentioned above, I see this the least in practice. Spleen and Liver involvement are far more frequent. However, TCM practitioners need to understand why and how fire can arise in the Heart.

Longer-term emotional stagnation transforming into fire, as well as an attack of pathogenic fire-heat from the external environment, can cause hyperactivity of Heart fire. The latter often occurs on hot summer days when people are exposed to heat for too long and do not protect themselves sufficiently. In Chinese medicine, summer is associated with the fire element and with the Heart. It is a time of abundant energy. Not being adequately protected or being exposed to the sun for too long, without sufficient protection, results in the accumulation of too much heat (and fire). This can cause patients to feel anxious, restless, and unsettled. Patients can also experience fever, thirst, palpitations, insomnia, mouth ulcers, and constipation. Exuberant heat can also attack the skin to cause eczema due to the generation of blood-heat, and the skin would present with very red papules, erythema, eruptions, burning, crusting, and pus formation. In this case, cooling heat in the blood always comes first in treatment!

In addition, an improper diet with long-term overconsumption of hot and spicy food or red meat, and excessive drinking of alcohol can also transform into fire, which affects the Heart. Thus, patients need to be educated that what they eat can make a difference, and especially in which season they eat it. Eating food that is too hot in the summer is like adding fuel to the fire, a fact that should be easy to understand.

CLINICAL TIP: Whenever you see worsening of the skin in combination with restlessness and bad sleep, keep the Heart in mind.

Internal Pathogenic Factors

The main internal factors that can cause skin conditions like eczema are the seven emotions: anger, joy, worry, anxiety, grief, fear, and fright.[1]

anger	Liver
joy	Heart
worry	Spleen
grief (anxiety)	Lungs
fear (fright)	Kidney

Other internal factors besides emotions can be an improper diet, genetic disposition, too little sleep, or overstrain. After practicing TCM for many years and specializing in skin disorders, I consider emotions to be a major cause of illness and of the weakness leading to diseases, especially when it comes to the skin.

The understanding that emotions strongly affect our qì and our overall health is deeply rooted in TCM theory. TCM has always integrated the connection between body and mind on a completely different level than Western medicine. Of course, patients often observe the interrelationships for themselves, but get nowhere when trying to address them. This is precisely the shortcoming of conventional medicine: its sometimes superficial approach to very complex issues such as skin conditions. Symptoms are viewed and, more importantly, treated in isolation; other crucial factors such as emotions and life circumstances are not taken into account. And this is exactly what many patients no longer want—superficial treatment through medicine that does not help them in the long term and also causes side effects.

It is clearly stated in the *Huáng Dì Nèi Jīng* that an overindulgence in the five[2] emotions can create imbalances within our body. Emotions are potential "internal pathogens" with the ability to imbalance the function of our organs. Each organ is related to one of the five emotions, and each emotion affects a specific organ system. This unbalancing effect can occur when an emotion is experienced very intensely, suddenly, or when any emotion is held over an extended period.

- Anger makes qì rise quickly and has a negative impact on the Liver.

- Excessive joy, meaning a state of overexcitement, can adversely affect the Heart qì.

- Worry, related to the Spleen, depletes this organ's qì, affecting the digestive process, causing stagnation of qì and retention of food.

- Sadness affects the Lung and depletes qì.

- Fear corresponds to the Kidney. This emotion depletes the essence, the basis for qì, which is stored in the Kidney.

Emotions are what makes us human and truly alive, and feelings are certainly a natural and good thing. Yet, viewing emotions from the TCM perspective, they must be in balance and flow to avoid an adverse effect on our well-being.

Too much anger and frustration, but also worry, overthinking, and thinking in mind loops are the main patterns I see in practice. In contemporary work contexts, many people are overwhelmed by their workload but still believe an ideal that tells them that hard work is recognized and will lead to success. They tend to lose connection with their needs or purposefully ignore them in order to fulfil what they assume is expected. And, of course, their own health suffers badly as a result.

Clinical Anecdote

This case from my practice illustrates the impact emotions and stress can have on the skin, but also how effectively Chinese herbs work.

A woman in her mid-fifties came to see me because of serious hand eczema. The skin on her hands was open, burning, oozing, and extremely painful. She couldn't touch anything and her skin easily became infected due to the open lesions. Gloves were not an option, because they would tear her skin over and over. She was a kindergarten teacher by profession. She was already experiencing stress from her job, her home life with many private family issues and then Covid-19 came on top of this. Her worries caused the internal pressure to further increase. She said that when she had time off, the skin improved, but as soon as kindergarten started again, it got worse. I gave her herbs as a decoction and as a hand bath. The herbs did wonders for her skin. In times of serious stress her skin got worse, but it was not as bad as before, and her skin would heal faster. I could not take away the stress at the kindergarten, nor could I resolve her private issues, but I was able to give her Chinese herbs which helped her skin. She now only comes to see me for prevention when she has a very small skin lesion on her hands.

Another point worth mentioning, as it exerts considerable influence: our society is unfortunately fixated on the concept of being perfectly beautiful all the time, as propagated on social media and glossy magazine covers. The idea that physical beauty and perfection are a normal thing in our society, and those who are seemingly "unattractive" are that way by their own fault, can cause a lot of unnecessary distress. In truth, not many people can live up to an abstract and photoshopped beauty standard. Apart from the fact that everyone sees beauty differently, it can be really hard for people with skin diseases to accept themselves.

For me, it has always been very important to reassure my patients not to feel stigmatized because of their skin conditions. I tell them that a person's beauty is reflected in their intellect and heart, and the way they take care of themselves. I always encourage them to have more confidence, and remind them that healthy, bright, and kind-hearted people are the ones considered truly beautiful. A conversation with your patients is always very important and helpful, and often an excellent start to treatment. We as TCM practitioners work differently; we take our time for the things that are important, and that includes talking about emotions.

External Pathogenic Factors

It is common knowledge, a kind of world wisdom passed on from generation to generation, that we must dress warm and keep our feet dry in winter. This piece of advice that we receive as children, and then pass on to our own children—simply stating that we should always dress appropriately for the weather—is deeply reflected in the Chinese wisdom that pathogenic factors are related to the weather. According to TCM theory, external causes, also called the "six exogenous pathogenic factors,"[3] are: wind (*fēng* 风), cold (*hán* 寒), summer-heat (*shǔ* 暑), dampness (*shī* 湿), dryness (*zào* 燥), and heat (*rè* 热) (fire, *huǒ* 火). Under normal circumstances, when it is strong and resilient, the human body can adapt to climatic conditions and variations. If the harmonic relationship between human beings and nature is broken, however, the body is unable to adapt to quickly changing weather or a different climate in a new location. This can either occur when the body's resistance is too weak, or in the case of abnormal or unseasonal weather patterns, as these exceed the body's ability to adapt. In both cases, the consequence is that the six natural climatic factors become pathogenic factors and cause an outbreak of disease. Climate change poses a particular challenge here, as adaptation has to happen even faster, and the weather phenomena are becoming more and more extreme. It certainly does not make it any easier for us humans to stay healthy.

Although the weather can have a huge impact on the skin, when discussing eczema, I do not see the external climatic factors as the primary cause, but rather as secondary factors that can worsen the condition—in particular heat and damp (humidity). Heat patterns are characterized by an acute onset, red and burning skin lesions manifesting in erythema and papules. Damp patterns are characterized by a slow onset, heaviness, and erosive oozing. When damp combines with heat, the occurrence is more intense, manifesting in redness, a burning sensation, intense itching, and oozing. All specific characteristics are explained in detail in the "Dampness-Heat" pattern in Chapter 6.

Medication and Chemicals

Certain drugs and chemicals can also lead to eczema. Skin reactions are among the most common undesirable side effects of medication. The spectrum ranges from mild rashes to serious skin reactions. In my practice I repeatedly see skin reactions after taking diuretics or ACE inhibitors for treatment of high blood pressure, heart problems and more. Thus, when seeing a patient with eczema accompanied by extreme itching all over the body, TCM practitioners should never forget to ask about additional medication.

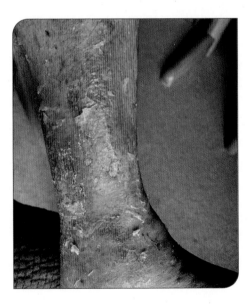

This picture presents a serious skin reaction on the patient's legs after taking the ACE inhibitor, Torasemide.

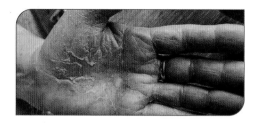

This picture shows an eczema reaction on a cleaner's hands after wearing latex gloves. Patients with sensitive skin whose job requires them to wear latex or nitrile gloves can develop hand eczema due to the substances inside. Thus, when skin reactions appear at a fixed location, such as the hands, the practitioner needs to ask about any contact with potential allergy inducing substances.

Diet and Food

I cannot stress enough the importance of nutrition and, as mentioned previously, that improper diet is one of the main reasons for the development of eczema. Therefore, a brief summary of the factors that can cause skin diseases such as eczema due to improper eating habits and lifestyle seems appropriate. The TCM view on diet, food, and eczema is detailed further in Chapter 10.

Times have changed, societies have changed, and so have dietary and lifestyle habits. I have already mentioned that many people do not recognize or live according to their needs and limits. This also applies to nutrition. The feeling of hunger is often ignored because people do not have time to eat–at least this is what they think. This eventually results in irregular eating habits. Even worse is skipping meals just to be slim in order to fit some surreal ideal of beauty. In my practice, I see a lot of women with eating disorders, either current or in the past. It seems almost too obvious to mention that this disordered eating has damaged their Spleen and Stomach over a long time. Yet it is crucial to explain and make them aware how important these organs are in TCM, how they can damage their own organs, and conversely how they can support them. The opposite is not a rarity either: some people eat carelessly, while watching television or writing emails, for example. They do not even pay attention to how food tastes, and how much and what they consume. People often do not eat mindfully.

As to what people eat: patients never cease to surprise me when they describe their eating habits. Many people consume meat, fast food, and unhealthy sweets in excess. Numerous conversations with patients in my practice confirm this. Thus, I am convinced that many diseases–including eczema–stem from the same negative influences: an unhealthy diet, overeating, and, as mentioned above, mindless eating, leading to a lifestyle that has an excess of illness-promoting factors, plus a deficiency of health-promoting factors. In so-called prosperous societies, some people's living and eating habits unfortunately have little to do with providing the body with the nutrition it needs, and more with constant consumption. I very often use the term "measure and middle" in practice to remind patients of a balanced diet and way of life. Less excess in life means a healthier one!

Another major issue is food production. Over the last few decades, food manufacturers have introduced many highly processed foods containing artificial colorings, preservatives, sweeteners and flavour enhancers, and modern agriculture uses many chemicals[4]–the effects are highly debatable and often criticized. Meat production and treatment of animals have also been criticized for many years; not only for the lack of animal welfare but also for the effects hormones and medications may have on consumers. All of this is certainly not to make our food healthier, but rather for the manufacturer's further profit. Many patients have no idea what their food actually contains, and I encourage them to read the ingredients. Often, I also explain what certain abbreviations mean to make them more aware of what is detrimental to their health. From my practice, I can report that patients often show reactions to cheap sweeteners and flavour enhancers.[5] Therefore, when talking to patients, TCM practitioners must explain how essential a proper diet is. Awareness of eating well to promote health is crucial.

Endnotes

1   The seven emotions are external manifestations of the functional activities of the five *zàng* organs. Intense disturbances in emotional states will lead to the onset of diseases relating to these organs.

2   For clarification between the five and seven emotions mentioned, the text says "The five yīn-organs of the human body produce five kinds of essential qì, which bring forth joy, anger, grief, worry, and fear." So these are the "main" emotions.

3   According to TCM theory, exogenous pathogenic factors are the six variations in the climate of the seasons. Please do not confuse concepts between the

modern ideas of weather or climate and the Chinese ideas of external pathogenic factors.

4   For example, insecticides, fungicides, pesticides, just to name a few. Many have side effects and can harm our health.

5   For example, E621: Monosodium glutamate (MSG), also known as sodium glutamate. It is commonly added to Chinese food, canned food, instant soups, and processed meats. A lot of patients report adverse reactions to foods containing MSG, be it headache, nausea, flushing, or bloating and diarrhoea.

6

Syndrome Differentiation and Treatment of Eczema According to Traditional Chinese Medicine

S KIN CONDITIONS are not as superficial as they may seem. Even though we have a diagnosis and a name for the skin disease, the presentation is different in each patient. In eczema for example, while one patient has more itching, the other will have a weeping rash. This means that our treatment results are only as good as our ability to make a precise TCM diagnosis and adapt the treatment plan and prescription to the patient. In TCM, there is no one standard treatment and this makes the significant difference compared with conventional medicine. The strength of TCM dermatology lies in a holistic approach with individualized and natural treatment tailored to the needs of each individual patient. This leads our discussion to the topic of syndrome differentiation according to TCM.

As mentioned before, precise syndrome differentiation is a vital requirement for effective treatment. In TCM, this process is called *biàn zhèng* (辨证). In practice, when explaining it to my patients, I often compare this process to very meticulous detective work. All clinical information is gathered by the four main diagnostic TCM methods:

- inspection (observation): appearance and localization of the skin lesion, patient's complexion, posture, and of course, tongue diagnosis

- auscultation (listening): voice, patient's report—symptoms and history

- olfaction (smelling): body odour or smelly breath, for instance

- palpation (feeling): consistency and mobility of the lesion, pain on touch, and pulse diagnosis according to TCM.

> CLINICAL ADVICE: Whenever you feel an irregular pulse (it may feel like your heart skipped a beat, added a beat, or is "fluttering"), please advise your patient to consult their general practitioner or cardiologist. It would be negligent to not refer out for issues beyond our scope of practice.

When treating a skin disease, always place the focus on the skin first! Make sure to use daylight while inspecting the skin, as there are color nuances on the skin that are difficult to see in less optimal lighting conditions.

After examining the skin, more data is gathered through questioning the patient, and details including the location, clinical presentation, onset/trigger, and duration, as well as the accompanying symptoms such as pain, discharge, and any sensations of burning, itching, or heat on the lesion, are evaluated. Don't forget to ask about the aggravating or alleviating factors. Let me give you a list of key factors that I have observed in practice:

- stress

- alcohol and/or nicotine

- diet with hot, spicy, oily foods

- too many sweets

- climate, especially hot and humid weather

- bad digestion, such as constipation

- medication, antidiuretics for example[1]

- menstrual cycle (in women).

Checking the tongue and pulse is another essential part of TCM diagnosis which can also provide prompts for further questioning, directing us towards symptoms the patient forgot to mention. It is a common experience in clinical practice that patients often add essential information only when somehow reminded of it. Since a successful treatment relies on accurate syndrome differentiation, the complex process of gathering all the information and making a correct diagnosis according to TCM is essential and cannot be replaced. Again, each patient presents with a different origin of the disease and suffers from different accompanying symptoms. We work holistically, always keep the big picture in mind!

> CLINICAL TIP: Methods like inspection, palpation, and olfaction may seem easy, but one gets more information than you might think, and above all more information about the patient than they will notice and report themselves. What is meant by this? Things you can see while feeling the patient's pulse: circulation of the skin, yellow fingertips from nicotine abuse, excessive chewing of fingernails and cuticles, and even deliberate self-harm, such as self-cutting. While taking the pulse, you can also feel very easily if the patient has cold hands and arms, or a dry and rough skin. Things you can smell while examining the patient: do they drink alcohol or coffee? Do they smoke cigarettes or other substances such as marijuana, for instance? And, of course, you can also evaluate their personal hygiene by their smell. All of this gives us clues about patient's way of life and emotional state. The latter mentioned points are often an indicator of emotional disorders. In conclusion, often we don't have to ask, we can see so many things without asking. Take your time and, of course, be attentive.

This is a simple overview of how I work in clinical practice during the initial consultation, step by step:

1. Initial overall impression (start)[2]

2. Skin check

3. Accompanying symptoms

4. Pulse diagnosis

5. Tongue diagnosis

6. Formulating the TCM diagnosis and explaining it to the patient

7. Information for the patient on diet, skin care, and herbal preparation

8. Answering potential questions from the patient

9. Writing the TCM prescription.

Clinical Anecdote

I am sharing a short story from my own practice to highlight all the information you can gain from a patient's tongue and pulse. A man aged around 50 years old came for treatment of urticaria. He had a red face, was sweating profusely and appeared nervous. I thought his nerves were due to trying something new, as he had never tried TCM before, however when I was close enough to feel his pulse, I could smell marijuana, and I noticed the thick yellow coating on his tongue. It wasn't until the end of our consultation, when I asked him about nicotine, coffee, and alcohol consumption, that he mentioned smoking marijuana every day, for relief from depression. He didn't want to take psychotropic drugs any more because he wasn't doing well on them and suspected that they have also been a trigger for his urticaria.

In Chinese medicine, marijuana is categorized as having a pungent taste and a hot, toxic nature. It enters into the Liver meridian and dispels wind, activates blood and opens collaterals, relieves pain and stops bleeding. It is often used for pain caused by wind-damp, trauma, and hemorrhage.[3] However, it seems pretty obvious that a hot toxic herb is absolutely inappropriate for someone who already has damp-heat, and so I explained the Chinese medicine perspective on marijuana and how it may be aggravating his skin. It's now up to him to decide whether he continues the marijuana. My job is to inform patients as best as I can but the decision is up to the patient; ultimately they are responsible for their own actions.

Practical Advice in the Use of Chinese Herbs

In eczema, as for most other skin conditions, I have found decoctions of raw herbs to be the most effective form of treatment in TCM. It has to be clearly explained that the herbs won't taste good in order to prevent the patient's illusion that a Chinese herbal decoction could resemble in any way a pleasant-tasting "wellness tea." Once prepared for the worst scenario, they will come back to their next appointment and say "You were so right! That tea was the most horrible taste adventure ever but you know what, after just one week I got used to it and now I don't find it so bad anymore." Decoctions are not a delight for taste buds. However, the decoction's purpose is to work, not taste. Patients usually tolerate them once the benefits are explained.

My practical hint for very bitter formulas as well as for taste-sensitive patients is to recommend the addition of honey to the decoction, which makes it taste a little less bitter and more tolerable. They can also have a small cookie straight after to neutralize the bitter taste. Patient satisfaction is very important for compliance with Chinese herbal medicine. It is better to drink a decoction with a little honey in it instead of drinking nothing. Patients can also drink a sip of tea or juice. You can advise the patient that a lukewarm or warm decoction will taste more tolerable than drinking it cold, especially when a formula contains a lot of very bitter herbs. Additionally, keep in mind that bitter decoctions should never be consumed cold, as the cold and bitter herbs will affect the Stomach and patients may feel uncomfortable after drinking it. One hint for making cold and bitter herbs more tolerable for patients with a weak digestion is to use *páo zhì* 炮制. This traditional preparation process, which changes and enhances the therapeutic effect of medicinal plants, has already been explained in detail in Chapter 3, under the heading "Chinese Herbal Treatment Options in Chinese Medical Dermatology." However, dry frying (*chǎo*) can be used to minimize the bitter and cold nature of herbs that easily harm the Spleen and Stomach. This preparation method reduces their cold properties and makes them more tolerable for the digestive system, and any qualified TCM pharmacy will be able to prepare it.

CLINICAL TIP: Never forget that we are the specialists. Patients seek our advice and usually they have tried many things beforehand. I have seen so many good results in patients with eczema. Thus, raw herbs are always best, don't deviate from them! Why should we recommend something less effective to our patients.

How This Chapter Is Structured

In order to keep this section as clear and practical as possible, I will not subdivide the different eczema types (according to conventional medicine). In TCM, we treat what we see and it makes no difference whether it is, for example, nummular eczema, seborrheic eczema, or dyshidrotic eczema. The TCM syndrome/pattern the patient presents with is more important than the subtype of eczema they have, as the syndrome/pattern is what we are treating. However, the modifications of the basic formulas for each pattern are of great importance, and I will go into these in great detail. The ability to flexibly modify formulae to fit your patient is what makes a good TCM doctor!

THERE ARE THREE WAYS TO MODIFY A FORMULA: 1. modification of the ingredients, 2. modification of dosages, 3. modification of the application form, such as decoction, pill, or granules.

In this chapter, I will cover the most common syndromes seen in practice, enabling you to treat patients regardless of their eczema subtype. However, I will make one exception: Contact dermatitis will be covered in a separate section, as this is distinguished by two particular TCM patterns, which are predominantly seen in this condition. Please note, there are always exceptions as well. Thus, these remarks can be applied to all eczema subtypes, even if it is not contact dermatitis. I will also cover an extra section for eczema in children (infantile eczema). While the patterns and the respective formulas are very similar, it is recommended to use different dosages and slightly different modifications when treating children. For this reason, infantile eczema will be discussed separately at the end of this chapter. As already mentioned, an extra part of this book will be dedicated to neurodermatitis (see Chapter 7).

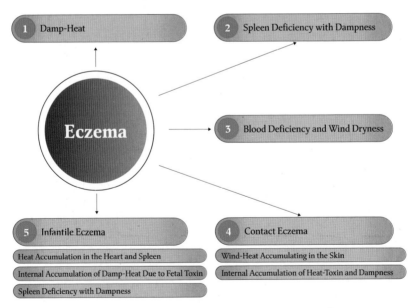

THE MOST COMMON TCM SYNDROMES OF ECZEMA[4]

My aim is to enable you to work independently in your practice, recognize the difference between patterns to identify your patient's presentation, and immediately write a prescription. I will primarily focus on the use of classical formulas and moderate dosages, which are affordable for patients, along with the use of external topical formulations (ointments, washes, compresses, and pastes). Exact instructions on how to prepare and how to apply the external topical treatments for the skin will be discussed in Appendix I. Each TCM syndrome will be accompanied by pictures of the tongue and skin.

Dampness-Heat (*Shī Rè* 湿热)

Damp-heat diseases can be divided into "externally induced" and "internally induced" damp-heat diseases. Each category has different etiologies and signs.

Externally induced damp-heat is caused by an invasion of exogenous dampness together with warmth or a heat-pathogen. The body is invaded by exogenous summer-heat and dampness mainly during late summer or early autumn. Externally induced damp-warmth diseases can also be caused by an improper diet with too much hot, spicy, and oily food, but also by an over-consumption of seafood. TCM believes that eczema patients should avoid seafood because it is suspected that excessive consumption of seafood like lobster, shrimp, oysters, crabs, or mussels can aggravate eczema by triggering allergic reactions and increasing inflammation. From the traditional TCM viewpoint, seafood is classified as *fā wù* 发物. These products always tend to generate heat and fire inside the body and injure fluids. In case of red-colored skin lesions as seen in eczema, heat is already predominant. When *fā wù* food is consumed, it adds even more heat to the pre-existing heat, and thus makes the skin rash worse. These products should be avoided in any case. Very simply said: Do not add fuel to the flames! Please note that *fā wù* will be described in detail in the section on diet in Chapter 10. From a modern perspective, please be aware that fish is also considered a problem when it's not fresh because it has higher histamine levels compared to fresh fish. If a person eats fish with a high level of histamine, the response may resemble an allergic reaction, with a skin rash for example.

However, internally induced damp-heat is usually caused by a dysfunction of the Spleen and Stomach in their transportation and transformation functions, and an improper diet also contributes to this pattern. As a result, foods and fluids will accumulate in the middle *jiāo*. Chronic retention of dampness easily transforms into heat, and it is often combined with toxins. In skin disorders, damp-heat accumulates in the skin and causes redness and pustules.

> CLINICAL TIP: You will find that these patients often have unhealthy lifestyles: eating lots of hot and spicy foods, smoking, and drinking alcohol. These patients often also have oily skin on the face.

Characteristics

Damp-heat is characterized by an acute onset and often a short duration. The skin lesions are polymorphic,[5] symmetric and appear as erythema, multiple, dense millet-size papules, papulovesicles, erosion, exudation (usually yellowish), and crusting. The lesions can spread all over the body, although damp-heat has the tendency to be more severe on the lower part of the body due to the heavy nature of dampness. The lesions have an indistinct border. Furthermore, the patient feels a sensation of heat on their skin with intense itching.

> CLINICAL TIP: The skin lesions will vary depending on the predominance of heat or dampness. If there is more heat, the lesions are more reddish in color; if there is more dampness, the papules and/or papulovesicles appear more yellowish.

Other symptoms may include fever, irritability, a dry mouth and throat, thirst, constipation, and a yellow urine, but also a heavy sensation in the chest, loss of appetite, fatigue, a heavy feeling in the lower limbs or vaginal discharge. Please note that not all of these symptoms need to occur but you will find that they are often present. Rare but sometimes seen is a yellowish facial color, which does not only occur in patients with Spleen qì deficiency from a TCM point of view.

The tongue is red with a greasy, yellow coating and the pulse is slippery and/or rapid.

Treatment Principle

Clear away heat, eliminate dampness, relieve itching (qīng rè, qū shī, zhǐ yǎng 清热祛湿止痒).

Representative Formula

The treatment is chosen based on the location of the affected region.
If damp-heat is more located on the upper part of the body, use:

Lóng Dǎn Xiè Gān Tāng (Gentian Decoction to Drain the Liver).

If damp-heat is more located in the lower part of the body, especially the legs, use:

Bì Xiè Shèn Shī Tāng (Dioscorea Decoction to Leach Out Dampness).

Ingredients
Lóng Dǎn Xiè Gān Tāng (Gentian Decoction to Drain the Liver)

lóng dǎn cǎo	Gentianiae, Radix	3–6 g
huáng qín	Scutellariae, Radix	9–12 g
zhī zǐ	Gardeniae, Fructus	9–15 g
chái hú	Bupleuri, Radix	9 g
mù tōng	Akebiae, Caulis	9 g
chē qián zǐ	Plantaginis, Semen	9–12 g
zé xiè	Alismatis, Rhizoma	9–12 g
shēng dì huáng	Rehmanniae Glutinosae, Radix	9–15 g
dāng guī	Angelicae Sinensis, Radix	9 g
gān cǎo	Glycyrrhizae Uralensis, Radix	6 g

Bì Xiè Shèn Shī Tāng (Dioscorea Decoction to Leach Out Dampness)

yì yǐ rén	Coices, Semen	15–30 g
huá shí	Talcum	9–15 g
bì xiè	Dioscoreae, Rhizoma	9–20 g
fú líng	Poriae Cocos, Sclerotium	9–12 g
huáng bǎi	Phellodendri, Cortex	6–10 g
mǔ dān pí	Moutan, Cortex	9–12 g
zé xiè	Alismatis, Rhizoma	12–15 g
tōng cǎo	Tetrapanacis, Medulla	6 g

First Reference

Lóng Dǎn Xiè Gān Tāng is a relatively recent formula. The first reference to the formula can be found in *Yī Fāng Jí Jiě* (Medical Formulas Collected and Analyzed, 1682, Qīng Dynasty), written by Wāng Áng. Over 700 prescriptions are listed in this book. Wāng Áng says that *Lóng Dǎn Xiè Gān Tāng* can clear heat from the organs, and he lists the following syndromes where it can be used:

1. Heat excess in the Liver and Gallbladder

2. Liver fire rising

3. Damp-heat in the Liver.

First reference to *Bì Xiè Shèn Shī Tāng*: *Yáng Kē Xīn Dé Jí* (Collected Experiences on Treating Sores, 1806), written by Gāo Bǐng-Jūn.

Formula Analysis
Lóng Dǎn Xiè Gān Tāng

As mentioned above, if damp-heat is mainly located in the upper part of the body, *Lóng Dǎn Xiè Gān Tāng* is the formula of choice. A formula like *Bì Xiè Shèn Shī Tāng* would definitely not be sufficient in this case, because heat is predominant, not dampness. "*Lóng Dǎn Xiè Gān Tāng* cools heat without causing stasis, dispels pathogenic qì and causes it to descend without hurting the normal qì. It is an excellent formula for treating the symptoms and underlying mechanisms associated with Liver and Gallbladder heat excess."[6] It relieves damp-heat from the Liver channel–and this is exactly what we need here because heat always tends to move upwards–by draining dampness and promoting urination to leach out heat via the lower *jiāo*. The clearing and purging method utilizes bitter-cold herbs, accompanied by nourishing, soothing, and dispersing herbs corresponding with the Liver's yīn nature and its yáng function. The main ingredients of the formula are: *lóng dǎn cǎo*, *huáng qín* and *zhī zǐ*. *Lóng dǎn cǎo* serves as chief herb because it accomplishes the primary functions of the formula. *Huáng qín*, *zhī zǐ* and *chái hú* are the three deputies within the formula. *Mù tōng*, *chē qián zǐ*, *zé xiè*, *shēng dì huáng* and *dāng guī* serve as assistants. *Gān cǎo* works as an envoy within the formula. But let's analyze the formula in more detail.

Lóng dǎn cǎo is extremely bitter in flavor and extremely cold in nature. This makes the herb highly effective not only in purging excess fire from the Liver and Gallbladder, but also in draining damp-heat from the Liver channel. *Huáng qín* and *zhī zǐ* assist *lóng dǎn cǎo* in draining fire and expelling dampness. Bitter herbs such as *lóng dǎn cǎo, zhī zǐ* and *huáng qín* are usually classified as having a heat purging effect or a heat clearing effect. To be precise, *lóng dǎn cǎo* and *zhī zǐ* purge heat and *huáng qín* clears heat from the Liver channel. *Zhī zǐ* is an effective herb for draining the Liver. It also resolves constrained heat and directs damp-heat downwards, leading it out through the urine.[7] In general it is said that if an emotion like anger sets Liver fire ablaze, the Liver fire needs to be cleared with herbs like *huáng qín*. In more serious situations, however, herbs that strongly purge Liver heat such as *lóng dǎn cǎo* are needed to eliminate the fire.

The Liver, like its associated element wood, has an innate desire to expand and disperse. *Chái hú* disperses heat due to constrained Liver qì. It soothes Liver qì and leads the other herbs to the Liver channel. Since *chái hú* has a pungent flavor, it can directly disperse stagnation. Thus, it is generally recommended for conditions characterized by a stagnation of qì. When it is combined with *huáng qín*, it can clear Liver fire, which is caused by Liver qì stagnation. *Mù tōng* (please see below regarding the herb's toxicity), *chē qián zǐ* and *zé xiè* drain heat from the upper burner and remove damp-heat via the urine. As the Liver fire needs a pathway to leave the body, this combination of urination-promoting herbs paves the way. It is an option to remove draining herbs like *mù tōng* and *chē qián zǐ* from this formula, and thus make it more suitable for treating fire without damaging the yīn as much. If damp-heat increases, these herbs can be returned to the formula. Blood and yīn are easily consumed when fire-heat is in excess in the Liver. Moreover, the components of the prescription are almost all bitter, cold, and drying, and herbs like *chái hú* also tend to damage the yīn. Thus, *dāng guī* and *shēng dì huáng* are included to nourish and protect blood and yīn while eliminating fire-heat. *Dāng guī* supplements and quickens the blood without causing stasis, while *shēng dì huáng* cools and nourishes blood and boosts yīn. *Gān cǎo* harmonizes the prescription because it mediates the extreme properties of the other components. It tonifies and harmonizes the Stomach and it is used as an envoy and guiding herb in the prescription as it enters all 12 channels.

CAUTIONS

Because of their bitter and cold nature, *lóng dǎn cǎo, huáng qín* and *zhī zǐ* can easily harm the Spleen and Stomach and should therefore be used with caution in patients with Spleen deficiency or deficiency-cold syndrome. To minimize the bitter and cold character of these three herbs they can be dry-fried (*chǎo*). This preparation reduces their cold properties and makes it more tolerable for the digestive system.

Mù tōng, while previously a common ingredient for treating various kinds of skin diseases, has been found to be nephrotoxic. The toxicity is due to the herb's aristolochic acid,[8] which in addition to being a potent nephrotoxin is also a known carcinogen.[9] Considering an increased risk of renal failure and urinary tract cancer from prolonged intake and ingestion of large doses, *mù tōng* is no longer used and alternative herbs like *tōng cǎo* are used instead.

Bì Xiè Shèn Shī Tāng

If the lower body is more affected with eczema than the upper body, damp-heat has sunken downwards due to the heavy nature of dampness. In such a case, a formula like *Lóng Dǎn Xiè Gān Tāng* would not be sufficient because dampness is predominant, not heat. *Bì Xiè Shèn Shī Tāng* is the best choice if lesions of eczema are seen on the legs and the patient shows signs of both damp and heat, because it is formulated mainly for damp-heat diffusing downward. The main functions of *Bì Xiè Shèn Shī Tāng* are resolving dampness, clearing heat and promoting urination. But let's go into more detail.

Yì yǐ rén strengthens the Spleen, promotes urination and leaches out dampness. It clears heat, expels pus, and clears damp-heat. *Huá shí* also clears heat and promotes urination. It can expel damp-heat through the urine. Do not forget to wrap *huá shí* in a small cloth bag, otherwise the talcum will stick to the pot rim when boiling and/or sink as sediment to the bottom of the pot after boiling. Inform your patient to leave the herb in the bag for cooking, as I have often noticed that patients think they have to take it out. *Bì xiè* separates the pure from the turbid, it consequently resolves turbid dampness in the lower *jiāo* and clears damp-heat from the skin. It is frequently used with *huáng bǎi* and *yì yǐ rén* to treat skin lesions on the lower part of the body caused by damp-heat. *Fú líng* strengthens the Spleen, promotes urination, resolves dampness and transforms phlegm. Combined with *zé xiè*, it facilitates the removal of stagnant water and leaches out dampness that might be causing oedema, swelling and heaviness throughout the body, particularly in the lower limbs. *Huáng bǎi* effectively drains damp-heat, especially from the lower *jiāo*. It drains fire and eliminates toxicity. *Mǔ dān pí* clears heat, cools the blood, drains pus and reduces swelling. *Zé xiè* promotes urination and leaches out dampness through the Bladder. It clears blazing ministerial fire in the Kidneys by draining damp-heat from the lower *jiāo*. And finally, *tōng cǎo* also promotes urination and clears heat. Because of the cold and draining properties of these herbs, this formula should be used with caution in patients with qì and yīn deficiencies.

Modifications

If the skin lesions are markedly fresh red, use *Lóng Dǎn Xiè Gān Tāng* in combination with *Huáng Lián Jiě Dú Tāng* (Coptis Decoction to Relieve Toxicity) to work more strongly on clearing away heat and toxin, removing heat from the blood, purging pathogenic fire, and nourishing yīn. This formula contains: *huáng lián, huáng qín, huáng bǎi* and *zhī zǐ*. You just add *huáng lián* and *huáng bǎi*, as *huáng qín* and *zhī zǐ* are already ingredients in *Lóng Dǎn Xiè Gān Tāng*.

For itchy skin lesions, add *dì fū zǐ* and/or *bái xiān pí*, 9–12 g of each. Bái xiān pí is very effective in stopping itching but should be used with caution if given as a single herb or for long periods of time, especially in patients with poor Liver function.[10] Alternatively, one may consider using *xú cháng qīng*, 9–12 g. It dispels wind and can thus alleviate itching. It can be used alone for this purpose but also in combination with *dì fū zǐ* and *bái xiān pí*.

> CLINICAL TIP: In general, once itching and scratching is stopped, the skin lesions heal better. Thus, focus on stopping itching!

If a stronger action of draining heat and removing damp-heat via the urine is required, add *dàn zhú yè*, 6–9 g, to support *zé xiè*. If yellowish pus and exudation are predominant, add *tǔ fú líng* at a dose of 15–30 g, depending on the severity of the lesion. It is a perfect herb for reducing redness, pain and swelling, due to its heat clearing, dampness resolving, and detoxifying effect. If this is still not enough, and the skin is burning and feels hot and painful, add *bái huā shé shé cǎo*, 9–12 g, to increase the inflammation-reducing effect. This herb is often used in treating abscesses, toxic sores, ulcerations and swellings because it cools heat, resolves toxicity and clears dampness through the urine. From a modern point of view, when the skin lesions are infected with bacteria, such as Staphylococcus aureus or streptococci, add *yú xīng cǎo*, 15 g. *Yú xīng cǎo* is known for its anti-bacterial and anti-inflammatory effects.[11] For deep red skin rash with many blisters filled with pus, discharge and crusting, add *pú gōng yīng*, 15–20 g, *zǐ huā dì dīng*, 9–12 g, and *jīn yín huā*, 12–15 g, +/- *lián qiáo*, 9–12 g. Together with *yě jú huā* and *tiān kuí zǐ* they form *Wǔ Wèi Xiāo Dú Yǐn* (Five Ingredient Decoction to Eliminate Toxins). Used in combination, *pú gōng yīng, zǐ huā dì dīng*, and *jīn yín huā* strongly clear heat and resolve toxicity, but also cool the blood and reduce swellings. Caution: As with all bitter and cold herbs, if taken at too large a dose, or for too long a time, the Spleen and Stomach may be harmed. Therefore, they should only be taken when a strong heat clearing and toxicity relieving effect is required, and when this is no longer needed, reduce their dosages or remove them.

For constipation, add *dà huáng*, 6–9 g. Practical hint to the use of *dà huáng*: Many books and colleagues prefer to decoct this herb for a shorter time, adding it later in the cooking process. I personally cook it together with all other herbs, which is absolutely fine. Due to the longer cooking process, the laxative action is slightly reduced, but the heat clearing effect still remains. I recommend informing the patient that *dà huáng* has a purgative effect, and advise them to start their herbs on the weekend to make sure they tolerate it well. It is also useful to advise the patient not to start the first dose shortly before leaving the house for work, rather to wait at home a while to see how fast any purgative effect occurs. It could be very uncomfortable for the patient to need to use a toilet while sitting on the train on their way to work, for example. If you find the patient's constitution is too weak for using raw *dà huáng*, the herb can be prepared as *(zhì) dà huáng* (mixed with rice wine and steamed, then dried in the sun) or *(chǎo) dà huáng* (roasted). Both methods make it more tolerable for patients with a weak digestion.

Last but not least, consider using *Lóng Dǎn Xiè Gān Tāng* and *Bì Xiè Shèn Shī Tāng* together, with modifications of course, when eczema is located on the legs and also on the upper part of the body. And because there are always multiple options, I would like to give you two more examples of formulas that can also be used for damp-heat, namely *Èr Miào Sǎn*[12] (Two-Marvel Powder) and *Sān Miào Wán*[13] (Three-Marvel Pill). Both formulas will certainly not be strong enough on their own and must be modified, but they can be a good starting point for damp-heat formulations for eczema, especially in the lower body regions such as the legs.

FOOD FOR THOUGHT: Because TCM is so flexible and the possibilities are so numerous, I would like to end by sharing one more formula in this section: *Qīng Rè Shèn Shī Tāng*[14] (Clearing Heat and Draining Dampness Decoction). It contains *huáng bǎi, huáng lián, zé xiè, fú líng, cāng zhú, bái zhú,* and *gān cǎo.* As you can see, there are many similar herbs between these formulas, in alternative combinations. Be flexible! Always choose the formula which suits your patient best.

Suggestions for External Treatment

There are so many options for external applications. To keep it simple and practical for you, I have chosen formulas in which all the primary herbal ingredients are readily available. I think it makes little sense to list formulas where the main herbs are not available in many countries due to species protection regulations or other reasons.

In this pattern, damp-heat, it is most important to work with herbal washes or wet compresses. Remember, in TCM we have a standard rule: Wet to wet, dry to dry! What does this mean? Whenever a discharge absorbing action is needed, always prepare the topical formula as a wash, wet compress, or an ointment. In this case the discharge has to be drained, not occluded. A thick and hardly spreadable cream would prevent this and keep inside what should be discharged. Instead of pathogens exiting the body, they are trapped and move transversely back into the body, and this can certainly worsen an inflammatory process.

For acute eczema and damp-heat with exudation it is recommended to clear heat, reduce inflammation, astringe, and promote epidermal recovery, with formulas like:[15]

- *Huáng Bǎi Róng Yè* (Phellodendri Cortex Solution)
- *Sān Huáng Xǐ Jì* (Three Yellow Cleanser Formula)
- *Shé Chuáng Zǐ Tāng* (Cnidium Fruit Decoction)
- *Sì Huáng Gāo* (Four Yellow Cream)[16]
- *Wǔ Huáng Gāo* (Five Huang Cream)[17]
- *Zào Shī Xǐ Gāo* (Damp-Heat Eliminating Ointment).

Examples for individually tailored herbal washes or wet compresses:

Please note that the following (and all) suggestions for external use should serve as examples, and can be adjusted according to your own preferences and, of course, to the patient's individual needs. Herbs can be replaced as required and dosages adjusted. Be flexible!

Standard Preparation

In general, 100 ml of water per 10 g herbs should be used for boiling. For example, if you have three herbs weighing 10 g each, use 300 ml of water. If you want a more concentrated wash, use less water, while if you want to work more mildly, use more water. Soak the herbs in water for about 20 minutes. Bring them to a boil, and then reduce the heat to a low flame allowing the herbs to simmer slowly for approximately 20 minutes, then strain the liquid.

Application Frequency and Time

Wash the affected area or apply as a wet compress two or three times a day, for about 15–30 minutes per application. Frequency of use depends on the severity of the skin lesions.

Commonly used herbs for herbal washes or wet compresses for this TCM pattern are: *huáng bǎi, huáng qín, huáng lián, dà huáng, kǔ shēn,* and *dì fū zǐ.* It is also always helpful to inform patients that there are many different possibilities and herbal combinations for external applications, and their wash can be adapted very flexibly if needed. Here are several examples of frequently used and effective combinations in this pattern:

huáng bǎi	Phellodendri, Cortex	10–15 g
huáng qín	Scutellariae, Radix	10–15 g
huáng lián	Coptidis, Rhizoma	10 g

Tǔ fú líng, 15 g, can be added to enhance the heat clearing process, and reduce redness and swelling. This combination should be boiled with about 300 ml of water. When adding *tǔ fú líng,* use 350–400 ml water.

huáng bǎi	Phellodendri, Cortex	10 g
huáng qín	Scutellariae, Radix	10 g
dì fū zǐ	Kochiae Scopariae, Fructus	10 g
kǔ shēn	Sophorae Flavescentis, Radix	10 g
+/- shé chuáng zǐ	Cnidii, Fructus	10 g
+/- bái xiān pí	Dictamni Radicis, Cortex	10 g

kŭ shēn	Sophorae Flavescentis, Radix	15 g
dì fū zĭ	Kochiae Scopariae, Fructus	15 g
bái xiān pí	Dictamni Radicis, Cortex	15 g
shé chuáng zĭ	Cnidii, Fructus	15 g

dà huáng	Rhei, Radix et Rhizoma	10 g
huáng băi	Phellodendri, Cortex	10 g
huáng qín	Scutellariae, Radix	10 g
kŭ shēn	Sophorae Flavescentis, Radix	10 g

Please see above for the calculation of the water volume. The amount of water required for boiling depends on how many herbs you are going to use and how concentrated you want to work. It goes without saying that the ratio also depends on how large the skin lesions are.

Simple examples of frequently used and effective stand-alone herbs in this pattern:

- *pú gōng yīng* (Taraxaci, Herba) 30 g

- *tŭ fú líng* (Smilacis Glabrae, Rhizoma) 30 g.

These herbs can be used individually, but if a stronger approach is needed, I tend to prefer combinations as mentioned above. Stand-alone herbs are often not enough here.

CLINICAL TIP: Any thick crusts or scales that are present must be left to fall off naturally. They should never be peeled off after any external application (or at any other time).

Please always pay attention to superinfections.[18] The yellower and thicker the crusts are, the more likely the presence of an infection. Caution and close observation of the process is extremely important. This applies to all TCM patterns!

Example Pictures of the Tongue

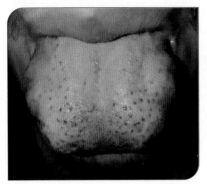

A red tongue with a thick
yellow coating.

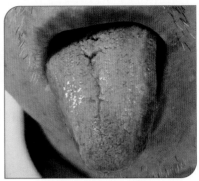

A red tongue with a thick,
greasy yellow coating.

Example Pictures of the Skin

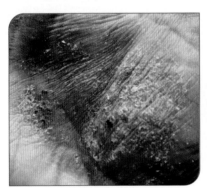

Hand eczema: More heat
than dampness.

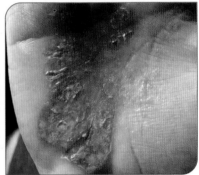

Hand eczema: More
dampness than heat.

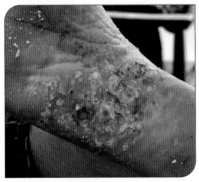

Foot eczema: Polymorphic skin
lesions with exudation and crusting.

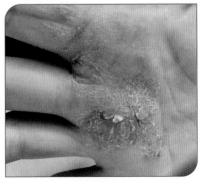

Hand eczema: Reduced redness
of the skin and crusting.

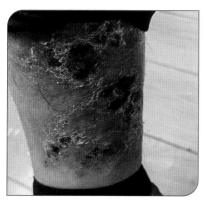

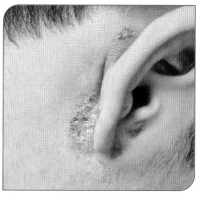

Eczema on the lower leg:
Intense red skin lesions.

Eczema around the ear: Thick skin
lesions due to weeping and crusting.

Spleen Deficiency with Accumulation of Dampness (*Pí Xū Shī Kùn* 脾虚湿困)

In contrast to the previous pattern (damp-heat), this is no longer an acute stage. What we see here is a subacute stage of eczema. The characteristics of the skin are no longer as extreme, and both onset and progression tend to be a little slower. However, this does not mean that the treatment will progress more quickly. In my experience, it often takes longer to treat skin conditions that look mild than those in the severe or acute stage, however patients usually expect the opposite. It is worthwhile to match your patient's expectations to what is possible in practice. Let's now look at what the skin looks like in this pattern.

Characteristics

The onset is slow and the skin characteristics are milder. If the Spleen is weak and dampness is predominant, the skin lesions primarily manifest as pale red or dull red macules,[19] papules, a few vesicles, or papulovesicles. The skin may be itchy. If eczema is scratched, the skin oozes and becomes encrusted. The exudate[20] usually appears clear, which makes it significantly different from the pattern before it. Needless to say, when heat is present the exudate turns yellowish.

Accompanying symptoms can include fatigue, poor appetite, loose stool, and abdominal distension. Patients also tend to get a recurrent stuffy nose or blocked sinuses due to phlegm. They will often have phlegm in the throat in the morning, and struggle to get out of bed. Everything tends to be very sluggish and slow in the morning. These patients are often overweight, with a craving for sweets and a sallow facial complexion. Don't forget to ask about how they feel in the mornings, and whether they like to eat sweets. Differentiate whether they have cravings (if they are already full, but want to eat sweets), or if they are truly hungry. The craving for sweets is a typical sign of a weak Spleen.

The tongue is puffy and pale with teeth-marks and a thick greasy coating, usually white. The pulse is slow, soft,[21] and slippery.

> CLINICAL TIP: Pay special attention to the right *guān* (关) position of the pulse, which relates to the Spleen and Stomach in Chinese medicine. This position can be noticeably weak, but it can also be strong initially at the skin level, then disappear from the muscle level to the bone level. At the beginning you have the feeling that it is strong but then at the deep level it is no longer palpable. This also a clear sign that the Spleen is not stable.

Treatment Principle

Tonify the Spleen, eliminate dampness and nourish the skin (*jiàn pí, qū shī, yǎng fū* 健脾祛湿养肤).

Representative Formula

Modified *Chú Shī Wèi Líng Tāng* (Eliminate Dampness Decoction by Combining Calm the Stomach with Five Ingredient Powder with Poria).

Alternatively, you could use: *Shēn Líng Bái Zhú Sǎn* (Ginseng, Poria and Atractylodis Macrocephalae Powder).

Ingredients
Modified *Chú Shī Wèi Líng Tāng* (Eliminate Dampness Decoction by Combining Calm the Stomach with Five Ingredient Powder with Poria)

cāng zhú	Atractylodis, Rhizoma	(3 g) 10 g
hòu pò	Magnoliae Officinalis, Cortex	(3 g) 6 g
chén pí	Citri Reticulatae, Pericarpium	(3 g) 6 g

zhū líng	Polyporus	(3 g) 10 g
zé xiè	Alismatis, Rhizoma	(3 g) 10–15 g
fú líng	Poriae Cocos, Sclerotium	(3 g) 10–15 g
(chǎo) bái zhú	(dry-fried) Atractylodis Macrocephalae, Rhizoma	(3 g) 10 g
huá shí	Talcum (wrapped)	(3 g) 10 g
fáng fēng	Saposhnikoviae, Radix	(3 g) +/- 3 g
zhī zǐ	Gardeniae, Fructus	(3 g) 10 g
mù tōng	Akebiae, Caulis	(3 g) ---
ròu guì	Cinnamomi, Cortex	(0.9 g) ---
gān cǎo	Glycyrrhizae Uralensis, Radix	(0.9 g) 3 g
dēng xīn cǎo	Junci, Medulla	(3 g) 3 g

For the sake of completeness, I have provided the complete formula and dosages from the source text. The original dosages are listed in brackets, followed by the dosages which I recommend in clinic. When treating eczema, I recommend removing the following herbs from the original formula: *mù tōng*[22] and *ròu guì*. The modifications of this formula are very interesting and very diverse. If there is little heat, you hardly need heat-clearing herbs but if dampness mixes with the heat, you can add heat-clearing herbs proportionally as needed. Please see below for more information.

Shēn Líng Bái Zhú Sǎn (Ginseng, Poria and Atractylodis Macrocephalae Powder)

rén shēn	Ginseng, Radix	10 g
bái zhú	Atractylodis Macrocephalae, Rhizoma	10 g
fú líng	Poriae Cocos, Sclerotium	10 g
zhì gān cǎo	Glycyrrhizae Preparata, Radix	10 g
shān yào	Dioscorea, Rhizome	10 g
(chǎo) bái biǎn dòu	(dry-fried) Lablab Album, Semen	10 g
lián zǐ	Nelumbinis, Semen	5 g
yì yǐ rén	Rehmanniae Glutinosae, Radix	15 g
shā rén	Amomi, Fructus	5 g
(chǎo) jié gěng	Platycodi, Radix	3–5 g

The original formula contains *rén shēn*. Since *rén shēn* is a slightly warm herb and relatively expensive, *dǎng shēn* is usually used as a substitute when a deficiency pattern is not severe because of its lower price and neutral character. It goes without saying that in very severe conditions and when an immediate relief is required, *rén shēn* should be used because it is the most powerful herb to tonify the primal qì of the five organs and it revives from collapse.[23] However, from clinical experience, *dǎng shēn* is quite often sufficient for everyday clinical use, especially in the treatment of skin diseases.

First Reference
Chú Shī Wèi Líng Tāng originally appeared in *Yī Zōng Jīn Jiàn* (The Golden Mirror of Medical Tradition, 1742), written by Wú Qiān et al.

The first reference of *Shēn Líng Bái Zhú Sǎn* was in the *Tài Píng Huì Mín Hé Jì Jú Fāng* (Formulary of the Pharmacy Service for Benefiting the People in the Taiping Era, 1107–1110), written by the Imperial Medical Bureau.

Formula Analysis
Modified *Chú Shī Wèi Líng Tāng*
Chú Shī Wèi Líng Tāng is basically *Wèi Líng Tāng* (Calm the Stomach and Poria Decoction) plus herbs which gently but firmly drain dampness and clear heat to relieve occasional itching: *zé xiè, huá shí, fáng fēng, zhī zǐ, mù tōng*, and *dēng xīn cǎo*. Looking at the formula from another angle, we see that it is a combination of *Wǔ Líng Sǎn* (Five Ingredient Powder with Poria) and *Píng Wèi Sǎn* (Calm the Stomach Powder), plus *huá shí, fáng fēng, zhī zǐ, mù tōng*, and *dēng xīn cǎo*. When treating eczema, I recommend removing *mù tōng* and *ròu guì* from the original formula. *Mù tōng* because of its toxicity and *ròu guì* because we don't need to disperse cold and it can be too warming for inflamed skin. Considering *ròu guì*'s blood moving action, I would always prefer to select other herbs when treating skin conditions. However, the overall action of the formula is to dry dampness, regulate qì, harmonize the middle *jiāo* and clear heat. The modified version which is used in treating eczema is analyzed below.

Cāng zhú, hòu pò, and *chén pí* are all acrid, bitter, and warm herbs. In this prescription, they dry dampness, strengthen the Spleen and Stomach, and eliminate dampness. *Cāng zhú* is particularly effective at removing dampness from the lower *jiāo*. Together with *hòu pò* it also removes dampness obstructing the middle *jiāo*. *Hòu pò* promotes the movement of qì in the middle *jiāo*, descends qì and resolves stagnation. *Chén pí* as an aromatic herb also promotes the flow of qì. *Zé xiè*, sweet, bland, and cold, used in a relatively large dosage, leaches out dampness by inducing diuresis and can also cool heat. *Zhū líng* and *fú líng*, both sweet, bland, and neutral in nature, drain dampness by promoting urination. *Zhū líng* is particularly useful when dampness is retained for a long time, for example, with oedema in the legs. *Bái zhú*, bitter, sweet in flavor and warm in nature, tonifies the Spleen to reduce the production of dampness. *Bái zhú* is recommended to be used as *(chǎo)* (dry-fried) because this method of preparation strengthens the Spleen and harmonizes the Stomach, and is most appropriate when the transportive and transformative function is weakened, which is exactly the case in this pattern. *Huá shí* clears heat and resolves dampness. It is a wonderful substance in treating urinary problems, like cystitis or an irritable bladder. It can expel damp-heat through the urine and I often use it when patients have urinary bladder problems. Interestingly, in my practice I have found *huá shí* to be excellent when used as a preventive care for sensitive bladders, and following treatment for cystitis as a type of aftercare. Let's continue with *fáng fēng*. This herb expels wind-dampness and alleviates itching. When treating damp-eczema, one might wonder whether *fáng fēng* is truly essential in the formula. If there is less itching, just leave it out. *Zhī zǐ* is bitter and cold with a downward-directed action, and it can effectively clear heat, drain fire, relieve toxicity, and cool the blood. It is the perfect herb for draining heat from all three burners through the urine. In eczema, the redder the skin lesions, the higher the dosage should be. However, in cases of long-term use, *(chǎo) zhī zǐ* (dry-fried) is advisable, because the cold nature has been reduced making it more tolerable for the digestive system, while the heat-clearing effect is still ensured. *Gān cǎo* tonifies Spleen qì and moderates the effects of the other herbs. And finally, *dēng xīn cǎo*: it clears heat, from the Heart and Lungs in particular, it unblocks the fluid pathways and leads the heat downwards where it is expelled through the urine. Together with *huá shí* it is a good herb for treating damp-heat related to bladder infections. To modify this formula for the treatment of eczema, please see below.

Shēn Líng Bái Zhú Sǎn

Shēn Líng Bái Zhú Sǎn is a very effective formula when the Spleen and Stomach's transportive and transformative function is weakened, resulting in internally generated dampness. This should be treated by replenishing the qì, strengthening the Spleen, and eliminating dampness. This formula is particularly suitable for long-term eczema and when patients have diarrhoea.

In this prescription, *rén shēn, bái zhú*, and *fú líng* act together as sovereign herbs to tonify the Spleen and leach out dampness. Together with *zhì gān cǎo*, this combination is *Sì Jūn Zǐ Tāng* (Four Gentlemen Decoction). Remember, *rén shēn* is usually replaced with *dǎng shēn* nowadays. But let's go in depth: *Dǎng shēn* replenishes the qì and harmonizes the Spleen. *Bái zhú*, bitter, sweet in flavor and warm in nature, is a key tonic for the Spleen and dries dampness to improve the transportive and transformative function of the Spleen. *Fú líng*, sweet-bland in flavor, removes dampness and strengthens the Spleen. This action is reinforced when used together with *bái zhú*. It also moderates the cloying nature of *zhì gān cǎo*. *Zhì gān cǎo*, sweet in flavor and warm in nature, tonifies Spleen qì and moderates the effects of the other herbs. *Shān yào* and *lián zǐ* assist the sovereign herbs in strengthening the Spleen. *(Chǎo) bái biǎn dòu* and *yì yǐ rén* support *bái zhú* and *fú líng* to strengthen the Spleen, govern the transportive and transformative function, and drain dampness. These four herbs serve as minister herbs in this formula. You may have noted that *bái biǎn dòu* is used as *(chǎo)*, which means processed as dry-fried. Prepared in this manner, *bái biǎn dòu* tonifies without obstructing, and is thus particularly indicated to patients with a weak digestion.[24] *Lián zǐ* and *bái biǎn dòu* are, by the way, very effective for stopping diarrhoea. Let's continue with *shā rén*: it acts as an adjuvant herb with the functions of transforming dampness and promoting the flow of qì. *Jié gěng* disperses the Lung qì, unblocks the passage of water and leads the other herbs upwards to the Lung in order to strengthen the Lung qì. It thus prevents the Lung becoming deficient, which is a common sequela of Spleen deficiency.[25] Finally, when the Spleen qì is strong enough, it is able to perform its transforming and transporting function and eliminate dampness. However, when treating eczema primarily manifesting as pale red or dull red skin lesions as outlined above, *Shēn Líng Bái Zhú Sǎn* without modifications would certainly not be enough. The corresponding modifications will be discussed immediately below.

Modifications

For severe oedema, add *chì xiǎo dòu* 15–30 g. It treats dampness, reduces heat, and is particularly effective in treating leg oedema. For increased itchiness, add *dì fū zǐ* and *bái xiān pí*,[26] +/- *kǔ shēn* at a dose of 10–12 g to expel dampness and stop itching. If skin lesions are very swollen and red, add *chē qián cǎo* at a dose of 10–15 g. *Chē qián cǎo* is the entire Plantaginis herb and has very similar functions to the Plantaginis seeds (*chē qián zǐ*). While *chē qián cǎo* is not as effective at promoting urination, it is more effective at clearing heat and resolving toxicity.[27] If the entire herb is not available, as in Germany for example, replace it with *chē qián zǐ* using a similar dosage but remember to keep the seeds in a separate cloth bag to prevent them sticking on the cooking pot and/or making the decoction too gelatinous. For abdominal distension, *zhǐ shí*, 6–10 g, can be added. This is unripe bitter orange fruit, therefore the name "Aurantii immaturus, Frutctus." It promotes the flow of qì and reduces accumulation, and is a good herb for epigastric or abdominal pain and focal distension. If you want to strengthen this effect, combine *zhǐ shí* with *zhǐ ké*, the ripe Aurantii fruit. Used together, their ability to promote the flow of qì and break up clumps[28] is greatly enhanced. For constrained Liver qì with signs of mood swings or anger, frustration or depression, abdominal distension and bloating, distension and pain in the breasts, and irregular menstruation, for instance, add *chái hú* 10 g, *xiāng fù* 10 g, +/- *yù jīn* 6 g. And finally, in case of severe Spleen and Stomach qì deficiency, add *huáng qí* 10 g and *shān yào* 10 g. For lack of appetite, add *mài yá* 10 g.

Suggestions for External Treatment

For subacute eczema, the following prescriptions for external use are recommended–all with the function of drying dampness, alleviating itching, relieving heat if present (marked by redness of the skin lesions), and finally, of course, promoting skin healing:

- *Bái Zhú Gāo* (White Atractylodis Ointment)

- *Cāng Zhú Gāo* (Black Atractylodis Ointment)

- *Qīng Dài Sǎn* (Indigo Powder)[29]

- *Qū Shī Sàn* (Dispel Dampness Powder)

- *Sān Huáng Xǐ Jì* (Three Yellow Cleanser Formula)

- *Shé Chuáng Zǐ Tāng* (Cnidium Fruit Decoction).

Examples for individually tailored herbal formulas:

dì fū zǐ	Kochiae Scopariae, Fructus	15 g
shé chuáng zǐ	Cnidii, Fructus	15 g

This combination should be boiled with approximately 300 ml of water and used as an external wash. If the skin lesions are large, simply increase the dosages and use more water.

huá shí	Talcum	15–30 g
huáng bǎi	Phellodendri, Cortex	15 g

This combination should be used as powder when the skin lesions are oozing. In this case, grind the ingredients to a fine powder and apply topically on the affected skin lesions in order to absorb damp exudate for at least 15 minutes.

You can also use this as a wash. For application, grind the ingredients to a fine powder, then soak the powdered herbs in 300 ml water for 15–20 minutes. Bring the herbs to a boil and reduce to a low heat, allowing the herbs to simmer slowly for approximately 15 minutes. Strain the liquid. For application, use the liquid as a wash or a wet compress for 15–30 minutes, once or twice a day on the affected skin lesions.

gān cǎo	Glycyrrhizae Uralensis, Radix	30 g
huáng bǎi	Phellodendri, Cortex	30 g
bái zhǐ	Angelica Dahuricae, Radix	30 g
qīng fěn	Calomelas	30 g
(duàn) shí gāo	(calcinated) Gypsum Fibrosum	60 g
bīng piàn	Borneolum	6 g

Please note that not all the listed herbs are available everywhere. *Qīng fěn* for example is not available in Germany. This herbal combination with a few changes or additions can be also used in the former pattern "dampness–heat" (*shī rè*). You may have noticed that many of the mentioned formulas/combinations can be used in different patterns when modified. It's all a question of modification. Don't always stick rigidly to specifications or to notes from others. Be courageous and try things out. Mindless copying often doesn't lead to the desired goal.

huá shí	Talcum	15 g
huáng bǎi	Phellodendri, Cortex	15 g
shí gāo	Gypsum Fibrosum	15 g
huá shí	Talcum	15 g
huáng bǎi	Phellodendri, Cortex	15 g
bái fán	Alumen	5 g

Both used topically as a fine powder or as a wash. In case of a wash, these combinations are suitable for about 350 ml of water. The dosages of the herbs are variable. Be flexible! Adjust according to whether you need more focus on absorbing dampness, clearing heat or stopping itching. Please see above for cooking and application instructions. Again, quantities of dosages and water vary according to need and how concentrated you want your topical medicines.

One example of an effective stand-alone herb in this pattern:

- *huá shí* (Talcum) with dosages adjusted according to the size of the skin area which needs to be treated.

Apply it as a fine powder to the affected area to absorb dampness from skin lesions and close the skin.

Example Pictures of the Tongue

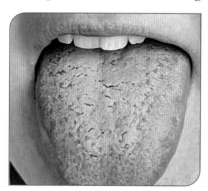
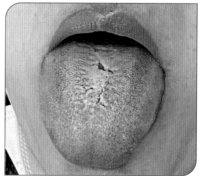

A puffy tongue with a
thick white coating.

A puffy and tooth-marked tongue
with a thick white coating.

Example Pictures of the Skin

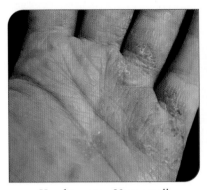

Hand eczema: Very small
blisters, erosions and crusts.

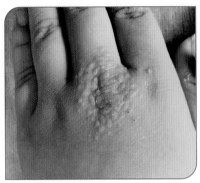

Hand eczema: Many pale
and dull red blisters.

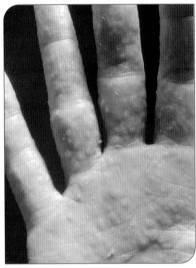

Hand eczema (dyshidrotic eczema):
Many small fluid-filled blisters on
the palms of the hands and fingers.

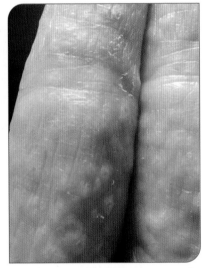

Hand eczema (dyshidrotic eczema):
Many small fluid-filled blisters
on the side of the fingers.

Blood Deficiency and Wind Dryness (*Xuè Xū Fēng Zào* 血虚风燥)

This is a chronic progression of eczema. It is well known that when the disease course is long, yīn and blood will be exhausted, which leads to pathogenic wind and blood stasis. At the very end, qì and blood have stagnated, which results in skin malnourishment. When the skin cannot be properly nourished, it becomes dry and rough. An excess of wind results in pruritus (itching) and later scaling. Thus, the longer the disease lasts, the more the blood stagnates and wind-dryness symptoms appear. But let's have a look how the skin presents in this pattern.

Characteristics

The skin is very dry[30] and usually appears dark in color or is hyperpigmented. The darker the skin lesions, the more blood stagnation is present. This gives you a hint that you need to add blood-moving herbs. Itching is severe, and usually worsens at night. The texture of the skin may be coarse or thick. Often, marks due to unconscious scratching (mainly during the night) can be observed. Patients often report that they do feel better after scratching. The patients' skin tends to be very sensitive to chemical substances, shampoo or shower gel for instance. Hot water often worsens the itching, too. Thus, this is also worth asking about.

Accompanying symptoms may include irregular menstruation with scanty blood, a dry mouth, constipation, dizziness, lassitude, and a pale and dull complexion.

The tongue is pale with a normal coating or a thin whitish coating. The pulse is thin, wiry, or rough.

Treatment Principle

Nourish blood and yīn, moisten the skin, dispel wind, and relieve itching (*zī yīn yǎng xuè, rùn fū, qū fēng zhǐ yǎng* 滋阴养血，润肤，祛风止痒).

Representative Formula

Dāng Guī Yǐn Zǐ (Chinese Angelica Drink).

Alternatively, you could use: *Sì Wù Xiāo Fēng Yǐn* (Eliminate Wind Drink with the Four Substances).

Ingredients
Dāng Guī Yǐn Zǐ (Chinese Angelica Drink)

dāng guī	Angelicae Sinensis, Radix	9–12 g
bái sháo	Paeonia Albiflora, Radix	9–12 g
chuān xiōng	Chuanxiong, Rhizoma	9 g
bái jí lí[31]	Tribuli, Fructus	9–12 g
fáng fēng	Saposhnikoviae, Radix	9 g
shēng dì huáng[32]	Rehmanniae Glutinosae, Radix	9–12 g
hé shǒu wū	Polygoni Multiflori, Radix	9 g
jīng jiè	Schizonepetae, Herba	9 g
huáng qí	Astragali, Radix	9–12 g
zhì gān cǎo	Glycyrrhizae Preparata, Radix	6 g

Sì Wù Xiāo Fēng Yǐn (Eliminate Wind Drink with the Four Substances)

shēng dì huáng	Rehmanniae Glutinosae, Radix	9 g
dāng guī	Angelicae Sinensis, Radix	9 g
jīng jiè	Schizonepetae, Herba	3–6 g
fáng fēng	Saposhnikoviae, Radix	3–6 g
chì sháo	Paeoniae Rubrae, Radix	3–6 g
chuān xiōng	Chuanxiong, Rhizoma	3–6 g
bái xiān pí	Dictamni Radicis, Cortex	3–6 g
chán tuì[33]	Cicadae, Periostracum	3 g
bò hé	Menthae, Herba	3 g
dú huó	Angelicae Pubescentis, Radix	3 g
chái hú	Bupleuri, Radix	3 g
dà zǎo	Jujubae, Fructus	2–3 pieces

First Reference

First reference of *Dāng Guī Yǐn Zǐ*: *Jì Shēng Fāng* (Formulas to Aid the Living, 1253), written by Yán Yòng-Hé.

First reference of *Sì Wù Xiāo Fēng Yǐn*: *Yī Zōng Jīn Jiàn* (The Golden Mirror of Medical Tradition, 1742), written by Wú Qiān et al.

Formula Analysis
Dāng Guī Yǐn Zǐ

This formula is a good choice when the skin becomes dry due to blood deficiency and needs to be nourished to alleviate itching (pruritus). In the formula, *dāng guī* and *hé shǒu wū* act as sovereign herbs, nourishing blood to moisten dryness. Only sufficient nutrient blood is able to effectively moisten the skin. *Bái jí lí, fáng fēng,* and *jīng jiè* dispel wind to relieve itching, acting as minister herbs in the formula. *Bái sháo, chuān xiōng, shēng dì huáng,* and *huáng qí* are all adjuvant herbs. *Bái sháo* and *shēng dì huáng* can help *dāng guī* and *hé shǒu wū* tonify blood. *Shēng dì huáng* also clears heat due to blood deficiency transforming into wind and dryness. *Chuān xiōng* promotes blood circulation; combined with *dāng guī* it nourishes and invigorates the blood and removes blood stasis, which encourages the production of fresh blood. The primary action of nourishing and circulating blood is clearly of higher priority than dispelling wind in this formula. Simply using wind dispelling herbs would definitely not be enough to relieve itching. *Huáng qí* tonifies Spleen qì and blood. By tonifying the Spleen qì, *huáng qí* augments the production of blood on a secondary level. Furthermore, *huáng qí* secures the exterior to prevent wind. *Zhì gān cǎo* tonifies Spleen qì to generate blood and moderates the effects of the other herbs. Please note, either *zhì gān cǎo* or *gān cǎo* can be used. *Gān cǎo* is the raw herb without honey preparation. Dry-frying the licorice in honey enhances its warming property. In eczema, which has a redder appearance, *gān cǎo* often seems to be the better choice.

CAUTIONS

Bái jí lí is slightly toxic because it contains potassium nitrite. Within the normal dosage range (6–15 g),[34] there should be no side effects. Overdosage, however, may cause symptoms such as general weakness, dizziness, nausea, vomiting, palpitations, rapid breathing, tachycardia, cyanosis, and allergic skin reactions.[35]

Sì Wù Xiāo Fēng Yǐn

When eczema presents as wind rash due to blood deficiency, it requires not only nourishing blood and yīn to moisten the skin, but also wind dispelling to relieve the itch. There are always multiple options for formulas, and in this presentation, we can use either *Dāng Guī Yǐn Zǐ* or *Sì Wù Xiāo Fēng Yǐn*, or another related formula. The information given in this book is to serve you as a guide, always use what seems most appropriate to you and form your own opinion.

Coming back to *Sì Wù Xiāo Fēng Yǐn*: This formula is basically a combination of two classic formulas, namely *Sì Wù Tāng* (Four Substances Decoction)[36] and *Xiāo Fēng Sǎn* (Eliminate Wind Powder). The two formulae in combination nourish the skin, expel wind and relieve itching, and eliminate dampness. *Sì Wù Tāng* in its "original description" includes *shú dì huáng, bái sháo, dāng guī,* and *chuān xiōng.* This combination is a classical simple and elegant prescription for treating blood deficiency while regulating the blood circulation. Taking a closer look at the individual herbs, *shú dì huáng* with its sweet flavour and rich character is the essential herb in this formula to nourish the yīn and supplement the blood. *Dāng guī* tonifies the blood and helps *shú dì huáng* enrich the blood, and also promotes the circulation of blood. *Bái sháo* nourishes the blood and astringes the yīn. Combined with *shú dì huáng* and *dāng guī,* the action of nourishing the yīn and blood is greatly enhanced. *Chuān xiōng* promotes blood circulation which clears blood stasis and encourages the production of fresh blood. When treating skin diseases, I prefer to use *shēng dì huáng* to replace *shú dì huáng.* If the lesions are redder and a blood cooling aspect is needed, *shēng dì huáng* is more suitable. If the lesions look relatively normal without redness, and blood tonifying is more necessary, *shú dì huáng* may be used. In general, either *shēng dì huáng* or *shú dì huáng* can be used up to 15 g but keep the dampness generating effect of *shú dì huáng* in mind. Adding a small dose of *shā rén* 3–5 g can counteract this effect. However, it is also possible to use *shēng dì huáng* and *shú dì huáng* in combination. In this case, I suggest using 9 g of each herb. You may notice that in *Sì Wù Xiāo Fēng Yǐn, chì sháo* is used instead of the usual *bái sháo,* from *Sì Wù Tāng? Chì sháo* is the better choice as it also cools and invigorates the blood, dispels blood stasis, and reduces swellings. It is, thus, often used to treat rashes and swellings from sores. This is a perfect example of how flexible TCM is, offering a variety of solutions for each individual need.

Moving on from *Sì Wù Tāng,* let's discuss the ingredients of *Xiāo Fēng Sǎn,* which makes up the second part within *Sì Wù Xiāo Fēng Yǐn. Jīng jiè* and *fáng fēng* can disperse wind and relieve itching (pruritus) due to their acrid and dispersing nature. These two herbs are commonly combined to expel wind to stop itching in skin rashes across a range of dermatological conditions. Doses of 3–6 g are absolutely sufficient for this. *Bái xiān pí* clears heat, expels wind and dries dampness. It is very effective in stopping itching. Please see above for cautionary advice for long-term use or as a single herb. *Chán tuì* releases the exterior to disperse wind-heat, vents rashes and stops itching. Please see below for cautionary advice for this herb. A small amount of *bò hé* (3 g) can disperse wind-heat and vent rashes. With *chán tuì,* for instance, it powerfully expels wind-heat, vents rashes and stops the itching. *Dú huó* dispels wind-dampness and releases the exterior. A dose of 3 g maximum is enough. *Dú huó* should be used with caution in patients with yīn or blood deficiency due its drying nature.[37] *Chái hú* can clear heat, relieve constraint due to its qì regulating action. *Chái hú* is often used for Liver qì constraint with symptoms such as emotional depression, stifling sensation in the chest and irregular menstruation due to Liver blood deficiency and obstruction, an effect that is enhanced in combination with *bò hé* as seen in *Xiāo Yáo Sǎn* (Rambling Powder).[38] And let us not forget, when combined with *dāng guī* and *chuān xiōng* as part of *Xiāo Yáo Sǎn*,[39] *chái hú* can also harmonize the blood. *Dà zǎo* completes this formula by nourishing the blood, moderating and harmonizing the harsh properties of the other herbs within the formula. In addition, *dà zǎo* is also capable of calming the spirit, in cases where a patient is irritable or restless.

CLINICAL TIP REGARDING THE PRINCIPAL FORMULA *XIĀO FĒNG SǍN*[40]: "Consumption of foods, that are thought to stimulate the stirring of wind…, such as alcohol, coffee, spicy foods, and seafood, as well as smoking, may interfere with the actions of the herbs and should be avoided while taking this formula." This is helpful information for us but also for passing on to your patient, as they play an essential part in the success of the treatment.

CAUTIONS

When using *chán tuì*, please watch carefully for any unwanted reactions. There have been reported cases of preparations of this substance leading to abdominal pain and allergic reactions, including generalized pruritus, erythema, facial flushing, sweating, fever, hoarseness, and palpitations.[41] I refrain from using this substance in sensitive patients and those who say that they easily have allergic reactions to various kinds of external influences. I remember my Professor in China saying: Some patients say that they are even sensitive to water. So be very careful in the usage of *chán tuì*. *Chán tuì* should also be used with caution in women who are or might be pregnant, especially if they have a history of miscarriage.[42]

Modifications

During my time in China, I have seen many animal products used for herbal modification in this pattern, such as *wū shāo shé*, the black striped snake. Because these products are either not available (often due to species protection regulations) or just not commonly used outside of China, I will just mention those herbs which I frequently use in my clinic and which are readily available.

In this pattern, don't forget to add some blood moving herbs when using *Dāng Guī Yǐn Zǐ* or *Sì Wù Xiāo Fēng Yǐn* as the base formula. When the blood is deficient, please always keep in mind that moving qì and blood is also necessary in order to prevent stasis. However, when there are skin lesions that usually appear dark in color or hyperpigmented, blood moving herbs are definitely indicated. When we move the blood, it is able to regenerate. In order to build blood, one ought to add *jī xuè téng* 12–15 g to the original formula. A word on the difference between *dāng guī*, the entire root of the herb, and *dāng guī wěi*, which are the fine lateral roots of the herb. As explained above, *dāng guī* is most tonifying, but less effective in promoting the movement of blood compared to the single parts of the herb. *Dāng guī wěi*, in contrast, is considered to be most effective in moving the blood.[43] Please note that *dāng guī* itself is considered to have a warming nature. *Dāng guī wěi*, in contrast, is more cooling and can be selected in the treatment of skin conditions when a blood moving and cooling action is required.[44] Although *dāng guī* is a very popular herb in TCM Dermatology, we should know the differences and choose the right part of the herb depending on what effects we require.

CLINICAL TIP: A colleague recently asked me why working night shifts for a long time will eventually cause blood stasis. There are two common reasons. First, the blood cannot be replenished and nourished during the night. In an already existing blood deficiency this is the worst which can happen because there is no time for the deficient blood to rebuild, and in later stages, the more deficient the blood is the more stagnant it becomes. Second, during the night yáng qì and its moving action is weak, which can cause qì and blood stagnation. In patients with blood deficiency who work in a profession requiring night shifts, you have to respect this but you can explain the theory behind this mechanism and that this information is useful for their diagnosis.

For extreme itch, depending on which of the formulas mentioned above have been chosen, herbs like *fáng fēng, jīng jiè, dì fū zǐ, bái xiān pí, xú cháng qīng,* and *chán tuì* are quite effective. *Sì Wù Xiāo Fēng Yǐn,* for example, already contains most of these herbs. *Dāng Guī Yǐn Zǐ* in comparison contains less of the above herbs to improve itching, so some should be added to the prescription. In regard to substances such as *quán xiē* (scorpion), I would refrain. I have seen the use of scorpion many times in China but, as already mentioned, some substances are not available or common outside of China, and scorpion falls in this category. If the patient is suffering from restlessness and sleeplessness, add *hé shǒu wū* 10–15 g, *yè jiāo téng* 30 g, or *lóng chǐ* (dragon teeth) 15 g. All of these herbs calm the *shén* 神 (spirit). Furthermore, many patients report that the itch gets worse once they have gone to bed, and sleep can be interrupted or delayed due to unconsciously scratching at night because the skin is so itchy. By using these herbs, one can calm the spirit but also reduce itching, especially at night. Patients will then not scratch as much, and sleep will improve.

> PRACTICAL TIP: To prevent eczema itching at night, advise your patients to wear cotton gloves to bed. This makes it more difficult to scratch in response to unconscious itching, and this way they avoid scratch marks on the skin. As we all know, scratching/itching the skin happens automatically. Keeping their fingernails short will also protect the skin from scratching. Often patients in conversation with me don't even notice when they scratch themselves. How should they then be aware that they do it at night?

If the patient is constipated, add *huǒ má rén* 9–12 g. This herb nourishes and moistens the Intestines and can, thus, unblock dry constipation[45] due to a lack of fluids. *Huǒ má rén* also nourishes yīn and clears heat. Another alternative for constipation due to dry Intestines and/or blood deficiency is to add *hēi zhī má* 9–12 g. As previously mentioned, the longer the disease lasts, the more the blood stagnates, resulting in dark colored or hyperpigmented skin lesions. The darker the skin lesions are, the more blood moving herbs must be added. In this case, I recommend using additional herbs to increase the blood stasis transforming action, such as *táo rén* 9–12 g and *hóng huā* 3–6 g, or *dān shēn* 12 g. All these herbs invigorate blood and break up blood stasis. If the patient is yīn deficient, the dosage of *shēng dì huáng* can be increased to 15 g and *mài mén dōng* 9 g can also be added. Both herbs benefit the yīn, moisten dryness, and clear heat.

Suggestions for External Treatment

For chronic eczema with dark colored, dry and itchy skin, herbs are recommended which moisten the skin and enrich the yīn, as well as reducing itching. The following formulas and individual combinations fulfil these actions:

- *Rùn Jī Gāo* (Flesh Moistening Ointment)

- *Yăng Xuè Rùn Fū Yĭn* (Nourish the Blood and Moisten the Skin Drink)

- *Qīng Liáng Gāo* (Clearing and Cooling Ointment)

- *Zĭ Sè Xiāo Zhŏng Fĕn* (Purple Powder to Reduce Swelling).[46]

Examples of individually tailored external herbal formulas:

dāng guī	Angelicae Sinensis, Radix	25 g
zhì gān căo	Glycyrrhizae Preparata, Radix	25 g

This is a very simple combination to moisten the skin and is usually given as an ointment or cream. Please see Appendix I for detailed instructions and explanations for making your own ointments and creams. If this combination is not enough, the next combination might be suitable:

dāng guī	Angelicae Sinensis, Radix	15 g
gŏu qĭ zĭ	Lycii, Fructus	15 g
sāng shèn	Mori, Fructus	15 g
dān shēn	Salviae Miltiorhizae, Radix	15 g

This combination is usually used as an ointment or cream. It nourishes the yīn, invigorates the blood and moistens the skin. To support the the yīn-enriching and skin moistening effect, *băi hé* can be added. *Bái jí lí* can be added to reduce itching.

bái jí lí	Tribuli, Fructus	25 g
zĭ căo[47]	Arnebiae Seu Lithospermi, Radix	25 g

This is another simple but effective choice for external treatment. *Bái jí lí* is used to stop itching and *zǐ cǎo* is used if the skin lesions are dark-purple, for its blood-invigorating action. This herbal combination can be used as an external wash and as an ointment or cream. For thicker and drier lesions, I recommend using an ointment or a cream.

jīng jiè	Schizonepetae, Herba	15 g
fáng fēng	Saposhnikoviae, Radix	15 g
huáng jīng	Polygonati, Rhizoma	15 g
chuān xiōng	Chuanxiong, Rhizoma	10 g
chì sháo	Paeoniae Rubrae, Radix	10 g
+/- *yě jú huā*	Chrysanthemi Indici, Flos	10 g

This combination can be given as either an external wash or as an ointment or cream. In the case of a wash, this combination is suitable for about 500–600 ml of water, depending on whether *yě jú huā* is added. *Yě jú huā* can be added to support the skin healing and in particular when the lesions are located on the face.

Example Pictures of the Tongue

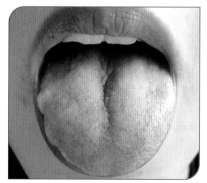 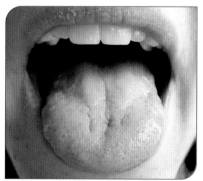

| A pale and puffy tongue with toothmarks. This indicates blood deficiency combined with weakness of Spleen qì. | A pale, puffy tongue with toothmarks and lips. When the skin cannot be properly nourished, it becomes dry. |

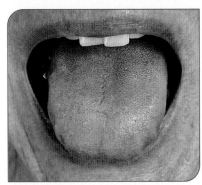

A slightly purplish tongue with purplish lips, which indicates stagnant blood. If there is not enough blood, it tends to stagnate.

Example Pictures of the Skin

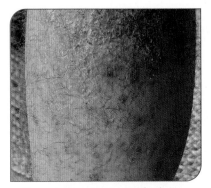

Long-term eczema on the lower leg. Continuous scratching leads to cracks and bleeding.

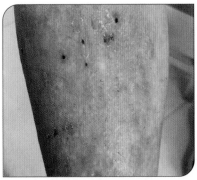

Long-term eczema on the lower leg. The skin lesions appear dark in color.

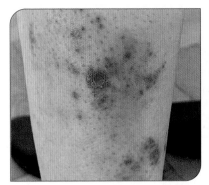

Eczema on the lower leg. The skin lesions appear purple-brownish in color and the skin is very dry.

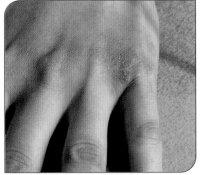

Eczema on the hand. The skin is very dry and scaly.

Contact Eczema

I am including an extra section on contact eczema, because the next two TCM syndromes are predominantly seen in this type of eczema. Exceptions prove the rule: these two patterns can occur in all other sub-types as well.

Please note that I will not differentiate between "irritant-toxic contact eczema," which is a non-allergic skin reaction, and "allergic contact eczema" in the TCM part of this book. However, regardless of the cause or type, contact eczema causes itching and skin rash. In general, irritant-toxic contact eczema is more painful than itchy. Symptoms usually subside after a day or two, once there is no more contact with the irritant. Allergic contact eczema usually causes itching rather than pain. Symptoms may take a day or more to become apparent and increase in intensity for two to three days after exposure. In both cases, the rash can vary in intensity and duration. It only develops where the skin and/or mucous membrane has come into contact with the irritant substance. The rash usually appears earlier on sensitive skin areas, such as between the fingers, and later on thicker areas of skin or areas that have had less intense exposure to the allergen.

Avoiding contact with the offending agent is the priority! When treating with TCM, always focus on the skin lesion first. The main focus is on clearing away heat and resolving dampness. That is the key to the success of any treatment.

Wind-Heat Accumulating in the Skin (*Fēng Rè Yùn Fū* 风热蕴肤)

In this pattern, the offending agents are generally classified as acrid, hot, and toxic substances. According to TCM, they stir wind and generate heat/fire inside the body, which spreads to the skin and flesh, manifesting as an acute and serious skin inflammation.

Characteristics

Contact eczema is characterized by sudden onset. The skin is red, swollen, usually dry and feels warm. The skin rash typically manifests as erythema or bright red, inflamed papules, which are painful, and severe itching and/or burning. Scratching tends to make the itch worse, not better. Accompanying symptoms may include constipation, dark-yellow urine, a dry mouth, thirst, restlessness, and blushing with a feeling of heat, which often occurs in this context.

The tongue is red with a thin yellow coating. The pulse is rapid and floating.

> CLINICAL TIP: In wind-heat patterns, the skin reactions are often found in the upper part of the body, primarily on the face. In contact eczema, this isn't the case, as it can appear almost anywhere on the body.

Treatment Principle

Clear heat, disperse wind, and relieve itching (*qīng rè shū fēng zhǐ yǎng* 清热疏风止痒).

Representative Formula

Modified *Xiāo Fēng Sǎn* (Eliminate Wind Powder).

Ingredients

jīng jiè	Schizonepetae, Herba	6 g
fáng fēng	Saposhnikoviae, Radix	6 g
niú bàng zǐ	Arctii Lappae, Fructus	10 g
+/- *chán tuì*	Cicadae, Periostracum	3 g
jīn yín huā	Lonicerae Japonicae, Flos	10 g
lián qiáo	Forsythiae, Fructus	10 g
shēng dì huáng	Rehmanniae Glutinosae, Radix	10–12 g
dāng guī	Angelicae Sinensis, Radix	10 g
shí gāo[48]	Gypsum Fibrosum	15 g
zhī mǔ	Anemarrhenae, Rhizoma	6 g
kǔ shēn	Sophorae Flavescentis, Radix	10 g
cāng zhú	Atractylodis, Rhizoma	6 g
tōng cǎo[49]	Tetrapanacis, Medulla	3 g
gān cǎo	Glycyrrhizae Uralensis, Radix	6 g

Please note that several versions of *Xiāo Fēng Sǎn* exist. When external wind-heat attacks the body, we see an acute and superficial process. In this case, to expel the external pathogenic factor we have to choose many herbs which strongly clear heat, disperse wind and eliminate dampness because of the swelling of the skin. Thus, I have selected the version above. It is also effective when the patient is constipated.

First Reference

This formula firstly appeared in the *Wài Kē Zhèng Zōng* (Orthodox Lineage of External Medicine,[50] 1617) by Chén Shí-Gōng.

Formula Analysis

Jīng jiè, fáng fēng, niú bàng zǐ and *chán tuì* unblock the pores and release the exterior by dispersing wind-heat. When the wind is dispersed, normally the itch is relieved. *Jīn yín huā* and *lián qiáo*, both acrid, cool, and fragrant, release the exterior, clear heat from the Lungs, and resolve toxicity. These two herbs are often used as a pair and can be seen in many skin prescriptions as well as in combinations for treating common cold with fever, cough, and headaches, for example within the popular formula *Yín Qiào Sǎn* (Honeysuckle and Forsythia Powder).[51] *Shēng dì huáng* and *dāng guī* nourish and invigorate the blood. They assist the blood, so to speak, by extinguishing the wind, and they moisten the dry skin. The theory behind this is as follows: When blood is sufficient, it can move. When blood moves freely, it can moisten the skin and naturally extinguish the wind. When there is insufficient blood, wind can invade. *Shēng dì huáng* also cools the blood to reduce the erythema. *Dāng guī* can gently moisten the Intestines caused by blood deficiency. The herb is often used when the patient is constipated and has difficulty voiding due to dry stools.

Shí gāo and *zhī mǔ* drain heat from the qì level, thus, preventing the condition progressing to a deeper level: the *yíng* (nutritive) or *xuè* (blood) level.[52] This herbal pair can be found in *Bái Hǔ Tāng* (White Tiger Decoction),[53] a very strong qì level-heat clearing and Stomach fire draining formula. As these two substances are very cold, be careful with patients who have a weak Spleen and Stomach. One may use *zhī mǔ* as *chǎo* or dry-fried, making it more suitable for patients with Spleen and Stomach deficiency. *Kǔ shēn, cāng zhú,* and *tōng cǎo* dry dampness and remove damp-heat from the body. *Kǔ shēn* in particular is a very common herb used in treating skin conditions to resolve toxicity. It is very effective in stopping the itch due to damp-heat, and I personally use it quite often in practice. *Cāng zhú* strongly dries dampness and strengthens the Spleen and Stomach. *Tōng cǎo* guides heat downward and out through the urine, unblocking the fluid pathways and facilitating urination.[54] All these actions are needed to relieve the swelling and reduce the inflammatory process of the skin. And finally, *gān cǎo*, to clear heat, resolve toxicity and harmonize the actions of the other herbs.

Modifications

For severe oedema, add more diuretic herbs in relatively high dosages, such as *dōng guā pí* 15–30 g, *fú líng* 15–30 g, or *zé xiè* 15–30 g. *Dōng guā pí* is particularly indicated if the patient is showing blisters on the skin. It is a gentle herb to facilitate urination, clear heat, and, thus, reduce swelling. If the wind-heat is severe and combined with (fire) toxin, one may add *pú gōng yīng* 15 g and *yě jú huā* 9–12 g. In this case, the lesions look more severe, with an intense red appearance, hot sensation, and are quite painful. Combined with *jīn yín huā*, *pú gōng yīng*, and *yě jú huā* are a part of the popular formula *Wǔ Wèi Xiāo Dú Yǐn*.[55] This formula is an excellent choice whenever skin lesions are marked by swelling, erythema, inflammation, and pain due to internal heat and toxin. It effectively clears heat and relieves toxicity. If the skin lesions are located on the upper parts of the body, especially on the face, add *jú huā* 9–12 g. Please note, if you already added *yě jú huā* to the formula, you don't need to add *jú huā* and vice versa.

For intense itching, add *bái xiān pí* 9–12 g. Please see above for cautionary advice for long-term use or as a single herb. In regard to animal substances such as *quán xiē* (scorpion) or *jiāng cán* (silkworm), I would refrain. These products are commonly used in China but, as already mentioned, some substances are not available or common outside of China, and both substances fall into this category. Considering that the script already contains *chán tuì*, one should be mindful of how many animal products one wants to use in a prescription, and exercise caution due to the potential for an allergic reaction.

A short spotlight on guiding herbs in Chinese medicine: You may have noticed that there are special herbs which convey the formula to the corresponding affected area of the body. These herbs are called "guiding herbs." Some examples[56] that have frequently shown good results are:

Affected Body Region	Guiding Herb
face (head)	*jú huā, yě jú huā, méi guī huā*
upper limbs	*sāng zhī*[57]
(heat affecting the) upper body	*fú píng*
upper back	*gé gēn*
lower back	*xù duàn*
chest	*chén pí*
legs	*niú xī,*[58] *mù guā*

Suggestions for External Treatment

- *Lóng Dǎn Cǎo Cā Jì* (Gentian Liniment)
- *Qīng Dài Sǎn* (Indigo Powder)
- *Qīng Liáng Gāo* (Clearing and Cooling Ointment)
- *Sān Huáng Xǐ Jì* (Three Yellow Cleanser Formula)
- *Shī Zhěn Sǎn* (Eczema Powder)

Examples for individually tailored herbal formulas:

In order to treat serious skin inflammation, one must use herbs which strongly clear heat, remove toxins, settle swelling, and alleviate itching. Commonly used herbal combinations for herbal washes or cold wet compresses for this TCM pattern are:

mǎ chǐ xiàn	Portulacae, Herba	15 g
pú gōng yīng	Smilacis Glabrae, Rhizoma	15 g
huáng bǎi	Phellodendri, Cortex	15 g
yě jú huā	Chrysanthemi Indici, Flos	15 g
kǔ shēn	Sophorae Flavescentis, Radix	15 g
gān cǎo	Glycyrrhizae Uralensis, Radix	15 g
+/- *dì yú*[59]	Sanguisorbae, Radix	15 g

Boil with about 750 ml water. Use a bit more water if *dì yú* is added. Increase the doses of the herbs and the volume of water if the skin lesions are larger and more liquid is needed. Use as cold compress on the affected skin area for about 20–30 minutes each time, 2–3 times a day. If there is no exudate, this combination can be also used as a paste or ointment. Please see Appendix I for how to make ointments and pastes.

dà huáng	Rhei, Radix et Rhizoma	15 g
huáng bǎi	Phellodendri, Cortex	15 g
huáng qín	Scutellariae, Radix	15 g
kǔ shēn	Sophorae Flavescentis, Radix	15 g

Boil with about 500 ml water. Use as a cold compress on the affected skin area for about 20–30 minutes each time, 2–3 times a day. Increase the doses of the herbs and also the volume of water if the skin lesions are larger and thus more liquid is needed. If there is no exudate, this combination can also be used as a paste or ointment.

Frequently used and effective stand-alone herbs in this pattern:

- *huáng lián* (Coptidis, Rhizoma) 30 g

- *huáng bǎi* (Phellodendri, Cortex) 30 g

- *dà huáng* (Rhei, Radix et Rhizoma) 25 g.

The dosages are intended for a wash with about 250 ml water depending on how concentrated you want the solution to be. Reduce the amount of water if you want to work in a more concentrated way. Use as cold compress on the affected skin area for about 20–30 minutes each time, 2–3 times a day. All three herbs can also be used as a paste or ointment when there is no erosion and no exudate.

Example Pictures of the Tongue

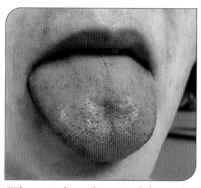

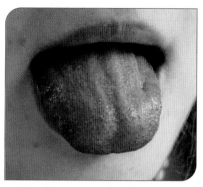

When wind combines with heat, the tip of the tongue is particularly red.

A red tongue with red spots on the tip and a thin white coating.

Example Pictures of the Skin

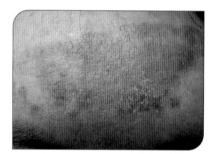

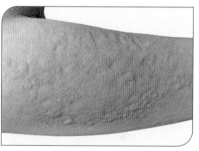

Contact eczema on the face.[59]

Contact eczema on the arm.[60]

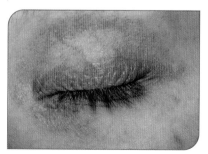

Contact eczema affecting the eyes.[61]

Internal Accumulation of Heat-Toxin and Dampness (*Shī Xié, Rè Dú Nèi Jù* 湿邪、热毒内聚)

In this pattern, a toxic substance invades the body, either due to constitutional deficiency or vulnerable skin and open interstices (*còu lǐ* 腠理). It is usually a combination of an external toxin which congeals with pre-existing internal dampness, forming excessive damp-heat (damp-toxin). When not expelled, it stagnates in the skin, flesh, and the interstices, causing severe inflammation of the skin.

Characteristics

When heat-toxins and dampness are combined together, the symptoms develop relatively quickly and a sudden onset of skin inflammation can be observed. The skin lesions appear swollen and bright red in color. The skin usually presents with papulovesicles, clusters of vesicles or pustules, erosions, oozing, and the formation of yellowish crusts. In severe cases, bullae or blood-filled blisters may appear. If they burst, the exudation usually looks reddish. It is generally a very painful process. The skin feels warm/hot, painful, and itchy and the patient often has a burning sensation on the skin. Accompanying symptoms may include fever, a sensation of heat throughout the body, a dry mouth, thirst, dark yellow urine, and constipation.

The tongue is red with a thin yellow coating. The thickness of the tongue coating depends on the degree of dampness present. The pulse is rapid and slippery.

Treatment Principle

Clear away heat and relieve toxicity, transform dampness and reduce swelling (*qīng rè jiě dú huà shī xiāo zhǒng* 清热解毒 化湿消肿).

Representative Formula

Huà Bān Jiě Dú Tāng (Maculae Transforming and Toxicity Removing Decoction, also called Rash Resolving and Toxicity Removing Decoction).[63]

Ingredients

xuán shēn	Scrophulariae Ningpoensis, Radix	12–15 g
zhī mǔ	Anemarrhenae, Rhizoma	6 g
shí gāo	Gypsum Fibrosum	15 g
rén zhōng huáng	Glycyrrhizae Extractionis Sedilis, Rulvis	6–9 g
huáng lián	Coptidis, Rhizoma	6–9 g
shēng má	Cimicifugae, Rhizoma	3–6 g
lián qiáo	Forsythiae, Fructus	9 g
niú bàng zǐ	Arctii Lappae, Fructus	9 g
gān cǎo	Glycyrrhizae Uralensis, Radix	6 g
dàn zhú yè	Lophatheri, Herba	3–6 g

Please note that are several formulas called *Huà Bān Jiě Dú Tāng*. The version mentioned above is the one that appeared in the original source text, while dosages are those which work best in my clinical experience. I will also share another version from the famous modern Chinese TCM skin specialist Prof. Zhào Bǐng-Nán[64] who mentioned the following version in his book *Zhào Bǐng-Nán Lín Chuáng Jīng Yàn Jí* (Zhào Bǐng-Nán's clinical experience set, 1975).

xuán shēn	Scrophulariae Ningpoensis, Radix	15 g
zhī mǔ	Anemarrhenae, Rhizoma	6 g
shí gāo	Gypsum Fibrosum	15 g
huáng lián	Coptidis, Rhizoma	6 g
lián qiáo	Forsythiae, Fructus	9 g
shēng dì huáng	Rehmanniae Glutinosae, Radix	12 g
líng xiāo huā	Campsis, Flos	9 g
gān cǎo	Glycyrrhizae Uralensis, Radix	9 g

Looking at these versions of the formula *Huà Bān Jiě Dú Tāng*, it can be said that both serve their purpose and are appropriate. Considering that contact eczema is a skin inflammation with severe signs and symptoms, it should be noted that both formulas must usually be modified to strengthen the mode of action. I will explain possible modifications below.

First Reference

While sources vary, this formula seems to have originally appeared in the *Wài Kē Zhèng Zōng* (Orthodox Lineage of External Medicine, Vol. 4: Miscellaneous Sores and Viruses,[65] 1617) by Chén Shí-Gōng. Interestingly, another source says it comes from the *Yī Zōng Jīn Jiàn* (The Golden Mirror of Medical Tradition, 1742), which was published more than a hundred years later. Thus, thinking logically, the first source makes the most sense.

Formula Analysis

The original formula contains many heat clearing and toxicity relieving herbs. *Xuán shēn* resolves toxicity, clears heat in the blood, and nourishes the yīn fluids. *Zhī mǔ* clears heat and drains fire, enriches the yīn, and moistens dryness. One may fry (*chǎo*) it to protect those with a weak Spleen and Stomach. *Shí gāo* clears heat in the qì level, drains fire, particularly Stomach fire, and should be used in large doses of at least 15 g. It strongly releases heat from excess and is often used together with *zhī mǔ* for high fever, heat in the qì level or excessive heat in the *yáng míng*.[66] The representative formula in this case is *Bái Hǔ Tāng* (please see above for ingredients). In the first version, one should consider that *rén zhōng huáng* is not used outside of China, and in fact I have never heard of it being used in modern China. Thus, you might look for a replacement. For better understanding, I will briefly explain the mechanisms of action of this substance. *Rén zhōng huáng* is produced by placing *gān cǎo* stored in a loose bamboo container into human faeces and leaving it there for an extended period of time. This "medical compound" can supposedly clear heat, cool blood, and remove toxicity. According to the texts it can theoretically be used for treating erysipelas, sores, polydipsia, high fever, macula, and ulcers due to heat-toxin. However, as already mentioned, we don't use it and my colleagues in China report that it is mentioned in references but also rarely used in practice. *Huáng lián* cools heat, drains fire, dries dampness, and resolves toxicity. Once the fire is drained, the toxin will disappear. As *huáng lián* is very bitter and very cold, I often use it dry-fried (*chǎo*), which moderates its cold property in order to protect the Spleen. *Shēng má, lián qiáo,* and *niú ang zǐ* disperse heat, relieve toxin, reduce swelling, and alleviate itching. *Gān cǎo* clears heat, relieves fire toxicity, and moderates and harmonizes the properties of other herbs, which are extremely cooling. *Dàn zhú yè* cools, generates fluids, and alleviates thirst.

ADDITIONAL INFORMATION: Looking at all ingredients of the formula, you will find that the following formulas or parts of them are included in *Huà Bān Jiě Dú Tāng*: 1. *Huà Bān Tāng* (Transform Maculae Decoction),[67] 2. *Bái Hǔ Tāng,* and a small part of 3. *Yín Qiào Sǎn.* Just to name a few.

Modifications

The range of modifications to this pattern are very diverse and quite similar to the options for the formula above, *Xiāo Fēng Sǎn.* To enhance the toxin removing action, one may add *jīn yín huā* 9–15 g, *pú gōng yīng* 15 g, and *yě jú huā* 9–12 g. As already mentioned above, these herbs form a part of *Wǔ Wèi Xiāo Dú Yǐn.* Using *huáng bǎi* is another option. I recommend using this herb dry-fried (*chǎo*) to reduce its potential to damage the Spleen and Stomach. For severe toxicity, *huáng bǎi* can be also used in addition to *jīn yín huā, pú gōng yīng,* and *yě jú huā.* For intense itching, add *bái xiān pí* 9–12 g. For profuse yellow exudation, add *tǔ fú líng* with a dose of at least 15 g. I also recommend adding herbs such as *mǔ dān pí, chì sháo,* or *dān shēn.* Never forget the "blood aspect." Regarding addressing the blood aspect, I recommend blood cooling and heat clearing, as well as blood moving and transforming stasis. Extreme heat exhausts yīn and blood, which inevitably leads to blood stasis. One or two of these herbs in a relatively high dose (9–15 g) are enough to cool and regulate the blood. For extremely dry mouth and thirst, add *shēng dì huáng* 9–15 g in order to clear heat, cool blood, and nourish yīn. Don't forget, heat tends to scorch and injure the yīn and body fluids (*jīn yè* 津液) as a consequence. For severe oedema, one may add *huá shí* 12 g. Together with *gān cǎo,* this combination represents *Liù Yī Sǎn* (Six-to-One Powder), a formula which clears heat, relieves toxicity, promotes urination, and releases summer-heat. It is a very small formula and is usually combined with other herbs. As the name says, it uses six parts of *huá shí* to one part of *gān cǎo.* As the basic formula already contains *shí gāo,* the dosage of *huá shí* can be reduced. If the patient is constipated, use raw *niú bàng zǐ* in order to moisten the Intestines. If there is no constipation, the herb can be used as dry-fried (*chǎo*) to protect Spleen and Stomach, or for a milder effect in weak and elderly patients.

In addition to these recommendations of single herbs for modification, I would also like to mention an alternative formula for this pattern: *Pǔ Jì Xiāo Dú Yǐn* (Universal Benefit Drink to Eliminate Toxin), consisting of:

huáng qín	Scutellariae, Radix	9–15 g
huáng lián	Coptidis, Rhizoma	6–15 g
rén shēn	Ginseng, Radix	9 g
niú bàng zǐ	Arctii Lappae, Fructus	3 g
lián qiáo	Forsythiae, Fructus	3–12 g
bò hé	Menthae, Herba	3–6 g
(chǎo) jiāng cán	Bombyx Batryticatus (dry-fried)	2 g
xuán shēn	Scrophulariae Ningpoensis, Radix	6–10 g
mǎ bó	Lasiosphaera/Calvatia	3–9 g
bǎn lán gēn	Isatidis, Radix	3–12 g
jié gěng	Platycodi, Radix	6–9 g
gān cǎo	Glycyrrhizae Uralensis, Radix	6 g
jú hóng	Citri Reticulatae rubrum, Exocarpium	6 g
chái hú	Bupleuri, Radix	6–9 g
shēng má	Cimicifugae, Rhizoma	2 g

This is another perfect example of how flexible TCM is, offering a variety of solutions. *Pǔ Jì Xiāo Dú Yǐn* clears heat, eliminates fire toxin and disperses wind-heat. For modifications, please see above. However, when using this formula for someone who is constipated, I would use *(chǎo) dà huáng* 9 g instead of raw *niú bàng zǐ*.

> **FOOD FOR THOUGHT:** From the TCM point of view, cortisone can only suppress inflammation, and cannot eliminate fire toxin. A strong heat clearing and fire eliminating formula always works better in the long run!

Suggestions for External Treatment

- *Huà Dú Sǎn Gāo* (Toxicity Transforming Powder Paste)[68]

- *Jiě Dú Xǐ Yào* (Detoxifying Lotion)

- *Qīng Dài Sǎn* (Indigo Powder)

- *Qū Shī Sǎn* (Damp-Removing Medicinal Powder)

- *Sì Huáng Sǎn* (Four-Yellow Powder)

- *Xīn Sān Miào Sǎn* (New Three Marvels Powder)

Examples for individually tailored herbal washes or wet compresses:
Cold wet compresses or washes work best here. Also consider using powders in order to absorb damp exudate. Thick creams are not recommended. In this pattern, the discharge has to be drained, not occluded, and a thick and hardly spreadable cream will tend to worsen the inflammatory process.

Although there are various formulas to choose from, you can also choose between different combinations. Frequently used herbal combinations for a wet compress or wash are:

pú gōng yīng	Taraxaci, Herba	15 g
dì yú[69]	Sanguisorbae, Radix	15 g
gān cǎo	Glycyrrhizae Uralensis, Radix	15 g

This combination is suitable for 400–450 ml of water, depending on how strong a solution you require. If you want to work with a very concentrated liquid, use less water and vice versa, if you want to work more mildly, use more water. For application, apply as a wet compress or wash the affected area two or three times a day, for about 15–30 minutes each time.

The function of this combination is to clear heat, absorb discharge, and relieve itching. It is suitable for any form of rash in which red, thick, swollen, inflamed, and very painful lesions are present.

kǔ shēn	Sophorae Flavescentis, Radix	15 g
dì fū zǐ	Kochiae Scopariae, Fructus	15 g
bái xiān pí	Dictamni Radicis, Cortex	15 g
shé chuáng zǐ	Cnidii, Fructus	15 g

huáng bǎi	Phellodendri, Cortex	15 g
huáng qín	Scutellariae, Radix	15 g
huáng lián	Coptidis, Rhizoma	10 g

chē qián zǐ	Plantaginis, Semen	15 g
dì fū zǐ	Kochiae Scopariae, Fructus	15 g
huáng bǎi	Phellodendri, Cortex	15 g

These combinations are suitable for 350–450 ml of water. For application, apply as a wet compress or wash the affected area two or three times a day, for about 15–30 minutes each time. A maximum of three to four herbs in combination are enough. However, *jīn yín huā*, *pú gōng yīng,* or *tǔ fú líng* can be added in order to increase the heat clearing process, reduce redness and swelling. Don't forget to increase the amount of water proportionally.

You may also choose herbs to use as a fine powder and apply topically to the affected skin lesions for at least 15 minutes, at least two times a day to absorb damp exudate.

huáng bǎi	Phellodendri, Cortex	25 g
(duàn) shí gāo	(calcinated) Gypsum Fibrosum	50 g

huá shí	Talcum	15–30 g
huáng bǎi	Phellodendri, Cortex	15 g

huá shí	Talcum	15 g
huáng bǎi	Phellodendri, Cortex	15 g
qīng dài	Indigo Naturalis	5 g

As with all powders, they can also be used as a cold wet compress or a wash. Please see above on how to make a wet compress or a wash. For application, use the liquid as a wet compress or a wash for 15–30 minutes, two or three times a day on the affected skin lesions. Keep in mind, the wet compress should always be cold.

Example Pictures of the Tongue

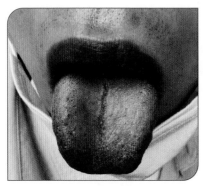
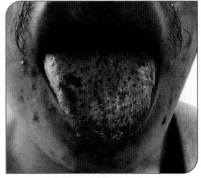

A very red tongue with a yellow coating.

A red tongue with a yellow coating.

Example Pictures of the Skin

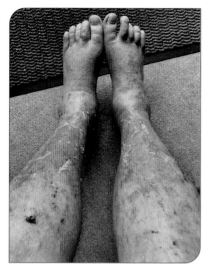
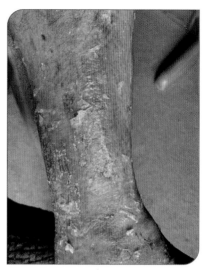

The skin is intense red, itchy, swollen, and burning, feels hot and painful.
Erosions and peeling of the skin (desquamation) can be seen.

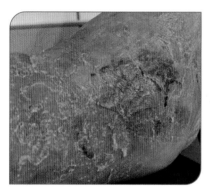
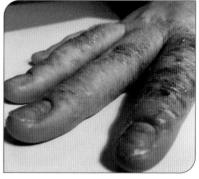

The skin is intense red, itchy, swollen, and burning, feels hot and
painful. Erosions with weepy exudate and crusts can be seen.

Infantile Eczema

Infantile eczema, also called childhood eczema, can affect children of any
age. It often starts at birth or in the weeks immediately afterwards. It mainly
affects the face, cheeks, forehead, and the scalp. Topical corticosteroids are
the primary treatment for childhood eczema in conventional medicine. In
severe cases, oral steroids may be given. Attempting to eliminate the skin
inflammation at all costs and as fast as possible by using medicines with

so-called "suppressive effects" is definitely not the best strategy for the long-term health of the child. Chinese herbal medicine offers gentle and effective solutions.

In this paragraph, I discuss the four main TCM syndromes of infantile eczema. While not the only patterns of eczema seen in children, these four syndromes are most commonly seen, but can also affect adults. It's important to note that treatment for children should be gentler than when working with adults. Lower doses are used, and sometimes internal herbal options are limited, as children do not always tolerate the taste of decoctions. Fortunately, TCM also offers external applications, such as wet compresses or washes, as another option for treatment.

> CLINICAL TIP: To make wet compresses more tolerable for babies and young children, repeatedly dab the areas, let them dry and dab them again. This way you don't have to leave them on the skin, which is often very difficult to do with babies.

In Chinese, infantile eczema is described as *năi xuăn* 奶癣. The Chinese character *năi* can be translated as "milk" or "breast," and the character *xuăn* refers to "tinea" or "dry ulcer." In general, when talking about *năi xuăn* it means an itchy rash that commonly affects infants or young children, a rash that is definitely not persisting until adulthood. In modern language, *năi xuăn* is synonymous with "milk crust," or "cradle cap."[70] This name comes from its visual appearance: the scales on the little one's head often form a crust that resembles burnt milk. Note: Milk crust itself has nothing to do with an intolerance to dairy products. However, milk crust or cradle cap can develop into neurodermatitis (ND), but this does not happen in every case.

What are the major causes of infantile eczema according to TCM?

- Innate weak constitution[71] / insufficiency of *zhèng qì* 正气.[72]

- Impairment of the Spleen's and Stomach's function.

- Fetal toxicity[73] and an internal accumulation of dampness and phlegm.

- An exogenous attack of wind, damp, and heat.

Another factor I have observed in my practice: if the child has had previous vaccinations, we are likely to see lingering pathogenic factors—a vast subject I will not address further here but definitely a valuable topic for in-depth research.

However, treatment in TCM doesn't just involve giving Chinese herbs to the child. It also involves educating the parents in prevention, proper diet for their child and health education, which means sharing health-related knowledge, skills, and behavior.[74]

Heat Accumulation in the Heart and Spleen (*Rè Yùn Xīn Pí* 热蕴心脾)

This syndrome occurs frequently in children, and is less common in adults, at least according to my clinical experience. Both the Heart and the Spleen can be affected by heat at the same time. The main causative factors are generally extended pent-up constraint or an improper diet with long-term overeating of hot and spicy foods, both leading to the transformation of heat and, if this occurs for a long time, into fire, accumulating in the Heart and Spleen and also steaming upwards along the channels.

Characteristics

This pattern is characterized by facial erythema, papules, scales, and crusts due to erosion and damp exudate. The exudate appears yellow because of the heat; thus the crusts appear yellowish, too. The lesions may spread to the trunk and limbs, feel warm or hot and swollen, and are usually quite itchy.

Accompanying symptoms can include palpitations, thirst, mental restlessness, insomnia, mouth ulcers, and a general feeling of heat indicating heat in the Heart, and in more severe conditions, Heart fire. Please note, heat and fire lie along a continuum and differ only in their severity, with heat at the mild end and fire at the more extreme end. Heart fire is a more intense form of Heart-heat. When the Spleen has heat, symptoms like thirst, dry stools, yellow urine, and burning epigastric and/or abdominal pain may be present. These signs also reflect heat in the Stomach, which is usually seen in combination with heat in the Spleen.

The tongue is red with a thin yellow greasy coating. The pulse is overflowing, especially at the left *cùn* (寸) position, which reflects the Heart and/or the right *guān* (关) position, which reflects the Spleen; and slightly rapid.

Treatment Principle

Clear heat from the Heart and Spleen, remove dampness and reduce itching (*qīng sàn xīn pí jī rè, qū shī zhǐ yǎng* 清散心脾积热，祛湿止痒).

Representative Formula

Sān Xīn Dǎo Chì Yǐn (Three Kinds of Plumula for Clearing the Heart and Promoting Urination).[75]

Ingredients

zhī zǐ xīn	Gardeniae, Fructus	9 g (12g)
lián zǐ xīn	Nelumbinis, Semen	9 g (12g)
lián qiáo xīn	Forsythiae, Fructus	9 g (12g)
shēng dì huáng	Rehmanniae Glutinosae, Radix	9 g (12–15 g)
dàn zhú yè	Lophatheri, Herba	3 g (6 g)
mù tōng	Akebiae, Caulis	3 g (6 g)
chì xiǎo dòu	Phaseoli, Semen	9 g (12 g)
huáng qín	Scutellariae, Radix	9 g (9–12 g)
chē qián zǐ	Plantaginis, Semen	9 g (12g)
chē qián cǎo	Plantaginis, Herba	9 g (12g)
+/- chán tuì	Cicadae, Periostracum	3 g (6 g)
gān cǎo	Glycyrrhizae Uralensis, Radix	3 g (3–6 g)
dēng xīn cǎo	Junci, Medulla	3 g (3–6 g)

Please note that the sources here vary. Some sources mention this formula with *xuán shēn*, some with *fú líng, bái zhú,* and *shān yào,* and some even mention it with *bái sháo.* This is one version of the formula.[76] Because it all depends on adjusting the formula to fit the individual needs of the patient, either combination is fine. The dosages mentioned above are the recommended doses for children and infants. The dosages for adults and adolescents are mentioned in brackets for your reference.

First Reference

This is a modern empirical formula created by Xú Yí-Hòu[77] (徐宜厚) from Wǔhàn, Húběi province, China.

Formula Analysis

This formula is basically a modification of *Dǎo Chì Sǎn*[78] (Guide Out the Red Powder), a traditional formula fulfilling the action of clearing heat/fire from the Heart, promoting urination and nourishing yīn, with the addition of a number of herbs supporting the Spleen, removing dampness, and reducing itching. Please note, that *Sān Xīn Dǎo Chì Yǐn* mentions three herbs with the addition of "*xīn*" (心): *zhī zǐ xīn, lián zǐ xīn, lián qiáo xīn*. In Chinese, this means the "centre," in terms of plants it means the core or kernel. However, in practical use this is usually not differentiated, at least in my experience, and so *zhī zǐ, lián zǐ,* and *lián qiáo* can be used.

Within this formula, *shēng dì huáng* cools the blood and nourishes yīn in order to subdue Heart fire. The original formula mentions *mù tōng*, which not only clears Heart fire but also directs heat in the Intestine to go downward. *Shēng dì huáng* and *mù tōng* are the sovereign herbs in *Dǎo Chì Sǎn* and in combination they have the effect of nourishing yīn to subdue the fire without retaining any pathogens. However, as mentioned before *mù tōng* is no longer used and other herbs are substituted, which will be mentioned immediately below. *Dàn zhú yè* serves as a minister herb in the formula, clearing heat from the Heart as well as inducing diuresis due to its bland nature, directing the Heart fire to go downward. *Gān cǎo*, acting as adjuvant and guiding herb, can clear heat, relieve toxicity and harmonize the actions of the other herbs in the formula.[79] So far, this explanation is about Dǎo Chì Sǎn, a small but very well-known prescription.

Let's continue to elaborate on the other herbs included in the modified extended formula, *Sān Xīn Dǎo Chì Yǐn*. *Zhī zǐ, lián zǐ, lián qiáo,* and *dēng xīn cǎo* clear heat from the Heart and eliminate irritability. *Dēng xīn cǎo, chē qián zǐ,* and *chē qián cǎo* expel heat by facilitating the water pathways and guiding heat out of the body through the urine. Let me explain the difference between *chē qián zǐ* and *chē qián cǎo* at this point. As previously mentioned, while *chē qián zǐ* are the Plantaginis seeds, *chē qián cǎo* is the entire Plantaginis herb. Both have basically the same functions. *Chē qián zǐ* is a little more effective at promoting urination and *chē qián cǎo* at clearing heat and resolving toxicity. While *chē qián cǎo* is more diffuse and tends to go into the flesh, cooling and clearing damp and fluids generally from the flesh level, *chē qián zǐ* is more specifically for facilitating urination, and the better choice when there is obvious oedema or poor urine flow, and for urinary tract infections.[80]

Chì xiǎo dòu reduces swelling and fire toxicity in this formula and is often used for swollen toxic sores and itchy wind rash.[81] *Huáng qín's* coldness clears heat and resolves toxicity, while its bitterness dries dampness. Because its aroma is light and clearing, *huáng qín* penetrates both above and below, reaching all the organs internally, and externally reaching the muscles, flesh, and the skin.[82] The latter is of particular importance in the treatment of eczema. Be careful, as the bitter and cold nature of *huáng qín* and *zhī zǐ* can easily harm the Spleen and Stomach and these herbs should therefore be used with caution in patients with Spleen deficiency. To minimize their bitter and cold nature they can be dry-fried (*chǎo*). This preparation reduces their cold properties and makes it more tolerable for the digestive system. And finally, *chán tuì*, light and dispersing, leads the other herbs to the superficial part of the body, disperses wind and clears heat. It vents rashes and alleviates itching.

Cautions

Mù tōng and *chán tuì*: Please note the cautionary advice mentioned earlier in this book regarding allergic reactions. While everyone has their preference, I'm personally very careful with animal products when treating infants and children. I've also noticed that many parents don't want to see these products in their child's formula. Consider whether *chán tuì* is needed, and if you think it is the best choice, I advise you to explain this to the parent, emphasizing that it's the discarded cicada shell not the cicada itself. *Chì xiǎo dòu*: Overdosage can induce miscarriage, so it should be avoided in pregnant women. Allergic reactions in both children and adults have also been reported, including pruritus, flushing, urticaria, nausea, vomiting, and palpitations. The herb should be used with other herbs that tonify the Spleen, and consumption ceased once the goal is achieved.[83]

Modifications

If you prefer a smaller formula for children, containing fewer herbs, you might use *Dǎo Chì Sǎn* in combination with *Xiè Huáng Sǎn* (Drain the Yellow Powder), consisting of the following ingredients:

shēng dì huáng	Rehmanniae Glutinosae, Radix	9 g (9–12 g)
dàn zhú yè	Lophatheri, Herba	3 g (6 g)
mù tōng	Akebiae, Caulis	3 g (6 g)
gān cǎo	Glycyrrhizae Uralensis, Radix	3 g (6 g)
shí gāo	Gypsum Fibrosum	10 g (15 g)
zhī zǐ	Gardeniae, Fructus	9 g (9–12 g)
fáng fēng	Saposhnikoviae, Radix	3 g (6 g)
huò xiāng	Agastachis, Herba	3 g (3–6 g)

This formula is another option for treatment, and as you can see, the quantity of herbs is nearly halved. Sometimes, large formulas can overwhelm children. Thus, shorter formulas can be more suitable in some cases. These are the dosages I recommend for younger children and infants. Please find the doses for adults in brackets for your reference. For other modifications, please see immediately below.

To fortify the Spleen and protect the Stomach, add *bái zhú* 9 g. If stools are loose, use *bái zhú* as *chǎo* (dry-fried). When the stools are dry, use (*shēng*) *bái zhú* (unprepared). *Gǔ yá* 9 g and *mài yá* 9 g can also be added to further strengthen digestive function. Both are best used as *chǎo* (dry-fried). *Gǔ yá* and *mài yá* are similar in action and are often used as a pair, to promote digestion, invigorate spleen and increase the appetite due to Spleen and Stomach deficiency. When treating adults, the doses of these three herbs can be increased to 12 g. For lesions appearing on the face, use *yě jú huā* 9 g. It is a wonderful herb for treating skin conditions on the face. To strengthen *shēng dì huáng's* action in nourishing yīn and clearing heat, one may add *mài mén dōng* 9 g and *xuán shēn* 9 g. When treating adults, the doses can be increased up to 12 g. To support *huáng qín* and enhance the heat clearing and fire purging action of the formula, add *huáng lián* 3 g. Using *huáng lián* as *chǎo* (dry-fried) will make it more tolerable for the digestive system. When treating adults, the dosage can be increased to 6 g, where needed.

Suggestions for External Treatment

In this pattern, the formulas and combinations for external treatment are essentially the same as described for "Dampness-Heat" in Chapter 6. One difference, however, is that I recommend working a little more gently, using lower dosages or more water with the same dosages.

A short note for individually tailored herbal washes or wet compresses: In general, the lesions can be rinsed or carefully washed with cool boiled water. It can cool the skin and soothe skin irritation. 100% cotton should be used for both the washcloth and the gauze. Another option is to use fresh organic green tea in a low concentration. The green tea should be cold and handled with care, especially if the lesions are on the face. Always check first to ensure that the infant/child tolerates the substance. Don't forget, the skin on the face is more sensitive than other areas on the body. Other possible herbal washes with single herbs might consist of *huáng lián, huáng bǎi*, or *yú xīng cǎo*, for example. As already mentioned, in children I recommend repeatedly dabbing the affected areas with the herbal solution, let them dry and dab them again. This way, children and babies will tolerate the external treatment. In adults, we can work as usual with cold wet compresses or powder when damp exudate drying function is needed. The application time in adults can be extended up to 30 minutes. When the rash is located on the face, which we see in this pattern quite commonly, I always recommend adding *yě jú huā* or *jú huā* as it is not only used for its heat clearing and toxicity relieving action, but also for guiding other herbs to the face.

Example Pictures of the Skin[84]

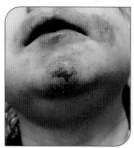 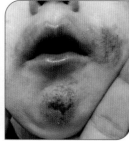 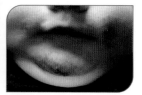

Red, itchy, hot, and painful skin around the infant's mouth.

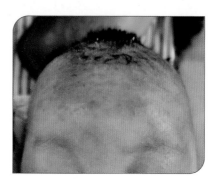

Red, hot, and swollen skin on a baby's face.

Internal Accumulation of Damp-Heat Due to Fetal Toxin (*Tāi Dú Suǒ Zhì Zhī Shī Rè Nèi Jù* 胎毒所致之湿热内聚)

As mentioned above, when a pregnant woman smokes, drinks alcohol or overconsumes hot, spicy, or oily foods, the baby will be born with intrauterine toxins which will cause—in this case—eczema. Interestingly, according to my clinical observations, these children will often develop allergies later in life. Whenever you have a pregnant patient, advise her to avoid hot and spicy food, alcohol, coffee, and cigarettes. One would think that this information should be known; however, I notice again and again that many women are not aware of this and, in some cases, even their gynecologists do not caution them about it. I advise every pregnant woman in my practice about the possible negative effects on their baby and of course on themselves.

Characteristics
The skin lesions are mostly symmetrical and appear as fresh red patches, papules, and/or papulovesicles, showing erosion with yellowish exudation and crusting. The skin feels hot with intense itching. The child may have fever, irritability, bad breath, thirst and poor appetite, scanty urine, and constipation.

The tongue is red with a greasy, yellow coating and the pulse is slippery and/or rapid.

Treatment Principle
Cool blood, clear fire, eliminate dampness, and relieve itching (*liáng xuè qīng huǒ, qū shī zhǐ yǎng* 凉血清火，祛湿止痒).

Representative Formula
Xiāo Fēng Dǎo Chì Tāng (Eliminate Wind and Guide Out the Red Decoction).

Ingredients

shēng dì huáng	Rehmanniae Glutinosae, Radix	6–10 g (9–12 g)
mù tōng	Akebiae, Caulis	3 g (3–6 g)
gān cǎo	Glycyrrhizae Uralensis, Radix	3 g (3–6 g)
fú líng	Poriae Cocos, Sclerotium	6–10 g (15–20 g)
jīn yín huā	Lonicerae Japonicae, Flos	6–10 g (15–20 g)
niú bàng zǐ	Arctii Lappae, Fructus	9 g (10 g)
bái xiān pí	Dictamni Radicis, Cortex	6–10 g (10 g)
dēng xīn cǎo	Junci, Medulla	3 g (3–5 g)
+/- huáng lián[85]	Coptidis, Rhizoma	1–2 g (3–5 g)
bò hé	Menthae, Herba	1–2 g (3–5 g)

These are the dosages I recommend for children and infants. For adults, I have mentioned the doses in brackets for your reference.

First Reference

Xiāo Fēng Dǎo Chì Tāng was first mentioned in the book *Yī Zōng Jīn Jiàn* (The Golden Mirror of Ancestral Medicine, ca. 1736–1743), written by Wú Qiān et al.

Formula Analysis

The first four herbs are basically *Dǎo Chì Sǎn* in combination with *Xiāo Fēng Sǎn*. Detailed explanation and analysis of the formulas are given earlier in the chapter. As mentioned before, *mù tōng* is no longer used and is usually substituted by other herbs, for example *tōng cǎo* 3 g. When a stronger heat clearing effect is needed, one ought to use *dàn zhú yè* 3 g instead of *tōng cǎo*. *Fú líng* promotes urination, leaches out dampness, strengthens the Spleen, and harmonizes the middle *jiāo*. *Jīn yín huā* clears heat, resolves fire toxicity, and is quite effective in treating swellings and sores. The dosage determines its function. In smaller doses (9–12 g in adults), it is best for dispersing wind-heat while larger doses—up to 20 g (in adults)—are very effective for heat toxin, sores, and abscesses. In this pattern "Internal Accumulation of Damp-Heat Due to Fetal Toxin," I definitely recommend using large dosages of *jīn yín huā* in this formula, 9–12 g for children and infants, and 15–20 g for adults. *Niú bàng zǐ* disperses wind-heat but also clears and drains heat toxin, and vents rashes. It is ideal for red swellings, erythema, and acute maculopapular rashes or when there are unexpressed rashes in which the skin rash remains below the surface. Due to its cold and slippery nature, *niú bàng zǐ* is able to promote the movement of both stool and urine. It is thus especially indicated when patients have constipation and scanty or difficult urination. Used together with *gān cǎo*, the fire draining and toxicity draining effect is boosted, while *gān cǎo* moderates *niú bàng zǐ's* potential undesired effects such as diarrhoea, when unprepared.[86] *Bái xiān pí* clears heat, resolves fire toxicity, expels wind, dries dampness, clears damp-heat, and effectively stops itching. Whenever there is much yellowish exudation with crusting, oozing skin, and itchiness, *bái xiān pí* is a good choice. Let's continue with *dēng xīn cǎo*: it clears heat in the Heart and Lungs, promotes urination and leads heat and dampness downward and out of the body through the urine. It is particularly useful and often used for infants or children with a restless sensation of heat in the chest, nightmares, night terrors, and dark, burning urine due to heat.[87] These are all accompanying symptoms which often appear in addition to the skin rash in this pattern. *Huáng lián*, a frequently used herb in skin conditions with signs of heat and fire, clears heat, drains dampness, drains fire, and resolves fire toxicity. In children and also in adults I tend to use it in its prepared form as (*chǎo*), dry-fried. This method of preparation moderates its cold property to avoid damaging the Spleen and Stomach. In infants, I recommend omitting *huáng lián* because it is too cold and too bitter for babies. Especially in infants and children, working cautiously and gently is recommended. And finally, *bò hé*: in this formula, it is used to disperse wind-heat and vent rashes. What is meant by that? When the rash is expressed to the surface as a means of venting the wind and heat, the rash can heal faster. As *bò hé* benefits the head and eyes, it is also good at relieving headaches when there is fever.

Cautions

Mù tōng and *bái xiān pí*: Please note the cautionary advice about this herb, mentioned earlier in this book.

Modifications

Regardless of whether children or adults are affected, the modifications are also many and varied here. The dosages included here correspond to those for children. Increase the dosages for adults if necessary.

To increase the heat cooling and dampness drying effect, add *huáng qín* 6 g. It works mildly and the taste is not that bad, which is particularly important when treating infants and children. Usually, *huáng qín* alone should do, but in some cases, this is just not enough, and you can consider adding *yú xīng cǎo* 9 g as well. However, in order to protect the Spleen and Stomach, use the herb as *chǎo* (dry-fried), which moderates any harmful effects from its cold and bitter nature. Please do not use *tǔ fú líng* when treating infants and children. Although it is quite effective in removing dampness and resolving toxicity for adults, it is too harsh for children. To eliminate dampness in infants and children, add *chē qián cǎo* or *chē qián zǐ* 9 g. If it is available, *chē qián cǎo* is preferred. To reduce itching, add *fáng fēng* and *jīng jiè* 3 g of each, or alternatively *chán tuì* 3 g. However, as already mentioned, *chán tuì* should be used with care especially in infants and children. If you decide to use it, inform the parents to give prompt feedback on potential side effects (mentioned earlier in this book, please see page 121). Again, especially in infants and children we have to work with care. If the child has a greasy tongue coating and more discharge, add *cāng zhú* 3 g. It dries dampness and strengthens the Spleen and Stomach. If the child shows oily crusts, especially on the head, add *dì gǔ pí* 6 g and *shān zhā* 6 g. Add *jú huā* 6–9 g if the child is quite irritated. It is a mild Liver calming herb, very well tolerated and has a good taste. If the Spleen is weakened, add *fú líng* 9 g, *bái zhú* 6 g, and *tài zǐ shēn* 9 g to strengthen the Spleen. Please do not use *dǎng shēn* as it might be too cloying for the digestion. To tonify the Kidneys and Spleen, add *shān yào* 9–12 g.

Suggestions for External Treatment

- *Jīn Huáng Sǎn* (Golden Yellow Powder)[88]
- *Qīng Dài Sǎn* (Indigo Powder)[89]
- *Sì Huáng Gāo* (Four Yellow Cream)[90]
- *Jiě Dú Xǐ Gāo* (Toxin Releasing Ointment)
- *Xīn Sān Miào Sǎn* (New Three Marvels Powder)
- *Zǐ Yún Gāo* (Purple Cloud Ointment)[91]

There are many choices for external treatments as well as simple individual tailored herbal washes. Herbs that strongly clear heat, resolve toxicity, invigorate the blood, reduce swelling and pain, but also herbs that absorb existing damp exudate, are the most suitable herbs in this pattern. The possible combinations are endless. Always keep in mind, these are just examples.

Frequently used herbal combinations in practice as a wash or as a wet compress are:

jīn yín huā	Lonicerae Japonicae, Flos	10 g
pú gōng yīng	Taraxaci, Herba	15 g
lián qiáo	Forsythiae, Fructus	10 g
yě jú huā	Chrysanthemi Indici, Flos	10 g
+/- *bái xiān pí*	Dictamni Radicis, Cortex	10 g

Boil with 350–450 ml water, depending on whether *bái xiān pí* is included. Herbs can be replaced as required, and dosages can be changed any time–be flexible.

yú xīng cǎo	Houttuynia Cordata Thunb., Herba	10 g
yě jú huā	Chrysanthemi Indici, Flos	10 g
jīn yín huā	Lonicerae Japonicae, Flos	10 g
pú gōng yīng	Taraxaci, Herba	15 g

huáng bǎi	Phellodendri, Cortex	10 g
huáng qín	Scutellariae, Radix	10 g
huáng lián	Coptidis, Rhizoma	10 g
+/- tǔ fú líng	Smilacis Glabrae, Rhizoma	15 g

wáng bù liú xíng	Vaccariae, Semen	15 g
míng fán[92]	Alumen	10 g
kǔ shēn	Sophorae Flavescentis, Radix	10 g

These combinations are boiled with about 350 ml water. Use a little less water when *tǔ fú líng*[93] is not added to the second combination.

mǎ chǐ xiàn	Portulacae, Herba	15 g
huáng bǎi	Phellodendri, Cortex	15 g

This combination should be boiled with about 250 ml of water. Use as a cold wet compress, or repeatedly dab the areas, let them dry and dab them again.

Simple examples of frequently used and effective stand-alone herbs in this pattern:

- *mǎ chǐ xiàn* (Portulacae, Herba) 15–20 g
- *pú gōng yīng* (Taraxaci, Herba) 20–30 g
- *shí gāo* (Gypsum Fibrosum) 15–30 g
- *yú xīng cǎo* (Houttuynia Cordata Thunb., Herba) 20–30 g
- *zǐ huā dì dīng* (Violae, Herba) 20–30 g.

The dosages specified are for a wash boiled using a single herb and about 150–250 ml water, depending on how concentrated you want to make it. Reduce the amount of water if you want the solution to be more concentrated. Use a cold wet compress or repeatedly dab the areas, let them dry and dab them again.

Example Pictures of the Skin

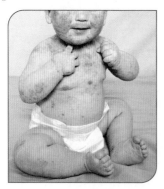 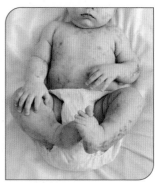

Symmetrical skin lesions that appear bright red, feel hot and painful.[94]

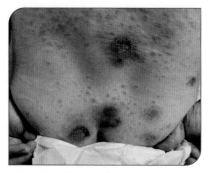

Bright red, inflamed skin lesions with light
crusts on a baby's back and buttock.

Spleen Deficiency with Accumulation of Dampness (*Pí Xū Shī Kùn* 脾虚湿困)

Characteristics

What we see here is a relatively subacute stage of eczema. This is not an acute stage and the characteristics of the skin are no longer as extreme. Both onset and progression tend to be a little slower. The skin lesions appear as pale red or dark and dull vesicles, showing mild erosion with thin crusting. As long as heat is present the exudate looks clear. The skin is usually itchy. The accompanying symptoms are those of Spleen deficiency with dampness, e.g., fatigue, poor appetite, loose stool, and abdominal distension. The only additional information one might keep in mind, because this is different in children compared with adults: as the Spleen is weak, the stool may contain undigested food residue.

The tongue is puffy and pale with teeth-marks and a greasy coating, usually white. Please note that the coating is generally different in children. It is not as thick as in adults. The pulse is slow, soft, and slippery.

Treatment Principle

Tonify the Spleen, eliminate dampness, and relieve itching (*jiàn pí, qū shī, zhǐ yǎng* 健脾祛湿止痒).

Representative Formula

Xiǎo Ér Huà Shī Tāng[95] (Children's Dampness Removing Decoction).

Ingredients

cāng zhú	Atractylodis, Rhizoma	6 g
fú líng	Poriae Cocos, Sclerotium	6 g
zé xiè	Alismatis, Rhizoma	6 g
chén pí	Citri Reticulatae, Pericarpium	6 g
(chǎo) mài yá	(dry-fried) Hordei Germantus, Fructus	9 g
huá shí	Talcum (wrapped)	6 g
gān cǎo	Glycyrrhizae Uralensis, Radix	1 g

First Reference

This formula comes from the book *Zhū Rén-Kāng Lín Chuáng Jīng Yàn Jí* (A Collection of Zhu Renkang's Clinical Experiences, 1979), written by Zhū Rén-Kāng.[96]

Formula Analysis

This is a mild and effective formula not only to tonify the Spleen and drain dampness, but also to clear mild heat, as dampness and heat often coexist when dampness has been accumulating for a long time. You will find this to be true in many skin conditions. Let's analyze the formula in detail: *cāng zhú* dries dampness and strengthens the Spleen and Stomach. *Fú líng* strengthens the Spleen, promotes urination and resolves dampness. Combined with *zé xiè*, it facilitates the removal of stagnant water and leaches out dampness that may cause oedema, swelling and heaviness throughout the body. This combination is particularly effective when oedema and swelling occurs mainly in the lower parts of the body, for example the lower limbs. *Chén pí* dries dampness and promotes the flow of qì. *Mài yá* reduces food stagnation, strengthens the Stomach, improves the digestion and the appetite. Keep in mind: for improving the digestion, always use *(chǎo) mài yá* (dry-fried). And finally, *huá shí* and *gān cǎo* in combination is known as *Liù Yī Sǎn* (Six-to-One Powder): it clears heat and resolves dampness.

Modifications

To increase the dampness transforming and Spleen and Stomach strengthening effect, one may add *hòu pò* 3–6 g. It also moves qì and removes dampness obstructing the middle *jiāo*. If you prefer to work more gently in infants, substitute *hòu pò huā* (Magnoliae Officinalis, Flos) 3 g. It works similarly but is milder than *hòu pò* and less drying. If there is severe heat present and the lesions turn intensely red, add *bái huā shé shé cǎo*[97] 6–9 g. It cools heat and resolves toxicity. Don't forget the blood moving aspect when severe heat is present. Add *(chǎo) mǔ dān pí* 6–9 g, which not only clears heat, cools the blood, drains pus and reduces swelling, but also gently invigorates the blood. However, if more heat is involved and the lesions are more painful and swollen, you might also add *jīn yín huā* 6–9 g and *lián qiáo* 6–9 g, or *(chǎo) huáng qín* 6–9 g. To strengthen the Spleen, add *tài zǐ shēn* 9 g. As already mentioned, do not use *dǎng shēn* in infants and children as it might be too cloying for their digestion. If dampness is mixed with heat, you might also consider using *yú xīng cǎo* 6–9 g, especially if the lesions become infected.

Suggestions for External Treatment

- *Bái Zhú Gāo* (White Atractylodis Ointment)

- *Cāng Zhú Gāo* (Dark Atractylodis Ointment)

- *Sān Huáng Xǐ Jì* (Three Yellow Cleanser Formula)

- *Shé Chuáng Zǐ Tāng* (Cnidium Fruit Decoction)

These are the external applications I recommend using in this pattern. The more that heat is involved, seen by the exudate turning yellow, the more appropriate the final three formulas are. If heat is predominant, the external treatment should be changed to suggestions described as for the "Dampness-Heat" pattern, please see Chapter 6 for more information. Please keep in mind, when working with children and infants it is advised to work with lower concentrations and shorter application times. This applies for cold wet compresses as well as when dabbing the skin areas.

Example Pictures of the Skin

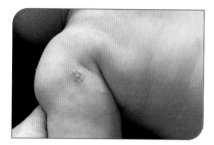 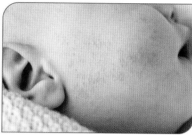

Pale red vesicles with very thin crusting.   98

Accumulation of Dampness-Heat with Spleen Deficiency
(*Shī Rè Nèi Jù Jiān Pí Xū Zhèng* 湿热内聚兼脾虚证)

I have already discussed damp-heat eczema in adults in Chapter 6. The longer the Spleen is weak and damp accumulates, the greater the tendency to generate heat. The skin characteristics and symptoms are nearly the same, however I recommend using some different formulas and lower dosages in infants and children.

Characteristics

The skin lesions appear as erythema, accompanied with erosion, copious yellowish exudation and crusting. Furthermore, the infant or child feels a sensation of heat on his/her skin with intense itching and always wants to scratch. Lots of discharge comes out after scratching. The infant or child will also have digestive problems such as poor appetite, loose stool, and abdominal distension. Other symptoms may include fever, irritability, a dry mouth and throat, thirst, and dark yellow urine.

The tongue is thick and red with teeth-marks, a greasy, yellow coating and the pulse is slippery and/or rapid.

CLINICAL TIP: As long as crusting, weeping, and erosion is present, the damp-heat has not yet resolved. Thus, draining dampness and heat is required.

Treatment Principle

Clear heat, eliminate dampness, relieve itching and strengthen the Spleen (*qīng rè, qū shī, zhǐ yǎng, jiàn pí* 清热祛湿止痒健脾).

Representative Formula

When working with adults I always recommend using *Lóng Dǎn Xiè Gān Tāng* because it is so effective. But when working with infants and children, we have to be cautious and work more gently. *Lóng Dǎn Xiè Gān Tāng* would definitely be too harsh in this case.

Thus, use: *Bì Xiè Shèn Shī Tāng* (Dioscorea Decoction to Leach Out Dampness) or *Èr Miào Sǎn* (Two-Marvel Powder).

Ingredients
Bì Xiè Shèn Shī Tāng

yì yǐ rén	Coices, Semen	6 g (15–30 g)
huá shí	Talcum	6 g (9–15 g)
bì xiè	Dioscoreae, Rhizoma	6 g (9–20 g)
fú líng	Poriae Cocos, Sclerotium	6 g (9–12 g)
huáng bǎi	Phellodendri, Cortex	3–6 g (6–10 g)
mǔ dān pí	Moutan, Cortex	6 g (9–12 g)
zé xiè	Alismatis, Rhizoma	6–9 g (12–15 g)
tōng cǎo	Tetrapanacis, Medulla	3 g (6 g)

Èr Miào Sǎn

huáng bǎi	Phellodendri, Cortex	3–6 g (9–12 g)
cāng zhú	Atractylodis, Rhizoma	6 g (9–12 g)

These are the dosages I recommend for children and infants. For adults, I have included the doses in brackets for your reference.

First Reference

Bì Xiè Shèn Shī Tāng: Yáng Kē Xīn Dé Jí (Collected Experiences on Treating Sores, 1806), written by Gāo Bǐng-Jūn.

Èr Miào Sǎn: Dān Xī Xīn Fǎ (Essential Teachings of [Zhu] Dan-Xi, 1481), written by Zhū Dān-Xī.

Formula Analysis
Bì Xiè Shèn Shī Tāng

Detailed explanations and analysis of this formula can be found in Chapter 6 This will not be repeated here. For modifications, please see below.

Èr Miào Sǎn

This formula is comprised of only two herbs in nearly equal amounts: *huáng bǎi*, acting as the sovereign herb, and *cāng zhú*, acting as the minister herb. It may be prepared as a powder or as a decoction. In infants and children, a powder can be useful because it can be mixed with meals. However, I always prefer giving this formula as a decoction when working with adults or older children, because, according to my clinical experience, raw herbs always work best. In this prescription, *huáng bǎi* bitter and cold, clears heat and dries dampness. It is an excellent herb for treating damp-heat, especially from the lower *jiāo*. *Cāng zhú* is effective in drying dampness and invigorating the Spleen with its pungent-aromatic and bitter-warm nature. The two herbs combined dry dampness and treat damp-heat pouring downward, disperse swelling and alleviate pain. In eczema, *Èr Miào Sǎn* can be given orally or applied topically with excellent results provided you see the following features: skin eruptions with pus, discolored yellow discharge, dark yellow urine and a yellow tongue coating. In the traditional preparation, both herbs are dry-fried (*chǎo*), which is intended to yield a more drying effect. I suggest using this formula when infantile damp-heat eczema is most severe on the legs.

Modifications

If the lesions are located on the upper part of the body, you might add *sāng yè* 6–9 g (10 g in adults), or *jú huā* 6–9 g (9–12 g in adults) if located on the face. In this case, when eczema is predominantly located on the upper parts of the body, I suggest omitting *huáng bǎi*. For eczema mainly found on the abdominal region, add *huáng lián* and *huáng qín* with 3–6 g each (use 10 g in adults). For eczema on the legs, add *niú xī* and *chē qián zǐ* 6 g of each (in adults: 10 g). If there is profound discharge, especially in infants and children, add *dōng guā pí* 10–15 g. In adults, this herb can be used with dosages up to 15–30 g because it is so mild. It gently clears heat and resolves dampness, thus it is a good choice in skin disorders with dampness and heat. To improve digestion in children, you might add *(chǎo) mài yá* and *(chǎo) gǔ yá* 9 g each. Please see the section on "Dampness-Heat" in Chapter 6 for other possible modifications. Don't forget to use low dosages in children and refrain from using harsh herbs, *tǔ fú líng* for instance.

Suggestions for External Treatment

- *Bài Jiàng Cǎo Gāo*[99] (White Flower Patrinia Ointment)

- *Qū Shī Sǎn* (Damp-Removing Medicinal Powder)

- *Xīn Sān Miào Sǎn* (New Three Marvels Powder)

- *Sān Huáng Xǐ Jì* (Three Yellow Cleanser Formula)

Apart from these combinations, all other suggestions for the damp-heat pattern in Chapter 6 are suitable. Always choose the combination that suits best.

Frequently used herbal combinations in practice as a wash or as a wet compress are:

huáng bǎi	Phellodendri, Cortex	15 g
gān cǎo	Glycyrrhizae Uralensis, Radix	10 g

huá shí	Talcum	15–30 g
huáng bǎi	Phellodendri, Cortex	15 g

If there is profuse discharge and ulceration, these combinations might be chosen. They can be given as either an external wash or as a cold wet compress. First herbal pair: Boil with about 150–200 ml water. Second herbal pair: Boil with about 250–300 ml water.

Use more water and increase the dosages if the skin lesion is larger and more liquid is needed. This applies for all other mentioned combinations, too. Use as a cold wash or cold compress (either with a gauze, washcloth or by dabbing) on the affected skin area for about 20 minutes each time, 2–3 times a day. If 20 minutes cannot be done because the child doesn't keep still, do inform the parents that a little is better than nothing. They should keep trying, even if they only can manage 10 minutes.

If there is less discharge but more heat involved, the skin lesions can be topically treated with *huáng lián*. A cold wet compress is best in this case. Furthermore, if there is almost no discharge, you can also work with sesame oil as an ointment. Be flexible!

Example Pictures of the Skin

Please see damp-heat eczema in adults in Chapter 6 for the appearance of the skin. The skin characteristics are nearly the same in infants and children.

Some final practical advice when treating children: No matter which syndrome presents, in infants and children it is necessary to avoid scratching and the use of warm/hot water when washing the infected skin areas. Always use cold water, as the lesions will most probably flare up with warmth or heat. Children are more sensitive and, especially with infants, it's harder to ask how it feels, does it burn, is it painful? We only see the negative effects when the infant cries or screams and this is obviously too late.

It is also suggested to postpone vaccinations during acute episodes of eczema. The general side effects of vaccination are mostly high fever and according to my experience, many patients claim that they experience headaches, aches, and pains in many body parts. TCM assumes that the vaccination process is perceived as an external pathogenic heat or toxic heat attacking the body. This means that those ill effects can be seen as signs that inflammation is rampant in the body. With this background, it does not make any sense to give "fire on fire," or in other words to make a "smouldering fire," the skin inflammation, burn even more. Thus, vaccinations and all other substances that increase heat[100] in the body are contraindicated. However, that should go without saying.

Endnotes

1 I have seen this several times in my practice.

2 Posture, appearance etc.

3 This is provided by the project of standardization of TCM terminology of the State (China) Administration of Traditional Chinese Medicine.

4 Source: Sabine Schmitz.

5 Occurring in several different forms.

6 Scheid, V., Bensky, D., Ellis, A., and Barolet, R. (2009) *Formulas & Strategies* (2nd Ed.). Seattle, WA: Eastland Press, p.200.

7 Bensky, D., Clavey, S., and Stöger, E. (2004) *Materia Medica* (3rd Ed.). Seattle, WA: Eastland Press, p.96.

8 Bensky, D., Clavey, S., and Stöger, E. (2004) *Materia Medica* (3rd Ed.). Seattle, WA: Eastland Press, p.285.

9 Han, J., Xian, Z., Zhang, Y., Liu, J., and Liang, A. (2019) "Systematic overview of aristolochic acids: Nephrotoxicity, carcinogenicity, and underlying mechanisms." *Frontiers in Pharmacology 10*, 648.

10 *Bái xiān pí* was involved in a series of cases involving Liver damage in skin disease patients in the UK and New Zealand. An allergic mechanism was suggested. Therefore, this herb should be used with caution in patients with atopic conditions, a history of Liver disease and a known poor Liver function. Source: Bensky, D., Clavey, S., and Stöger, E. (2004) *Materia Medica* (3rd Ed.). Seattle, WA: Eastland Press, p.199.

11 Wagner, H., Bauer, R., Peigen, X., Jianming, C., and Bächer, S. (1997) Chinese Drug Monographs and Analysis. Verlag für Ganzheitliche Medizin Dr. E. Wühr, Germany. Vol. 1, No. 6.

12 *Èr Miào Sǎn: huáng bǎi, cāng zhú.*

13 *Sān Miào Wán: huáng bǎi, cāng zhú, niú xī.*

14 清热渗湿汤: 黄柏, 黄连, 茯苓, 泽泻, 苍术, 白术, 甘草. This formula is rarely found in sources so to give you as much information as possible, I would like to mention the formula name and all ingredients for you in Chinese as well.

15 All boiling instructions and detailed explanations can be found in Appendix I.

16 Use as a wash or wet compress.

17 Use as a wash or wet compress.

18 Superinfection: an infection that occurs after, or on top of an earlier infection.

19 A flat, distinct, discolored area of skin usually less than one centimeter wide.

20 The fluid that has seeped out.

21 This pulse sensation gives the impression of being easily moved, as if your finger is floating on water. Why is that? It's because the dampness is obstructing the vessels plus the *qì* is unable to fill the vessels, giving it its soft quality.

22 Mainly due to its toxicity.

23 Bensky, D., Clavey, S., and Stöger, E. (2004) *Materia Medica* (3rd Ed.). Seattle, WA: Eastland Press, p.711.

24 Bensky, D., Clavey, S., and Stöger, E. (2004) *Materia Medica* (3rd Ed.). Seattle, WA: Eastland Press, p.740.

25 Scheid, V., Bensky, D., Ellis A., and Barolet, R. (2009) *Formulas & Strategies* (2nd Ed.). Seattle, WA: Eastland Press, pp.314–315.

26 For cautions of this herb, please see above.

27 Bensky, D., Clavey, S., and Stöger, E. (2004) *Materia Medica* (3rd Ed.). Seattle, WA: Eastland Press, p.280.

28 Bensky, D., Clavey, S., and Stöger, E. (2004) *Materia Medica* (3rd Ed.). Seattle, WA: Eastland Press, p.518.

29 Use as a wash or wet compress. Use when heat is also present.

30 No pus or exudation anymore compared to the previous TCM patterns.

31 Alternate name: *cì jí lí.*

32 Please keep in mind, if the lesions are redder and a blood cooling aspect is needed, *shēng dì huáng* is better than *shú dì huáng*. If the lesions are paler and the patient needs more tonification, *shú dì huáng* may be used.

33 It is an animal product and should not be used for vegetarians. While that should actually be clear, I just wanted to emphasize it.

34 Normal dosage range: Bensky, D., Clavey, S., and Stöger, E. (2004) *Materia Medica*

(3rd Ed.). Seattle, WA: Eastland Press, p. 975.

35 Bensky, D., Clavey, S., and Stöger, E. (2004) *Materia Medica* (3rd Ed.). Seattle, WA: Eastland Press, p. 976.

36 First reference *Sì Wù Tāng: Xiān Shòu Lǐ Shāng Xù Duàn Mì Fāng* (Secret Formulas to Manage Trauma and Reconnect Fractures Received from an Immortal, c. 846), Author: Daoist priest Lìn Dào-Rén.

37 Bensky, D., Clavey, S., and Stöger, E. (2004) *Materia Medica* (3rd Ed.). Seattle, WA: Eastland Press, p.324.

38 Bensky, D., Clavey, S., and Stöger, E. (2004) *Materia Medica* (3rd Ed.). Seattle, WA: Eastland Press, p.74.

39 *Xiāo Yáo Sǎn: chái hú, dāng guī, bái sháo, bái zhú, fú líng, zhì gān cǎo, shēng jiāng, bò hé.*

40 Taken from: Scheid, V., Bensky, D., Ellis A., and Barolet, R. (2009) *Formulas & Strategies* (2nd Ed.). Seattle, WA: Eastland Press, p.637.

41 Bensky, D., Clavey, S., and Stöger, E. (2004) *Materia Medica* (3rd Ed.). Seattle, WA: Eastland Press, p.54.

42 Bensky, D., Clavey, S., and Stöger, E. (2004) *Materia Medica* (3rd Ed.). Seattle, WA: Eastland Press, p.52.

43 Bensky, D., Clavey, S., and Stöger, E. (2004) *Materia Medica* (3rd Ed.). Seattle, WA: Eastland Press, p.753.

44 My notes from China.

45 Bensky, D., Clavey, S., and Stöger, E. (2004) *Materia Medica* (3rd Ed.). Seattle, WA: Eastland Press, p.245.

46 In chronic eczema, commonly used as an ointment.

47 Unfortunately, *zǐ cǎo* is not available in Germany. It is a very effective herb and it is used quite frequently in China and worldwide.

48 Please note that some sources advise to cook *shí gāo* for about 30 minutes before adding the other herbs, however I usually cook all the herbs together at once.

49 The original formula contained *mù tōng*. I have substituted this herb with *tōng cǎo* for safety reasons.

50 Also called: "True Lineage of External Medicine."

51 *Yín Qiào Sǎn: jīn yín huā, lián qiáo, niú bàng zǐ, dàn dòu chǐ, bò hé, jié gěng, jīng jiè, dàn zhú yè, lú gēn, gān cǎo.*

52 Four levels theory developed by Yè Tiān Shì (ca. 1667-1746, Qīng Dynasty), which describes the progression of *wēn bìng* (warm and febrile diseases) through the *wèi* (defence), *qì* (qi), *yíng* (nutritive), and *xuè* (blood) levels.

53 *Bái Hǔ Tāng: shí gāo, zhī mǔ, zhì gān cǎo, jīng mǐ.*

54 Bensky, D., Clavey, S., and Stöger, E. (2004) *Materia Medica* (3rd Ed.). Seattle, WA: Eastland Press, p.286.

55 *Wǔ Wèi Xiāo Dú Yǐn: jīn yín huā, pú gōng yīng, zǐ huā dì dīng, yě jú huā, tiān kuí zǐ.*

56 Collected information from my clinic hours in China and my Chinese dermatology seminar notes.

57 TCM works in analogies. *Sāng zhī* are the branches of the mulberry tree (Morus alba). Arms and legs can also be seen as branches of the body.

58 The name *niú xī* generally refers to *huái niú xī*. Both *chuān niú xī* and *huái niú xī* are capable of guiding the formula to the lower limbs. *Huái niú xī* more strongly tonifies the Liver and Kidneys, while *chuān niú xī* invigorates blood and expels blood more strongly.

59 When available. Otherwise, leave it out.

60 Source: Adobe Stock.

61 Source: Adobe Stock.

62 Source: Adobe Stock.

63 Some sources call this formula also "Erythema Resolving and Toxicity Removing Decoction" or "Erysipelas Resolving and Toxicity Removing Decoction."

64 Professor Zhào Bǐng-Nán (Chinese: 赵炳南, 1899–1984).

65 《外科正宗》卷之四 · 杂疮毒门.

66 This pattern is also called yáng brightness disease (*yáng míng bìng* 阳明病).

67 *Huà Bān Tāng: shí gāo, zhī mǔ, gān cǎo, xuán shēn, jīng mǐ, shuǐ niú jiǎo.*

68 Use as a wash or wet compress.

69 This herb is not available everywhere outside of China. In Germany, for example, it is not.

70 The term cradle cap, or in German Milchschorf, goes back to Adalbert Czerny (1863–1941), an Austrian pediatrician.

71 The constitution of a person determines the susceptibility to some pathogenic factors but also the tendency towards disease causing processes. A person with a weak constitution will usually be more susceptible to many kinds of diseases than a person with a strong constitution, who has a greater power of disease resistance.

72 *Zhèng qì* or healthy qì represents our ability to maintain health when challenged by external pathogens. It can also be called "anti-pathogenic qì." In modern language, the term *zhèng qì* can be equated with the innate immune system. An insufficiency of *zhèng qì* is most probably the basis for various diseases in later life, or the primary cause leading to a disease.

73 Fetal heat, acquired from parents. For example, when a pregnant woman smokes or drinks alcohol, the baby will be born with intrauterine toxins which will most likely cause frequent health issues like eczema or allergies in the child's later life. The literal translation in Chinese is: *tāi' ér dú sù* (胎儿毒素).

74 In general: healthy diet, sufficient sleep, maintaining a good work-life balance (more important when talking to adults), physical activity and so forth.

75 Also known as "Three-Pith Guide out the Red Powder."

76 Li, B., Shi, Y.J., Song, S.P., and Zhan C. (2010) "Xu Yi-Hou's experience in herbal administration for the differential treatment of skin diseases." *Journal of Traditional Chinese Medicine* 30, 3, 211–216.

77 Born in 1940, he is the former chief doctor and Professor at the Dermatology Department of Wǔhàn Hospital of Traditional Chinese Medicine. He is the author of the book *Dermatology in Traditional Chinese Medicine*, published by Donica Publishing Ltd (UK) in 2004.

78 *Dǎo Chì Sǎn*: *shēng dì huáng, mù tōng, dàn zhú yè, gān cǎo*.

79 *Dǎo Chì Sǎn* and *Sān Xīn Dǎo Chì Yǐn*.

80 My clinical notes from Steven Clavey's clinic in Melbourne, Australia.

81 Bensky, D., Clavey, S., and Stöger, E. (2004) *Materia Medica* (3rd Ed.). Seattle, WA: Eastland Press, pp.308–309.

82 Bensky, D., Clavey, S., and Stöger, E. (2004) *Materia Medica* (3rd Ed.). Seattle, WA: Eastland Press, p.132.

83 Bensky, D., Clavey, S., and Stöger, E. (2004) *Materia Medica* (3rd Ed.). Seattle, WA: Eastland Press, p.309.

84 In my practice, I mainly treat adults. Therefore, I will show pictures of the skin but not of the tongue.

85 To be omitted in infants because of its coldness and bitterness.

86 Bensky, D., Clavey, S., and Stöger, E. (2004) *Materia Medica* (3rd Ed.). Seattle, WA: Eastland Press, p.50.

87 Bensky, D., Clavey, S., and Stöger, E. (2004) *Materia Medica* (3rd Ed.). Seattle, WA: Eastland Press, p.288.

88 I recommend using as a wash or wet compress in case of existing exudation.

89 I recommend using as a wash or wet compress in case of existing exudation.

90 Use as a wash or wet compress.

91 May contain herbs that are restricted or forbidden in some countries.

92 Also known as *bái fán*.

93 Using *tǔ fú líng* topically in children is fine.

94 Source: Shutterstock.

95 Please do not confuse this formula with *Xiǎo Ér Huà Shí Tāng* (Xiao Er Hua Shi Decoction). Although they might sound similar, the ingredients are completely different: (*chǎo*) *shén qǔ*, (*chǎo*) *shān zhā*, (*chǎo*) *mài yá*, (*chǎo*) *bīng láng, é zhú, sān léng*, (*chǎo*) *qiān niú zǐ, dà huáng*.

96 People's Medical Publishing House (PMPH) Beijing, 1979.

97 Cautionary advice for the sake of completeness: Although we are working with children here, keep in mind that this herb should be used with caution during pregnancy when used in adults.

98 Source: Shutterstock.

99 Especially if the wounds don't heal for a long time.

100 Repetition: What else can bring heat into the body according to TCM? Too much coffee, alcohol, sugar, hot, spicy and oily food, but also cortisone or–very simply–mistakenly applied moxa treatment can be seen to bring heat into the body.

7

Neurodermatitis
(*Sì Wān Fēng* 四弯风)

What Is Neurodermatitis (ND)?

ND–also called "atopic eczema" or "atopic dermatitis"–is one of the most common skin diseases, not only in developed countries, but now also in low-income countries, and the numbers are increasing.[1] It is also one of the skin conditions I see most often in my practice. ND is characterized by its episodic nature, and dry skin, which can also be irritated, severely itchy, scaly, and inflamed. Together with hay fever, food allergies, and allergic asthma, ND is one of the so-called "atopic" diseases, which can occur individually or in combination over entire family generations. However, their pathogenesis is complicated. In the clinic, for example, we find that if both parents suffer from ND, the probability that their child will also be affected is very high.

Where Does the Term ND Come From?

ND gets its name from the French term "névrodermite." Two French dermatologists[2] assumed that the disease was caused by inflammation of the nerves. This was back in 1891. Today, we know that the two are not related. Rather, the causes of ND are seen as an interaction of various factors. Most important in this regard are the disturbed barrier function of the skin and the genetically determined tendency of the immune system to overreact to harmless environmental stimuli. Please also see the section on "Atopic Eczema" in Chapter 2.

The Definition of ND According to Traditional Chinese Medicine

As mentioned above, ND is a relatively "modern" name in conventional medicine. Writing this text in 2023, the name is just 132 years old. Perhaps it is of interest to know that, in conventional medicine, the field of dermatology itself is a product of internal medicine and surgery, and became an independent subject only in the second half of the 19th century. In contrast, TCM dermatology, as I have already mentioned in Chapter 3, can look back on more than 1000 years of knowledge and experience.

However, coming back to the term "ND," this name has nothing to do with TCM. The colloquial Chinese name of ND is *shén jīng xìng pí yán* 神经性皮炎 but this is not a medical term in TCM. Looking at the TCM classics, we can already find information that describes this skin disease in the *Zhǒu Hòu Bèi Jí Fāng* (Emergency Formulas to Keep Up One's Sleeve, c. 363 AD),[3] written by Gě Hóng. The earliest citation of ND was identified in this pre-Tang dynasty book by the term *jìn yín chuāng* 浸淫疮 (wet spreading sore/immersed sore). Other ancient names may include: *shè lǐng chuāng* 摄领疮 (collar sore/around the neck),[4] *niú pí xuǎn* 牛皮癣 (skin of an ox neck, dry and thick skin–now obsolete because this term is today used for psoriasis; however, this could be a reason why some sources still mention that ND belongs to the category of psoriasis), as well as *gān xuǎn* 干癣 (dry tinea) and *wán xuǎn* 顽癣 (stubborn tinea). The term *xuǎn* is synonymous with "tinea" or "dry ulcers," characterized by thickening of the skin, coupled with scaling and exudation. So much for the term "ND" in ancient books. Nowadays, the standard name for ND is *sì wān fēng* 四弯风, defined by the *Criteria for Diagnosis and Treatment of TCM Syndromes*, also known as Guidelines for Chinese Medicine Diagnosis and Treatment, published in 1994 by the State Administration of Traditional Chinese Medicine, China. As already mentioned, *sì wān fēng* means "wind of the four crooks" or "four bends of wind," after the lesions typical to ND. The term itself seems to originate from the *Wài Kē Dà Chéng* (Great Compendium of External Medicine, 1665), by Qí Kūn.

The Different Stages of ND

In clinic, we differentiate between the acute, subacute, and the chronic stages of ND. For the sake of clarity, in the illustrations below I will describe the symptoms/characteristics of acute and chronic eczema in detail for you. The subacute is an intermediate stage and occurs between acute and chronic ND. It is marked by mild to moderate inflammation that may come and go when left untreated. Whatever the stage, after almost two decades of seeing ND patients, the symptom that most bothers all patients–and most affects quality of life–is itching. ND sufferers often scratch themselves constantly, often unconsciously: seen in consultations or when asked, they confirm that they do so at night. Sleep disturbance is a related consequence among ND patients.

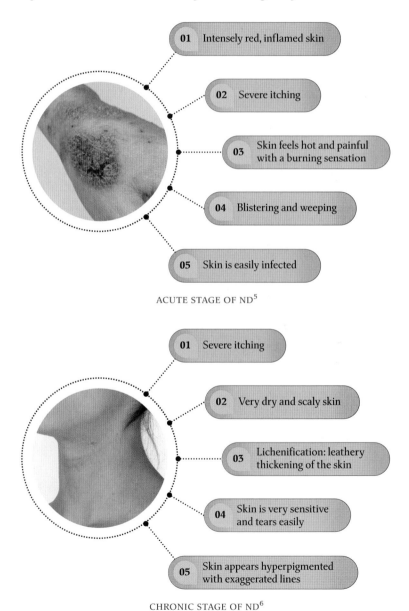

01 Intensely red, inflamed skin

02 Severe itching

03 Skin feels hot and painful with a burning sensation

04 Blistering and weeping

05 Skin is easily infected

ACUTE STAGE OF ND[5]

01 Severe itching

02 Very dry and scaly skin

03 Lichenification: leathery thickening of the skin

04 Skin is very sensitive and tears easily

05 Skin appears hyperpigmented with exaggerated lines

CHRONIC STAGE OF ND[6]

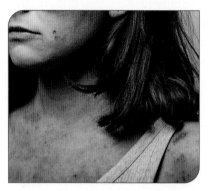
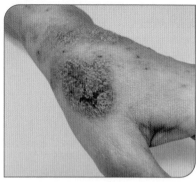

⁷   How the skin typically looks in practice at the acute stage.

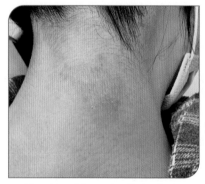
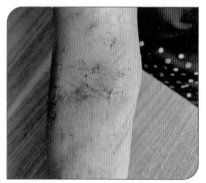

How the skin typically looks in
practice at the chronic stage.

Scratch marks due to repeated
scratching on itchy skin.

Reminder

The great advantage of TCM is its inherent flexibility. No matter the stage, we treat what we see and our treatment is based on the TCM syndrome differentiation. With insights from so many TCM doctors before us, obtained through the careful use of concepts and refined over centuries, a "modern" disease like ND can successfully be controlled and treated with TCM. In TCM, there is never a standard treatment. We have a completely different framework, and this is a main reason patients come to my practice. Most of them have an odyssey of doctors behind them.

Etiology and Pathogenesis of ND in Traditional Chinese Medicine

So far, we have briefly looked at the signs and symptoms, different terms and stages of ND. Let's now discuss in detail the etiology and pathogenesis of ND according to TCM.

Skin diseases that are rarely life-threatening are thought not to pose much of a problem for those that experience them. I think this is totally wrong. A skin disease like ND raises a whole new set of challenges because of the visibility of its symptoms—visibility that almost all of my patients experienced their whole life. Although ND is common in children, the condition is often seen later in life. I find this to be true, as I treat mainly adults in my practice. Don't forget, ND most commonly appears on the neck and face in adults. Thus, ND's visibility may attract attention in social situations, making the patient feel that they can't keep their condition private. Compared to acne spots, for example, it can be quite difficult to cover a large ND rash with make-up, if not impossible. As a consequence, patients often feel ashamed, but also stigmatized due to the presence of the rash, the scratching and the obvious scratch marks. How could they not, when images in magazines and on television always seem to be flawless and beautiful, and when the most discussed topic on social media is beauty? However, for those who have lived their whole life with the consequences of ND it is obvious that the effects are more than skin-deep. Clearly there are both social and psychological consequences of living with ND besides all the physical suffering, no matter if you are a child or an adult.

For me, ND is one of the most complex skin diseases I see in practice because it is a "multi-level" skin disease. Stop for a minute and think: you come into this world and from that minute on, a skin disease (among the other complaints within the framework of atopic diseases) will accompany you. Imagine how hard it is to be subjected to strict diets, special bedding and/or clothing, all the greasy creams and countless doctor visits from the moment you can think. You have done nothing to deserve it. Maybe it is just bad luck? Is it really? So, what does TCM think about it?

TCM considers ND to be mainly caused by:

- fetal toxicity

- congenitally weak constitution[8]

- predisposition towards attacks of external pathogenic factors, such as wind, dampness, and heat as a result of constitutional weakness

- internal pathogenic factors, such as wind or heat due to emotional disturbances

- Spleen and Stomach deficiency with dampness and heat

- unhealthy, predominantly spicy diet resulting in dampness and heat

- the recurrent and chronic course of ND can injure the yīn and blood, generating wind and dryness, resulting in skin malnourishment.

As mentioned earlier, the trends in ND are increasing significantly in industrialized countries. Therefore, it could possibly be related to other factors, such as:

- the environment, such as low humidity, low outdoor temperatures, indoor heating

- urbanization and industrialization, which may lead to an increase in aeroallergens (air pollution) and dietary allergens[9]

- excessive hygiene: associated with a reduced microbial exposure in early life[10]

- widespread use of antibiotics: they destroy the intestinal flora, thus affecting the immune system.[11]

These are the "common" theories of ND from the TCM point of view. In the following section, I would like to share my experiences in practice with you. After all my years of seeing patients with ND, the following aspect is the most important for me: fetal toxins the child receives intrauterine from the mother.

Fetal Toxins

There is a consensus that heat toxins can be transmitted from the mother to the baby when the mother consumes too much hot and spicy food during pregnancy, for example, or when she overconsumes alcohol or cigarettes. Another possible cause could be when the mother has a serious infection or a vaccination during pregnancy. No matter which of the reasons mentioned, toxic heat is passed to the child, and the toxins are then called fetal toxins.

Generally, I agree. According to my clinical observation, however, I like to expand this to "emotions" and call it "fetal toxins originating in emotions." What exactly do I mean by this? I am convinced that long-term maternal stress (according to TCM, most probably "Liver qì stagnation with excess heat" or "Heart fire") during pregnancy affects the fetus, exposing the child to an increased risk of vulnerability to skin issues, emotional problems or allergic reactions–to name just a few that play an enormously important role in this context. Consider that the child is born with a predisposition to develop ND: something must have happened during pregnancy (or even just before, or during conception) that caused it. The onset of ND usually manifests as an intensely pruritic, red rash, which is a clear sign of heat. A heat which was very likely to have been transmitted from the mother.

We know that, if one or both parents suffer from ND, the probability that the child will also be affected is very high. But what if that is not the case–when neither of them has ND? Then it gets more complicated, and that's exactly what I often experience in my practice. Let me give you a classic example: a turbulent marriage with constant, loud and aggressive arguments during pregnancy, even violence. This couple has three kids–all have ND since birth. How can this happen? The connection is very clear to me: "fetal toxins originating in emotions."

Let me share with you a passage from the classics that explains more clearly what fetal toxins mean. The information given in the text sets forth and supports my idea that fetal toxins are not exclusively, or for the most part, related to a bad diet, or the alcohol consumption of the mother during pregnancy. They are also triggered by emotions and can be transferred to the child. Let's have a look at what Chén Fù-Zhèng stated in the *Yòu Yòu Jí Chéng* (Complete Work on Children's Diseases, 1750):

> Fetal toxins are toxins due to the *Mingmén* ministerial fire of the mother and father. *Mingmén* is where the *jīng*-essence of male infants is stored, and where female infants have a link to the uterus. The Daoists call it the lower Dāntián. [As Zhōu Dūn-Yí (1017–1073) says in his *Tài Jí Tú Shuō* (Illustrated Explanation of Tai Ji)] "The essence of yīn yáng and the five elements combine miraculously and congeal." The liquid of pure essence is fused into a foetus. The fire of carnal lust can accumulate and become fetal toxin. Usually, a person is born into quietude: this is the nature of Heaven. Exposure to things creates movement: this is human desire. After the fetus is formed, its connection to the mother is particularly tight. So whenever fire from over-thinking arises in the Heart, fire from anger is generated in the Liver, fire from sadness and grief becomes pent-up in the Lungs, fire from sweets and fats accumulate in the Spleen, or fire from lust erupts from the Kidneys, then these "Five Fires of Desire" lurk in the mother's uterus, gradually knotting into fetal toxin. When fetal toxin

expresses, it could be as scabies (蟲疥), or erysipelas (流丹), or eczema (濕瘡), or boils (痈癤) or tubercular nodules (結核). It could manifest as sublingual inflammation, muteness, oral thrush or mouth ulcers.

Emotions as the Triggering Factor

ND, as one of the common dermatological diseases, can not only be caused by emotional stimuli but also triggered by emotions in later life. This can be seen if the skin shows flare-ups after arguments, stressful situations in the professional environment, or after difficult and exhausting psychotherapy sessions, when past traumas come up. I am sure all of you have seen this in your practice many times.

No matter the causative factor, ND may be triggered by many things, such as irritants, aeroallergens, food, microbial organisms, sex hormones, stress, sweating, and climatological factors[12] in the course of the disease. I would like to make it clear once again that emotions are not only a causative factor in the form of fetal toxins, but also a triggering or exacerbating one. For me, it is one of the most important factors; the one I see most often in practice, often in connection with an unhealthy lifestyle.

CLINICAL HINT: When working with ND patients, please don't forget to mention that setbacks caused by psychotherapy sessions are always possible. Most of them are, or have been, in psychotherapy, or are currently looking for a psychologist. Many of them realize that they themselves are part of the therapy and that old processes have to be worked through carefully. A TCM practitioner also works with and/or on emotions, but in a different way.

Other Psychological Aspects of ND Patients to Keep in Mind

This title reflects that working with ND patients can often be complex. They have a lifelong skin disease and, as already mentioned, have had an odyssey of doctors and cortisone prescriptions. Cortisone relieves ND only for a short moment. It never makes it go away because the root cause is not treated. More and more patients understand this and are looking for alternatives.

One could assume that a patient who receives help is incredibly happy about the healing process. Yes, that's usually the case—pure joy to finally put on short-sleeve T-shirts again, to go outside and be unafraid. That's what everyone would think first, right? In most cases it is like that, but not always. Let me tell you about a case from practice to illustrate another side of the story:

> A young woman in her early 30s with ND came to see me. The effects of a stressful job can often manifest as aggression and/or frustration, and this woman clearly wasn't happy with her life. I gave her a tailored prescription and "warned" her about the taste of the herbs as I always do. However, she drank the herbs I prescribed her only irregularly. Moreover, she outrightly rejected the external herbal application during her first and second visit, saying she had been trying external applications—such as cortisone and other greasy creams, moistening lotions etc.—for as long as she could remember. She made it very clear to me that she did not want to do this again. It was interesting that she was being unkind to a therapist who was happy to be there for her, to help her. Shortly thereafter, she discontinued her therapy. I only saw her twice.

One might think that a patient is happy to seek an alternative, and hope for relief. (Note, they always decide for themselves to come and seek treatment, either through their own research or, more often, via word of mouth.) Now, my question is: the woman obviously wasn't feeling comfortable in her skin but rejected a potentially effective therapy without giving it a chance. Why was this the case? I am asking this question because I want you to bear the following aspects in mind: a person behaves differently depending on the dynamics of the context in which they move, e.g. family setting. A human being is a self-contained system (body/mind/soul), which is always busy with the process of self-preservation. This means that behavior, no matter how constructive or destructive, has a functionality to maintain the "system" itself. In the case of the young woman, the patient suffers from ND—equally, the ND also has its functionality. Why the patient's system needs her skin disease should first be clarified on a psychological level. What is good about ND for her? The basic assumption is that her ND has a strong function, in the sense of the system being maintained. So, the primary solution for this patient does not seem to be to relieve the ND. A paradox, isn't it? Here are now two realities that collide—the patient's and the therapist's, and both equally have their justification. Think about it when something like this happens to you, and don't take it personally!

Hypotheses for Therapy Discontinuation[13, 14]

Here are a few example cases in which we might see therapy discontinued, along with potential reasons related to the functionality of a skin disease for the patient.

Hypothesis	Cause
The pace of treatment is too fast.	If there is no inner confidence in one's own resources, breaking old patterns could lead to the system being destabilized.
ND creates boundaries.	If a patient can't separate themselves internally, then ND does it for them. ND allows them to withdraw, which they otherwise cannot do.
The patient is dealing with strong emotions, like anger. These result primarily in a drive, they mobilize–and can lead to a person being increasingly goal-oriented and driven in the workplace.	The caring side comes up short, and if this is not allowed to be shown in the job or in the family, the (destructive, but functional) withdrawal–through which care can be experienced–succeeds through ND.
The patient's professional or social environment responds to ND.	Because they are dealing with ND, the person receives recognition, care, and closeness.
The patient is out of touch with their feelings. Their awareness of their emotions is poor, and they have little ability to categorize them.	ND creates a physical stimulus (itching, throbbing, etc.) and the person reacts with a counter-stimulus (scratching, pinching, etc.). This counter-stimulus can lead to feeling oneself. Feeling negative emotions is better than feeling none.
The patient doesn't come on their own motivation, but is carrying out an other's wishes by visiting the clinic.	Family or friend has recommended TCM, for example, so the patient appears in practice to avoid a conflict with the person placing the order.

I think it is very important for us to also address these aspects in our TCM therapy. Often they are neglected in training and education, even though it can make such a big difference in our interaction with patients. This is the reason why I have dedicated myself to this topic in such detail here.

Often patients come on an impulse, when the suffering is so great that the self-protecting mechanisms no longer work. It can, however, change so quickly that the previously arranged appointment might be cancelled or the aforementioned hypothesis might come into play again. We as TCM practitioners should meet the patient where they are and understand that the practitioner's solution might be far from being the solution for the patient. The symptoms we are trying to capture are so complex, especially with ND, that the practitioner should have confidence that the solution lies within the patient, and can be found at the right time, if they are willing to look for it. TCM supports this process with all the methods we have. What I mean to say is that if the patient is not ready for change, then our therapy cannot work as effectively as we want. We TCM therapists are not psychologists. However, it is part of the competence of a TCM doctor to consider all aspects.

The next chapter will deal in more detail with our core competence, namely TCM syndrome differentiation.

Endnotes

1   Urban, K., Chu, S., Giesey, R.L., Mehrmal, S., Uppal, P., Nedley, N., and Delost G.R. (2021) "The global, regional, and national burden of atopic dermatitis in 195 countries and territories: An ecological study from the Global Burden of Disease Study 2017." *Journal of The American Academy of Dermatology (JAAD International)* 2, 12–18.

2   Louis Anne Jean Brocq and Leonard Marie Lucien Jacquet.

3   Also known as the *Handbook of Prescriptions for Emergencies.*

4   Characterized by severely painful or itchy, symmetrical scaly plaques. The itch-scratch cycle causes the skin to become thick and leathery, typically on the neck.

5   Source: Sabine Schmitz.

6   Source: Sabine Schmitz.

7   Source: Shutterstock.

8   When a child has been having recurrent problems from birth because of a constitutional weakness.

9   Shams, K., Grindlay, D.J.C., and Williams, H.C. (2011) "What's new in atopic eczema? An analysis of systematic reviews published in 2009-2010." *Clinical and Experimental Dermatology* 36, 6, 573–578.

10 Gandini, S., Stanganelli, I., Palli, D., De Giorgi, V., Masala, G., and Caini, S. (2016) "Atopic dermatitis, naevi count and skin cancer risk: A meta-analysis." *Journal of Dermatological Science* 84, 2, 137–143.

11 Oszukowska, M., Michalak, I., Gutfreund, K., Bienias, W., et al. (2015) "Role of primary and secondary prevention in atopic dermatitis." *Advances in Dermatology and Allergology/Postępy Dermatologii i Alergologii* 32, 6, 409–420.

12 Morren, M.A., Przybilla, B., Bamelis, M., Heykants, B., Reynaers, A., and Degreef, H. (1994) "Atopic dermatitis: Triggering factors." *Journal of the American Academy of Dermatology* 31, 3 Pt 1, 467–473.

13 Can be applied to almost all chronic and complex skin diseases. Psoriasis is a very good example besides ND.

14 There are certainly many more aspects. The list does not claim to be complete.

≋ 8 ≋

Syndrome Differentiation and Treatment of Neurodermatitis According to Traditional Chinese Medicine

W E ALL KNOW that the treatment of ND in Western medicine is often confined to prescribing cortisone. That's the standard not just for ND, but for all types of eczema. In contrast, TCM offers personalized and "to the point" medicine. Results are most effective when an individual diagnosis is given to each patient, with the aim of resolving the root cause and not just masking the symptoms. TCM likes to work with analogies; thus, only when the roots of the tree are treated for a disease will the branches and leaves come back, and then the entire tree can grow and thrive.

In this part of the book, I will discuss the five most common TCM syndromes of ND I see in my practice. The first four syndromes relate more to adults, and I see the first three patterns most often in my practice. The last one relates mostly to children and infants. At this point, I would like to mention again that I mainly treat adults in my practice. However, if you treat more children in your clinic and they present with the first patterns I discuss, you must work more mildly and reduce the dosages. In this case, consider whether you really should use all the–sometimes very cold and bitter–herbs, as they can be too harsh for a child's digestive system. Preparations may have to be considered to reduce the coldness and bitterness of these herbs.

Please note that I have structured this part of the book a little differently to the first part (on eczema). The difference here, because I believe it makes more sense, is that external applications will be covered at the end of the ND part. I will list the recommendations for external treatment and examples for tailored herbal washes or wet compresses based on the appearance of the skin. Instead of being listed by TCM syndrome, they can be found at the end of the section on TCM syndrome differentiation. At the very end of this part of the book, I also discuss practical and helpful tips for dealing with ND patients, such as preventing triggering factors, how to deal with scratching, stress, and emotions, and explain differences in treating children and adults. But let's start now with TCM syndrome differentiation and the TCM syndrome that is seen very often in practice today–perhaps the most common one.

Heat Stagnation in the Liver Meridian (*Gān Jīng Yù Rè Zhèng* 肝经郁热证)

One of the most commonly seen patterns nowadays is Liver qì stagnation (*gān qì yù jié* 肝气郁结) with excess heat. My clinical experience shows that stress and emotional factors, like frustration and anger, are often the main causative factors for the onset or exacerbation of ND. People's living habits and personal environment play an important role in this pattern, and according to my clinical experience, addressing the Liver (*gān* 肝) is crucial when treating cases of ND with a clear emotional cause. Interestingly, TCM books discussing ND very often miss this very common syndrome of modern times, which is Liver qì stagnation with excess heat. However, I have frequently observed in clinic that ND markedly worsens after an upset, anger/rage, or stressful situations, be it in a professional or personal environment. Remember that ND is closely linked to early childhood experiences, so family factors definitely play an important role. It's really not uncommon for me to hear that there are ND flare-ups after family gatherings. Furthermore, patients often consume alcohol or cigarettes to cope with stressful situations. Alcohol, cigarettes, and also spicy food have been found to be negative factors, which can trigger or worsen heat in the Liver and thus exacerbate skin conditions, for example, ND.

Let me explain the patho-mechanism behind this pattern. The Liver is well-known for its desire to keep qì flowing smoothly within the body. So, what can make the Liver qì stagnate? Liver qì stagnation can easily arise from a number of causes, most commonly emotional problems or excessive emotions. This means that a person is either experiencing his or her emotions too intensely, showing up as anger for example; or to the contrary, repressing their emotions, seen a lot in frustration. Emotional imbalances can strongly impede the function of the Liver in regulating the smooth flow of qì. When not flowing properly, the Liver qì is overstimulated and accumulates, leading to stagnation. Don't forget: whenever a person's qì is not free, the mind is also not free. The qì is stuck and can't move forward and this will create even more anger or frustration. When blocked Liver qì cannot move freely and stagnates for a long time within the body, it will produce heat, and if this continues for too long, it gradually turns to fire. It may even cause blood stagnation, because fire tends to consume yīn and/or blood at a later stage. And if there is little blood it cannot flow well, thus it stagnates. Please see also the analogy I have described in Chapter 5, in the Liver section under the "Zàng Fǔ" heading. When looking at the skin, qì stagnation transformed into heat will manifest as fresh red, often warm or burning ND rashes with itching sensation.

The following case from my practice illustrates the emotional connection very clearly:

> A young man came to my practice without a specific reason, because a family member sent him to me. Interestingly, he didn't have much to report, but when I felt his pulse it was pretty tense. I was intrigued, because from the outside he appeared calm, so I asked him about his emotions. I always ask about the patient's stress levels or how stressed they feel, and how they assess their own emotions. This is completely independent of what I think and feel. I want to hear the patient's story. And so, it turned out that the young man told me that in his childhood he had severe ND with allergies and asthma. It was very stressful for him, he said. The longer he talked, the more he told me about his life and the problems he had to overcome. In his early 20s, he moved out of home to a completely different city, very far away from home. He told me that the very next day his ND was gone! And somehow, he felt liberated to be away from home and able to start living his own life. He felt free! Today, he reports, he only has minor ND issues now and then, and only when he has had contact with his family. Then ND flares up only briefly, mostly after arguments because his parents don't agree with his way of life. He always feels constraint and frustration afterwards. Doesn't this clearly show us how emotional triggers work and how the skin reacts to them? Just listen to your patients and you will find out a lot! You will also notice the more patients you see, the more stories and patterns repeat.

Characteristics

This pattern primarily appears on the neck and face, the forehead in particular. The neck represents the Liver area, please keep this in mind. If you see ND lesions on the neck you should definitely pay close attention to whether this patient is chronically angry and frustrated. Please keep also seasonal changes in mind, as the skin often gets worse in Spring. This is because according to TCM, Spring is the season of wood and of the Liver. The energy of the Liver desires growth and expression in various ways, so in Spring, the wood energy is striving for "growth" and "expansion." If this energy is not able to fulfil the forward movement and expansion it desires, the Liver will be impacted and the Liver qì will stagnate.

The ND usually appears bright red, often accompanied by a warm sensation, and it feels burning, dry, tight, and itchy. Other typical signs can be irritability, upsets, mood swings, a loud voice, insomnia or restless sleep with many dreams, a bitter taste in the mouth and dry throat, dry stool, or dark yellow urine. Women may present with menstrual irregularities, dysmenorrhea or breast distension. Female patients often report that their skin worsens before or during their period.

The tongue is red (especially on the edges, which reflect the Liver), indicating internal heat. The tongue coating is thin and yellow. The pulse is wiry, rapid and forceful, which indicates heat excess in the Liver channel.

Treatment Principle

Disperse stagnated Liver qì and drain excess heat from the Liver channel (*shū gān jiě yù, qīng gān jīng huǒ rè* 疏肝解郁，清肝经火热).

Representative Formula

Lóng Dǎn Xiè Gān Tāng (Gentian Decoction to Drain the Liver).

Ingredients

lóng dǎn cǎo	Gentianiae, Radix	6–9 g
huáng qín	Scutellariae, Radix	9–12 g
zhī zǐ	Gardeniae, Fructus	9–15 g
chái hú	Bupleuri, Radix	6–9 g

mù tōng	Akebiae, Caulis	6–9 g
chē qián zǐ	Plantaginis, Semen	9–12 g
zé xiè	Alismatis, Rhizoma	9–12 g
shēng dì huáng	Rehmanniae Glutinosae, Radix	9–15 g
dāng guī	Angelicae Sinensis, Radix	9 g
gān cǎo	Glycyrrhizae Uralensis, Radix	3–6 g

First Reference
The first reference of the formula can be found in *Yī Fāng Jí Jiě* (Medical Formulas Collected and Analyzed, 1682, Qīng Dynasty), written by Wāng Áng.

Formula Analysis
With ND, I recommend using *lóng dǎn cǎo* in relatively large dosages of 6–9 g for about two to three weeks. Then, gradually reduce the dose and modify the original prescription. I also tend to use *zhī zǐ* and *shēng dì huáng* in large dosages of up to 15 g if needed. For a detailed analysis of this formula, please see "Dampness-Heat" pattern in Chapter 6.

Cautions
Because of their bitter and cold nature, I tend to use *lóng dǎn cǎo, huáng qín* and *zhī zǐ* as dry-fried (*chǎo*) most of the time. This preparation reduces their cold properties and makes them more tolerable for the digestive system, reducing their potential to harm the Spleen and Stomach. And again, *mù tōng* is no longer used.

Modifications
One may add *huáng lián* to enhance the clearing action of the formula if a stronger action is needed. Only 3 g is required. As mentioned above, as soon as the heat (fire) is reduced, the dosage of *lóng dǎn cǎo* can be reduced to 3 g, for example, to protect the digestive system. If the skin appears fresh red, this indicates internal fire, add *mǔ dān pí* 9–12 g, especially at the beginning of the treatment. Unprocessed *mǔ dān pí* effectively clears blood heat, but it can easily harm the stomach. Particularly in cases of long-term use of this herb, (*chǎo*) *mǔ dān pí* (dry-fried) is advisable, because the cold property has been reduced making it more tolerable for the digestive system, but the blood

heat-clearing effect is still ensured. In addition, the combination of *mǔ dān pí* and *zhī zǐ* is perfect for treating fire due to Liver qì stagnation. *Mǔ dān pí* treats qì at the blood level. Its acrid nature is dispersing, and its coolness enables it to drain heat at the blood level. In contrast, *zhī zǐ* treats blood at the qì level. It clears fire from constraint at the qì level and it also has a blood-cooling effect. Thus, *mǔ dān pí* and *zhī zǐ*, used in combination, can resolve qì level constraint leading to heat as well as heat in the blood[1] as in the formula *Dān Zhī Xiāo Yáo Sǎn* (Moutan and Gardenia Rambling Powder).

To reduce itching and calm the Liver, add *bái jí lí* 9–15 g. For chronic itching, "wind herbs" such as *fáng fēng* and *jīng jiè* are often not as effective as *bái jí lí*. For insomnia, sleep disrupted by disturbing dreams, and shallow sleep, add *zhēn zhū mǔ* up to 30 g (decocted first) and *gōu téng* 9–15 g to sedate yáng and drain Liver heat. For constipation, add *dà huáng* 6–9 g. For menstrual pain with dark blood and blood clots, add *yì mǔ cǎo* 9–12 g. It regulates menstruation by invigorating blood and dispelling blood stasis. *Yì mǔ cǎo* goes to the *chòng* and *rèn mài*[2] as well as the Liver channel, and it is not only cool in temperature but also relieves toxicity. There are two other herbs which are very useful in this pattern: *mài mén dōng* 9–12 g to moisten the skin, clear heat, nourish yīn, and promote fluid production; and *jú huā* 9 g to clear and calm the Liver as well as subduing rising heat. Keep in mind that flowers should be considered for the treatment of ND lesions on the face. They are light in weight and thus can rise to the head while regulating qì and relaxing emotions. It also helps that patients love flowers and they make the formula look nicer, a useful effect for all patients, not just those "sensitive" to drinking bitter decoctions. All emotional aspects are very important in treating patients with ND.

If there is solely "heat stagnation in the Liver meridian," there is rarely damp exudation or pus involved. However, if yellowish exudation is present *Lóng Dǎn Xiè Gān Tāng* still works perfectly but can be slightly changed to boost the damp-heat clearing action. For example, add *dàn zhú yè* 6–9 g in order to support the damp draining and heat-clearing actions of *zé xiè*. If yellowish pus and exudation are predominant, add *tǔ fú líng* at a dose of 15–30 g. Damp exudate, crusts and erosions are an ideal breeding ground for infections with bacteria. Whenever the skin has become infected with bacteria, adding *yú xīng cǎo* 15 g, or the combination of *pú gōng yīng* 15 g, *zǐ huā dì dīng* 9–12 g, and *jīn yín huā* 12–15 g will clear heat and relieve toxicity in order to treat the infected skin.

Finally, another option for those who prefer a milder approach in a formula: *Dān Zhī Xiāo Yáo Sǎn,* also known as *Jiā Wèi Xiāo Yáo Sǎn,* is another option one may use in the treatment of heat stagnating in the Liver meridian.

The ingredients of *Dān Zhī Xiāo Yáo Sǎn* are:

chái hú	Bupleuri, Radix	9 g
dāng guī	Angelicae Sinensis, Radix	9 g
bái sháo	Paeonia Albiflora, Radix	9 g
bái zhú	Atractylodis Macrocephalae, Rhizoma	9 g
fú líng	Poriae Cocos, Sclerotium	9 g
zhì gān cǎo	Glycyrrhizae Preparata, Radix	4.5 g
mǔ dān pí	Moutan, Cortex	9–12 g
zhī zǐ	Gardeniae, Fructus	9–12 g
+/- bò hé	Menthae, Herba	3 g
+/- shēng jiāng	Zingiberis Recens, Rhizoma	3 g

First reference of *Dān Zhī Xiāo Yáo Sǎn: Nèi Kē Zhāi Yào* (Summary of Internal Medicine, 1529), written by Xuē Jǐ. The formula is basically *Xiāo Yáo Sǎn* (Rambling Powder), with the addition of *mǔ dān pí* and *zhī zǐ.* It is a traditional formula for heat arising from stagnated Liver qì. The formula is classically used to soothe the Liver, relieve qì stagnation, nourish blood, invigorate the Spleen and clear heat. Compared to *Lóng Dǎn Xiè Gān Tāng* it is relatively mild in action but with the right modification it can be quite suitable and effective, too.

In this formula, *chái hú* is a guiding herb for the Liver channel; it soothes and regulates the stagnated Liver qì. *Bái sháo* nourishes the blood and astringes the yīn. Combined with *dāng guī,* this yīn and blood nourishing action is more effective. *Dāng guī* additionally possesses the ability to regulate blood circulation. *Bái zhú, fú líng,* and *zhì gān cǎo* all strengthen the Spleen and replenish qì in order to generate blood as well as support the Spleen's transportive and transformative function. *Zhì gān cǎo* also harmonizes the formula by moderating the properties of the other herbs. A small amount of *bò hé* soothes stagnant Liver qì and clears heat stagnating in the Liver channel. *Shēng jiāng* soothes stagnant qì due to its pungent flavour and harmonizes the middle *jiāo.* Finally, *mǔ dān pí* and *zhī zǐ* used in combination can resolve qì level constraint leading to heat as well as heat in the blood.[3] In addition, if both herbs are used together, they are particularly useful if the patient has lesions on the face as a result of ascending heat, which follows the pathway of the Liver channel. In cases of long-term use, dry-fried (*chǎo*) *mǔ dān pí* and (*chǎo*) *zhī zǐ* is advisable, because the cold nature has been reduced, but the heat-clearing effect is still ensured. This makes it more suitable for the digestive system. If you think you need to enhance the heat clearing effect within this formula, add *huáng qín* 9 g, +/- *huáng lián* 3 g. Even *lóng dǎn cǎo* in small amounts of not more than 3 g can be used. But to be precise, if you modify *Dān Zhī Xiāo Yáo Sǎn* in this way you might directly consider using *Lóng Dǎn Xiè Gān Tāng* right from the start. For other modifications, please see above.

Example Pictures of the Tongue

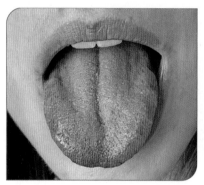 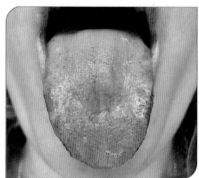

The tongue is red, especially at the borders, which correspond to the Liver in Chinese medicine. The tongue coating is thin and yellowish.

A red tongue with red spots, especially at the borders and a yellow coating.

Example Pictures of the Skin

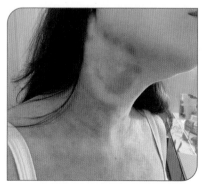 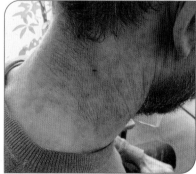

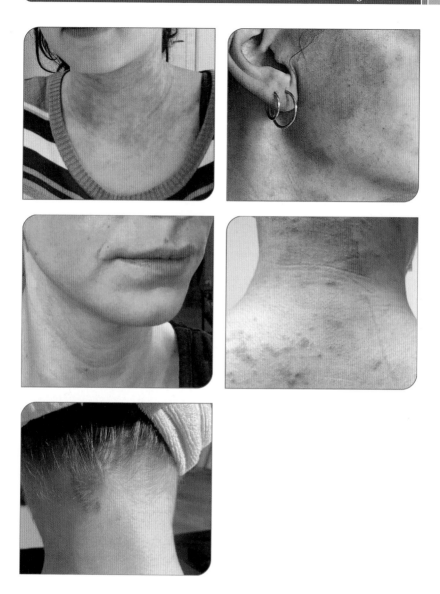

Wind-Heat (*Fēng Rè* 风热)

In this pattern, you may find that ND flare-ups occur more frequently or get worse in the spring months. Why does this happen? In Spring, the grasses and trees begin to sprout tender buds as the yáng energy in the soil rises and nature begins to flourish. Thus, allergies are also worse in Spring because pollens are the biggest trigger of allergies. However, Spring is also a season in which yáng easily becomes excessive, the climate changes frequently and also windy weather is more common during the Spring months. Wind is closely connected to the wood element, which represents the season Spring in TCM. Wind is characterized by itching and, thus, many skin diseases where itching is the predominant sign are noticeably increased or exacerbated in Spring. Moreover, it is not uncommon that ND patients present from birth with a history of allergic asthma for example, which suggests an underlying weakness of the Lung. According to TCM theory, the Lung controls the skin and pores. When the Lung is deficient, the pores do not close correctly and thus, this subsequent deficiency may allow wind-heat to enter the body manifesting in skin conditions such as ND but also hay fever or allergic asthma, as mentioned before. In this case, Lung deficiency is the "root" of the disease, whilst wind-heat rash may be considered its manifestation or "branch." Remember, in skin diseases we mainly treat the "branch" first. After the symptoms of the skin get markedly better, we can start to treat the "root." So how does the skin present in ND when wind-heat has entered the body?

Characteristics

Wind-heat ND primarily occurs on the neck and face but can also spread all over the body. It presents as bright red, dry and scaly patches which feel warm and are extremely itchy. The redness of the skin rash signifies heat, whilst the dry and scaly skin lesions point to the involvement of wind. Wind-heat is characterized by rapid onset and as mentioned above, it often occurs in spring in combination with hay fever and allergic asthma. Wind-heat may ascend to the face resulting in flushing of the face and a feeling of warmth. These patients report that cooling usually brings relief. All this may be accompanied by an aversion to heat, thirst, dark yellow urination, and dry stool.

The tongue has a red tip with a thin white or slightly yellow coating. The pulse is floating and rapid.

Treatment Principle

Dispel wind and release the exterior, clear heat and relieve itching (*shū fēng jiě biǎo, qīng rè zhǐ yǎng* 疏风解表, 清热止痒).

Representative Formula

Modified *Xiāo Fēng Sǎn* (Eliminate Wind Powder).

Ingredients

jīng jiè	Schizonepetae, Herba	10 g
fáng fēng	Saposhnikoviae, Radix	10 g
niú bàng zǐ	Arctii Lappae, Fructus	10 g
+/- *chán tuì*	Cicadae, Periostracum	6 g
jīn yín huā	Lonicerae Japonicae, Flos	10 g
lián qiáo	Forsythiae, Fructus	10 g
huáng qín	Scutellariae, Radix	10 g
shēng dì huáng	Rehmanniae Glutinosae, Radix	10–12 g
dāng guī	Angelicae Sinensis, Radix	10 g
+/- *shí gāo*[4]	Gypsum Fibrosum	15 g
zhī mǔ	Anemarrhenae, Rhizoma	6 g
kǔ shēn	Sophorae Flavescentis, Radix	10 g
tōng cǎo[5]	Tetrapanacis, Medulla	6 g
gān cǎo	Glycyrrhizae Uralensis, Radix	6 g

First Reference

This formula first appeared in the *Wài Kē Zhèng Zōng* (Orthodox Lineage of External Medicine, 1617) by Chén Shí-Gōng.

Formula Analysis

Please see the detailed analysis of this formula and description of herb actions in Chapter 6. The only difference is that I have replaced *cāng zhú* with *huáng qín* to boost the heat clearing action of the formula. I tend to use it dry-fried (*chǎo*) to reduce its cold properties and make it more tolerable for the digestive system.

> Please also review my clinical tip regarding foods to avoid while taking *Xiāo Fēng Sǎn* on page 121.

Modifications

For widespread red skin rash all over the body with extreme pruritus, add *mǔ dān pí* 10 g and *chì sháo* 10 g. These herbs cool the blood and clear heat. With regards to *mǔ dān pí* and long-term use, *(chǎo) mǔ dān pí* (dry-fried) is advisable, because the cold property has been reduced, making it more tolerable for the digestive system, while the blood heat-clearing effect is still ensured. For unbearable itching, add *bái xiān pí* with a dosage of at least 10 g. *Bái xiān pí* is very effective in stopping itching but it should be used with caution if given for longer periods of time. Please see the cautionary advice on pages 101 and 162. If the skin lesions are concentrated on the face, add *jú huā* 10 g. If the patient is constipated, add *huǒ má rén* 10 g. It nourishes and moistens the Intestines and can therefore unblock dry constipation. And finally, a small amount of *bò hé* (3 g) can be added to disperse wind-heat and vent rashes. It also helps when the patient has red eyes and headaches due to hay fever in spring.

Example Pictures of the Tongue

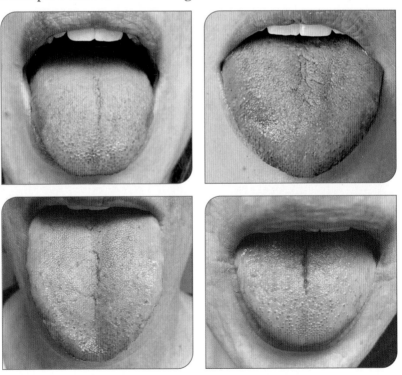

Different tongues with a thin yellow or white coating,
showing a red tip with or without red spots.

Example Pictures of the Skin

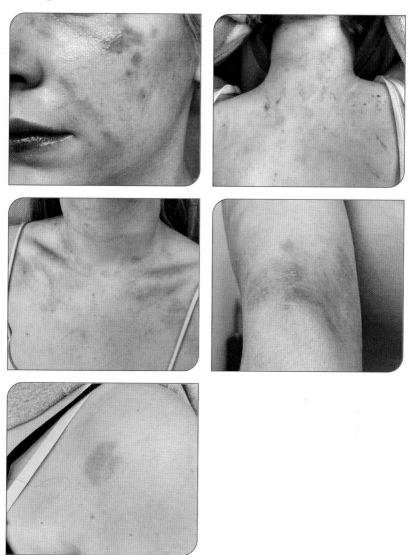

Blood Deficiency and Wind Dryness
(*Xuè Xū Fēng Zào* 血虚风燥)

I have described the pattern "Blood Deficiency and Wind Dryness" in detail already in Chapter 6. The skin appearance and accompanying symptoms are very similar, therefore we can basically work with the same formulas.

However, I would like to mention an alternative prescription for this pattern at this point and describe it in detail to demonstrate again how flexible TCM is.

Characteristics

ND has been present for a very long time at this stage, yīn and blood have been exhausted and the skin cannot be properly nourished, and thus becomes dry, thick, rough, and scaly. The skin looks greyish-white. The appearance of the skin can be compared with wood: deeply furrowed and dry like a dry bark of a tree. Furthermore, when blood is deficient then wind is generated, which results in pruritus (itching) and scaling. Thus, itching is a predominant sign in this pattern. Later on, qì and blood stagnate and this changes the skin lesions into a greyish or purplish color. In this pattern, the color of the lesions can range from pale red to grey or dark purplish, depending on whether the deficient blood has already become stagnant. In my opinion, the appearance of the color of the skin makes it relatively easy to choose the right herbs and/or formula. How to adjust the patient's prescription will be explained immediately below with the modifications.

Accompanying symptoms may include palpitations, insomnia, dizziness, forgetfulness, thirst, constipation, dry hair, dry nails and so on; and a pale and dull complexion. In women, we might observe a delayed cycle, irregular menstruation with scanty blood, or amenorrhoea.

The tongue is pale with a thin whitish coating. Please note that the tongue can also be swollen. This is because many patients who have blood deficiency also have a degree of dampness or phlegm which tends to make the tongue swollen. The pulse is deep and thready (thin), and if blood stagnation is present, the pulse can be also rough.

ONE MORE PRACTICAL HINT: In some cases, stasis spots on/underneath the tongue or dark bluish veins underneath the tongue can be found, which is a clear sign that blood stasis is present. Sometimes, the color is not very strong, so a precise observation in good daylight is essential, in order that these signs are not overlooked. Never forget to also check the veins underneath the tongue. For examples, please see immediately below.

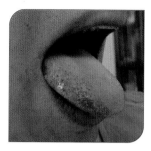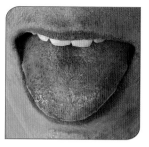

Examples of two pale and purple tongues, showing stasis spots.

Treatment Principle

Nourish blood and yīn, moisten the skin, dispel wind, and relieve itching (*zī yīn yǎng xuè, rùn fū, qū fēng zhǐ yǎng* 滋阴养血，润肤，祛风止痒).

Representative Formula

In this pattern, we have a range of effective formulas. I will mention my three favourites for treating this pattern:

- *Dāng Guī Yǐn Zǐ* (Chinese Angelica Drink)

- *Sì Wù Xiāo Fēng Yǐn* (Eliminate Wind Drink with the Four Substances)

- *Yǎng Xuè Dìng Fēng Tāng* (Nourishing Blood and Subduing Wind Decoction).

Ingredients
Dāng Guī Yǐn Zǐ

dāng guī	Angelicae Sinensis, Radix	9–15 g
bái sháo	Paeonia Albiflora, Radix	9–12 g
chuān xiōng	Chuanxiong, Rhizoma	9 g
bái jí lí	Tribuli Terristris, Fructus	9–12 g
fáng fēng	Saposhnikoviae, Radix	9 g
shēng dì huáng[6]	Rehmanniae Glutinosae, Radix	9–12 g
hé shǒu wū	Polygoni Multiflori, Radix	9 g
jīng jiè	Schizonepetae, Herba	9 g
huáng qí	Astragali, Radix	9 g
zhì gān cǎo	Glycyrrhizae Preparata, Radix	3–6 g

Please see Chapter 6 for detailed explanations and analysis of this formula.

Sì Wù Xiāo Fēng Yǐn

shēng dì huáng	Rehmanniae Glutinosae, Radix	9–12 g
dāng guī	Angelicae Sinensis, Radix	9–12 g
jīng jiè	Schizonepetae, Herba	3–6 g
fáng fēng	Saposhnikoviae, Radix	3–6 g
chì sháo	Paeoniae Rubrae, Radix	3–6 g
chuān xiōng	Chuanxiong, Rhizoma	3–6 g
bái xiān pí	Dictamni Radicis, Cortex	3–6 g
chán tuì	Cicadae, Periostracum	3 g
bò hé	Menthae, Herba	3 g
dú huó	Angelicae Pubescentis, Radix	3 g
chái hú	Bupleuri, Radix	3 g
dà zǎo	Jujubae, Fructus	2–3 pieces

Please see Chapter 6 for detailed explanations and analysis of this formula.

Yǎng Xuè Dìng Fēng Tāng

shēng dì huáng	Rehmanniae Glutinosae, Radix	12 g
dāng guī	Angelicae Sinensis, Radix	12 g
chì sháo	Paeoniae Rubrae, Radix	10–12 g
chuān xiōng	Chuanxiong, Rhizoma	8 g
tiān mén dōng	Asparagi, Radix	10 g
mài mén dōng	Ophiopogonis Japonici, Tuber	10 g
jiāng cán	Bombyx Batryticatus	15 g
hé shǒu wū	Polygoni Multiflori, Radix	8 g
mǔ dān pí	Moutan, Cortex	8 g

First Reference

This formula firstly appeared in the *Wài Kē Zhèng Zhì Quán Shū* (Complete Book of Patterns and Treatments in External Medicine, 1831), written by Xǔ Kè-Chāng.

Formula Analysis

Yǎng Xuè Dìng Fēng Tāng addresses long-term malnourishment of the skin causing symptoms such as dry skin, obvious scaling, itching, and severe itching. The first four herbs are basically *Sì Wù Tāng,* with *chì sháo* being used instead of *bái sháo.* Note that in many skin formulas *chì sháo* is the more suitable herb because of its blood invigorating and blood cooling effect. Please see Chapter 6 for detailed explanations and analysis of this formula. *Tiān mén dōng* and *mài mén dōng* together clear heat, nourish the yīn, and generate the fluids. *Jiāng cán* eliminates wind and stops itching. I have often seen this substance used in China to stop itching of skin lesions, however I refrain from using it as it is an animal substance. Those who feel uncomfortable using animal products could easily substitute *bái jí lí* (10–12 g). *Hé shǒu wū* nourishes blood to moisten dryness. Remember, sufficient nutrient blood is needed in order to effectively moisten the skin. *Hé shǒu wū* can also moisten the Intestines and is therefore quite helpful if the patient is constipated. *Mǔ dān pí* clears heat and cools the blood. Always keep in mind that when yīn and blood are exhausted, it inevitably leads to blood stasis. Thus, blood cooling and heat clearing as well as blood moving and transforming stasis is recommended in this formula to make it complete.

Modifications

For serious itching, as mentioned above, add *bái jí lí* 10–12 g. If the sleep is disturbed due to itching, herbs that calm the spirit are often effective, such as *yè jiāo téng* 30 g. Add this herb whenever sleep is problematic and the itching is due to dryness and blood deficiency. The herb tonifies and invigorates blood and, thus, *yè jiāo téng* is also effective when the lesions turn dark in color, indicating that blood stagnation is present. For improving sleep, you might also consider increasing the dosage of *hé shǒu wū* up to 12–15 g. In clinic, the name *hé shǒu wū* usually refers to the prepared drug *(zhì) hé shǒu wū.* Please keep in mind that if used for too long with high dosages, it can lead to loose stools and dampness within the body. To soften hard skin by tonifying and moving blood, add *dān shēn* 12 g and *é zhú* 6 g. Hard skin usually appears greyish or dark purplish in color. Thus, both herbs are perfect to treat blood stagnation as well. Because it is a chronic stage of the condition, it is recommended to also tonify the blood and Kidneys. *Nǚ zhēn zǐ* 10–12 g can be added as it tonifies Kidney and Liver yīn and clears heat from deficiency. If you prefer to direct the formula to the wrists and hands, add *sāng zhī* 3–5 g. TCM works in analogies. *Sāng zhī* are the branches of the mulberry tree (Morus alba). Arms and legs can also be seen as branches of the body. Thus, this herb is the guiding herb[7] for the upper limbs. For hay fever, think about adding *Cāng Ěr Zǐ Sǎn* (Xanthium Powder, prepared as decoction), consisting of *cāng ěr zǐ* 10 g, *xīn yí huā* 10 g, *bái zhǐ* 10 g and +/- *bò hé* 3–5 g. *Cāng Ěr Zǐ Sǎn* is a simple but effective choice to disperse wind and unblock nasal congestion. As ND belongs to the atopic conditions, hay fever is often present, especially in Spring.

MORE FOOD FOR THOUGHT: Because TCM is so flexible and the possibilities are so numerous, I would like to end by sharing one more formula, a very simple combination, in this section: *Sì Wù Tāng + Zēng Yè Tāng* (Increase the Fluids Decoction). This combination contains: *shú dì huáng* 12 g, *chì sháo* 9 g, *dāng guī* 12–15 g, *chuān xiōng* 6–9 g, *xuán shēn* 9 g, *mài mén dōng* 9 g, *shēng dì huáng* 12 g. As you can see, this formula has many similar herbs as already mentioned above, and is often overlooked due to its simplicity. There is not just one way in TCM. Be flexible!

Example Pictures of the Tongue

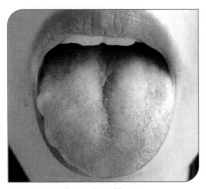

A pale and puffy tongue with tooth-marks.

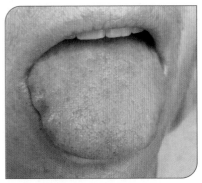

A pale and slightly purplish tongue with tooth-marks, which indicates blood and qì deficiency.

Example Pictures of the Skin

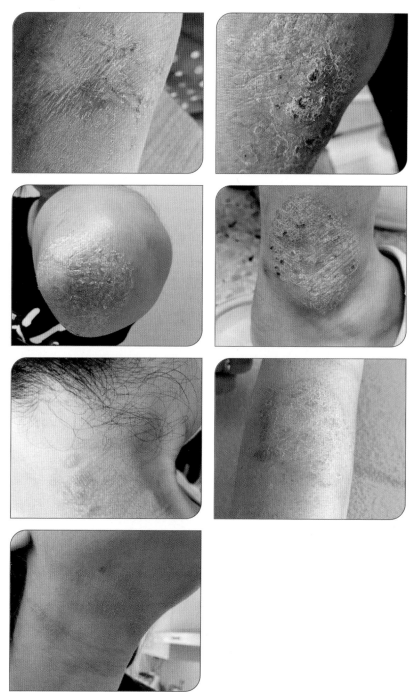

Fetal Toxin (*Tāi' Ér Dú Sù* 胎儿毒素)

I have already talked in detail about "fetal toxin" in Chapters 6 and 7. Please see this information for more background details on etiology and further explanations. As I have already explained in the "infantile eczema part" in Chapter 6 it can often develop into ND, although this does not happen in every case. Here, we talk about when infantile eczema has developed into ND in the child.

The description of ND due to "fetal toxin" refers to an itchy, bleeding, exudative, painful rash that occurs in infants/children due to fetal heat acquired in utero from parents. There are different names, which basically describe the same skin condition:

- *Tāi xuǎn* 胎癣, literally translated as "fetal tinea/dry ulcer"

- *Tāi liǎn chuāng* 胎斂疮, literally translated as "fetal accumulation sore."

To make it easier to understand: *tāi' ér dú sù* is the name for the TCM syndrome, the causative mechanism. The skin condition itself that you see in practice can be called either *tāi xuǎn*[8] or *tāi liǎn chuāng*. And for clarity, the Chinese name for "fetal toxin" is *tāi dú* 胎毒. So, whenever you hear these terms, you know straight away what they mean and you won't get confused.

Characteristics

As mentioned above, in this pattern the skin presents as an itchy, bleeding, exudative rash, which is very painful. The characteristics of the skin are essentially the same as in the "Internal Accumulation of Damp-Heat Due to Fetal Toxin" as explained in Chapter 6. The skin lesions appear as fresh red patches, papules, and/or papulovesicles, showing erosion with yellowish exudation and crusting. The skin feels hot with intense itching. The child may have fever, irritability, bad and restless sleep, bad breath, thirst and poor appetite, scanty urine, and constipation.

The tongue is red with a greasy, yellow coating and the pulse is slippery and/or rapid.

Treatment Principle

Cool blood, clear fire, eliminate dampness, and relieve itching (*liáng xuè qīng huǒ, qū shī zhǐ yǎng* 凉血清火，祛湿止痒).

Representative Formula
Xiāo Fēng Dǎo Chì Tāng (Eliminate Wind and Guide Out the Red Decoction).

Ingredients
Please see the earlier description of the formula in Chapter 6 on pages 149–51. This will not be repeated again at this point.

Formula Analysis
Please see Chapter 6 for a detailed elaboration of this formula.

Modifications
The modifications for *Xiāo Fēng Dǎo Chì Tāng* in this pattern are similar to those mentioned when talking about "Internal Accumulation of Damp-Heat Due to Fetal Toxin" in Chapter 6.

When more crusting, weeping and erosion is present, I recommend switching to either *Sān Xīn Dǎo Chì Yǐn* or *Lóng Dǎn Xiè Gān Tāng,* but with reduced dosages when working with children. These formulas have already been discussed in great detail in Chapter 6. Please visit these pages for an in-depth description. It all depends on the individual needs of the patient. Choose the formula that is best suited to the skin appearance, tongue and pulse presentation.

Example Pictures of the Skin

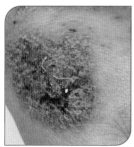
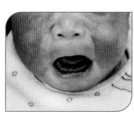
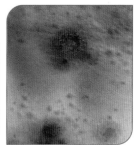

Please see "Internal Accumulation of Damp-Heat Due to Fetal Toxin" in

Chapter 6 for more pictures of the appearance of the skin. The skin characteristics are essentially the same.

Yīn Deficiency with Internal Heat
(*Yīn Xū Nèi Rè* 阴虚内热)

This is a chronic stage, and ND has been present for a very long time. Interestingly, I often see this pattern in women approaching 50 years of age, who are either going into menopause or are already in it. The prevailing yīn deficiency can intensify the skin disease. Of course, this pattern is not limited to women and can also occur in men, although I see it more often in women. However, it makes no difference for you, because in the end you must always treat the pattern you diagnose. The appearance of the skin, accompanying symptoms, tongue, and pulse will provide enough clues.

Please note again that I treat mainly adults in my practice. In my clinical experience, adults present with more Kidney yīn deficiency while children tend to have more Lung and Stomach yīn deficiency. In order to give you a fully comprehensive picture, I will also mention an alternative formula for treating children at the very end of this section.

Characteristics

The skin appears red. It's not a bright red, it appears more dark or deep red, which means that the heat runs deep inside. The skin feels warm, and is dry and scaly, showing cracks and/or transverse furrows, which easily tear. In this case, the skin feels very painful and burning, in addition to feeling tight. If the skin tears, the tear is an ideal breeding ground for infections. So please pay close attention to that and inform your patient about the potential for super-infections. The skin usually itches, especially at night. Unconscious scratching during the night also damages the skin, making the skin vulnerable to super-infections. Finally, I would like to mention that yīn deficiency can also be accompanied by dampness. I will describe this as a kind of sub-pattern at the end of this section and also reference the appropriate formula for it.

Accompanying symptoms may be dry lips, mouth, and throat, with thirst, especially at night. The patient wants to moisten the mucous membranes because they feel parched, due to the internal heat damaging the fluids. These patients love to have a glass of water beside their bed. They may also present with heat sensation within the body or hot flushes, tinnitus, dizziness, night sweating, heat in the five palms,[9] dark scanty urine, constipation but also mood changes like depression or anxiety. All these symptoms are signs of Kidney (and Liver) yīn deficiency. Please note, not all of these symptoms have to be present—they can be, but they don't have to be.

The tongue is usually small, red, and dry with a scanty coating or a thin yellow coating. In chronic and severe cases, the tongue has cracks. The pulse is thready (thin) and rapid.

Treatment Principle

Nourish and tonify yīn, clear heat, and moisten the skin (*zī yīn qīng rè rùn fū* 滋阴清热润肤).

Representative Formula

In this pattern, we also have a range of effective formulae. I will describe the most commonly used one in my practice when treating this pattern.

Liù Wèi Dì Huáng Wán (Six Ingredient Pill with Rehmannia) + *Zēng Yè Tāng* (Increase the Fluids Decoction).

Ingredients
Liù Wèi Dì Huáng Wán

shú dì huáng	Rehmanniae Preparata, Radix	24 g
shān zhū yú	Corni, Fructus	12 g
shān yào	Dioscorea, Rhizome	12 g
zé xiè	Alismatis, Rhizoma	9 g
mŭ dān pí	Moutan, Cortex	9 g
fú líng	Poriae Cocos, Sclerotium	9 g

Zēng Yè Tāng

shēng dì huáng	Rehmanniae Glutinosae, Radix	12 g
mài mén dōng	Ophiopogonis Japonici, Tuber	9 g
xuán shēn	Scrophulariae Ningpoensis, Radix	9 g

First Reference

Liù Wèi Dì Huáng Wán first appeared in *Xiǎo Ér Yào Zhèng Zhí Jué* (Craft of Medicinal Treatment for Childhood Disease Patterns, 1119) written by Qián Yǐ, a TCM classic on pediatrics.

First reference of *Zēng Yè Tāng*: *Wēn Bìng Tiáo Biàn* (Systematic Differentiation of Warm Pathogen Diseases, 1798), Author: Wú Jū-Tōng (Wú Táng).

Formula Analysis
Liù Wèi Dì Huáng Wán

In the ND yīn deficiency pattern, I mainly use *shēng dì huáng* instead of *shú dì huáng*. I have listed the original ingredients for your reference. If the ND lesions have a red hue and the blood cooling aspect is the priority, *shēng dì huáng* is definitely more suitable. However, *shēng dì huáng* and *shú dì huáng* can also be used in combination, in which case I suggest reducing the dosages to 9–12 g each. When using *shú dì huáng*, please also keep the dampness generating effect of the herb in mind. Adding a small dose of *shā rén* 3–5 g can counteract this effect. However, let's move forward in analyzing this formula.

In the formula, *shú dì huáng*–in ND, ideally *shēng dì huáng*–is used in a very large dose. It acts as sovereign herb and strongly enriches the Kidney yīn and essence. *Shān zhū yú* and *shān yào* act as minister herbs. *Shān zhū yú* nourishes the Liver and Kidney and restrains the Kidney essence, enabling it to replenish. *Shān yào* stabilizes the Kidney essence by strengthening the Spleen. To reinforce the Kidney essence and improve its function, the Spleen must function properly.[10] Keep in mind: The Spleen is the postnatal source of essence. These three herbs–*shēng dì huáng*, *shān zhū yú*, and *shān yào*–assist each other in nourishing yīn and replenishing the Kidney, and tonifying the Liver and Spleen. They can be called "the three tonics" in this formula. *Zé xiè* promotes urination and leaches out dampness through the Bladder. It also clears and drains Kidney fire, as well as preventing *shú dì huáng*–when used–from generating dampness. *Fú líng* is mild in its action of eliminating dampness from the Spleen. It helps *zé xiè* to discharge turbidity from the Kidney as well as helping *shān yào* to promote the Spleen's transportation and transformation function. *Mǔ dān pí* clears and drains Liver fire and counterbalances the warm and astringent properties of *shān zhū yú*. Thus, the three latter herbs can be also called "the three purgatives" within this formula.

Zēng Yè Tāng

Zēng Yè Tāng is a popular formula for increasing fluid to moisten dryness. This formula (with or without modifications) is quite often used for treating skin disorders with pronounced dryness accompanied by other systemic signs of dryness. I use it very often in combination with other formulas, like in this case with *Liù Wèi Dì Huáng Wán*.

Xuán shēn, mài mén dōng, and *shēng dì huáng* all benefit the yīn and moisten dryness. *Xuán shēn* with its bitter-salty flavor and cold nature, serves as sovereign drug and enriches the yīn, clears heat, increases fluids, and moistens dryness. *Mài mén dōng* and *shēng dì huáng* act as minister drugs in the formula. While *mài mén dōng* enriches the yīn and moistens dryness, *shēng dì huáng* nourishes the yīn and clears heat. Both herbs help *xuán shēn* to nourish yīn, clear heat, increase the body fluids, and moisten dryness.

Modifications

For insomnia due to itching, add *yè jiāo téng* 30 g. It calms the spirit and expels wind. Alternatively, *lóng gǔ* 15 g and *zhēn zhū mǔ* 15 g (boiled first before the other herbs are added) can be used. If the lesions appear intensely red, add *bái máo gēn* 15 g. Cold in nature and sweet in flavour, it cools the blood without any risk that it might injure the yīn or cause accumulation or stagnation.[11] For very thick skin lesions, invigorate the blood with *dāng guī* 9 g or *dān shēn* 9–12 g. If accompanied by more pronounced Liver and Kidney (yīn) deficiency, add *hàn lián cǎo* 9–12 g to tonify both Liver and Kidney while clearing heat. If the lesions are located on the wrists, add *sāng zhī* 3–5 g because this herb is the guiding herb for the upper limbs.

As mentioned above, I would like to offer an alternative formula if you are treating children, when nourishing the Lung and Stomach yīn is more important than Kidney yīn. The representative formula in this case is:

Shā Shēn Mài Mén Dōng Tāng (Glehnia and Ophiopogon Combination),[12] sometimes also called just: *Shā Shēn Mài Dōng Tāng*.[13]

Ingredients

shā shēn	Adenophonrae seu Glehniae, Radix	9 g
mài mén dōng	Ophiopogonis Japonici, Tuber	9 g
yù zhú	Polygonati Odorati, Rhizoma	6 g
sāng yè	Mori Albae, Folium	6 g

tiān huā fěn	Trichosanthis, Radix	9 g
bái biǎn dòu	Lablab Album, Semen	6 g
gān cǎo	Glycyrrhizae Uralensis, Radix	3–6 g

This formula clears and nourishes the Lung and Stomach yīn, generates fluids, and moistens dryness through the combination of sweet and cooling herbs. With regards to *shā shēn:* the most frequently used form of this herb is *běi shā shēn* (北沙参). You can, however, add both forms of the herb: *běi shā shēn* and *nán shā shēn* (南沙参) in combination, to support Stomach yīn and nourish fluids more strongly.

Additional Modification Suggestions for Children

Within this formula, I recommend adding *shēng dì huáng* 9–12 g in all cases. Children commonly have weaker constitutions, and their immune systems are disturbed in many cases. Thus, it is not unusual that children catch cold easily. They feel warm and dress too lightly in order to cool down. To support the immune system, add *jiǎo gǔ lán* 12 g. *Jiǎo gǔ lán* tonifies qì, strengthening endurance and lessening fatigue effect, as well as strengthening the patient's immunity; it is often used in patients with a poor constitution and weak immune system.[14] If this herb is not readily available or too expensive, as it can be in Germany, you might consider using *tài zǐ shēn* 12 g for this purpose. To further support the yīn nourishing and Lung heat clearing function, add *tiān mén dōng* 10 g. In combination with *mài mén dōng* it is very effective for yīn deficiency with heat signs in the upper burner, dryness, and thirst.

Example Pictures of the Tongue

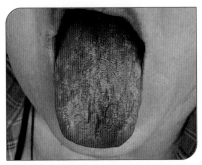

A dark red and slightly purplish tongue with a little coating.

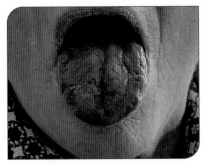

A red tongue with cracks. The color of the tongue indicates that heat consumes the yīn fluids and is turning into stasis.

Example Pictures of the Skin

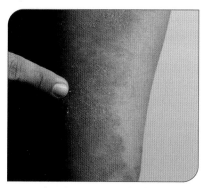

The skin appears dark red and is dry and scaly.[15]

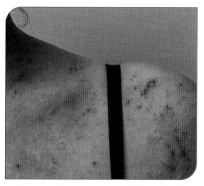

Dark red skin lesions. The skin is dry and shows scratching marks.[16]

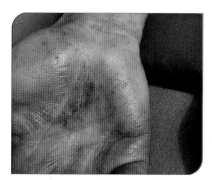

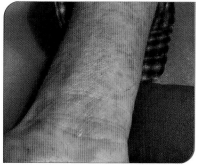

Dark/intense red skin that feels hot and burning, is painful and cracks easily.

As part of the modifications for yīn deficiency with internal heat, I have explained the treatment of children above. Now I will describe the presentation and corresponding treatment options when yīn deficiency is accompanied by dampness. This can be seen as a kind of sub-pattern, one seen more often in adults than in children.

Yīn Deficiency with Dampness (*Yīn Xū Jiā Shī* 阴虚夹湿)
Characteristics

This is a chronic form of ND and, in this case, the damp exudate has been part of the clinical picture for a very long time. The skin lesions appear dark, the skin scales and itches. Please note that, according to my experience, the itching is less intense than in the pattern of yīn deficiency with internal heat. Accompanying symptoms may be dry lips, mouth, and throat, but fatigue will also tend to be present.

The tongue is usually small, red, and has a thin yellow coating. The pulse is thready (thin) and rapid.

Treatment Principle

Nourish yīn and blood, clear heat, remove dampness, and moisten the skin (*zī yīn yǎng xuè, qīng rè qū shī rùn fū* 滋阴养血，清热祛湿润肤).

Representative Formula

I will discuss the two most commonly used formulae from my practice for the treatment of this sub-pattern:

- *Zhī Bǎi Dì Huáng Wán* (Anemarrhena, Phellodendron, and Rehmannia Pill)

- Modified *Zī Yīn Chú Shī Tāng* (Yin-Enriching, Dampness-Eliminating Decoction).[17]

Ingredients
Zhī Bǎi Dì Huáng Wán

shēng dì huáng	Rehmanniae Glutinosae, Radix	24 g
shān zhū yú	Corni, Fructus	12 g
shān yào	Dioscorea, Rhizome	12 g
zé xiè	Alismatis, Rhizoma	9 g
mǔ dān pí	Moutan, Cortex	9 g
fú líng	Poriae Cocos, Sclerotium	9 g
zhī mǔ	Anemarrhenae, Rhizoma	6 g
huáng bǎi	Phellodendri, Cortex	6 g

First Reference

The first reference of the formula can be found in the *Yī Fāng Kǎo* (Investigations of Medical Formulas, 1584), by Wú Kūn.

Formula Analysis

The first six herbs of this formula make up *Liù Wèi Dì Huáng Wán*, with the addition of *zhī mǔ* and *huáng bǎi*. Please see above for a detailed explanation of *Liù Wèi Dì Huáng Wán*. By adding the cool and bitter herbs *zhī mǔ* and *huáng bǎi*, the formula not only nourishes Kidney yīn and clears heat, but also strongly drains fire, and directs it downward. Although unpleasantly bitter, *huáng bǎi* strongly clears heat in the lower *jiāo*. Thus, *Zhī Bǎi Dì Huáng Wán* is a perfect choice whenever Kidney yīn deficiency with excess heat or damp-heat in the lower *jiāo* is present. Keep your eyes open, the tongue coating should be somewhat thicker than when using *Liù Wèi Dì Huáng Wán* alone.

Zī Yīn Chú Shī Tāng (modified)

shēng dì huáng	Rehmanniae Glutinosae, Radix	15 g
xuán shēn	Scrophulariae Ningpoensis, Radix	9 g
dān shēn	Salviae Miltiorhizae, Radix	9 g
dāng guī	Angelicae Sinensis, Radix	9 g
kǔ shēn	Sophorae Flavescentis, Radix	9 g
zé xiè	Alismatis, Rhizoma	9 g
fú líng	Poriae Cocos, Sclerotium	9 g
dì fū zǐ	Kochiae Scopariae, Fructus	9 g
shé chuáng zǐ	Cnidii, Fructus	9 g
gān cǎo	Glycyrrhizae Uralensis, Radix	3–6 g
+/- *zhī mǔ*	Anemarrhenae, Rhizoma	6 g
+/- *huáng bǎi*	Phellodendri, Cortex	6 g

First Reference

This formula comes from the book *Zhū Rén-Kāng Lín Chuáng Jīng Yàn Jí* (A Collection of Zhu Renkang's Clinical Experiences, 1979), written by Zhū Rén-Kāng.[18]

Formula Analysis

This formula is commonly used in chronic cases of eczema. Within this formula, *shēng dì huáng* nourishes yīn, clears heat, and cools blood. *Xuán shēn* enriches the yīn, drains fire, and can also soften hardness, which is useful when the skin becomes hardened after long-term disease. *Dān shēn* and *dāng guī* tonify and invigorate the blood. *Dān shēn* combined with *xuán shēn* effectively works to reduce swelling and, therefore, alleviates pain. *Kǔ shēn* clears heat, dries dampness, disperses wind, and stops itching. *Zé xiè* and *fú líng* function to remove water and leach out dampness, thus clearing any rash due to dampness. Finally, *dì fū zǐ* and *shé chuáng zǐ* stop itching, and *gān cǎo* tonifies the Spleen, clears heat and relieves fire toxicity. *Gān cǎo* also moderates and harmonizes the harsh properties of other herbs in the formula. To strengthen the heat clearing and fire draining effect, I recommend adding *zhī mǔ* and *huáng bǎi* to the formula.

Modifications

To modify both formulas, I recommend adding blood cooling and invigorating herbs such as *mǔ dān pí* 9–12 g and *dān shēn* 9–12 g. Depending on which herb is already present in the formula, add the other herb. In order to tonify the Spleen, add *bái zhú* 9 g. It is a key tonic for the Spleen and dries dampness to improve the transportive and transformative function of the Spleen. When the Spleen qì is strong enough, it is able to perform its transforming and transporting function and eliminate dampness. For all other choices for modification, please see above.

Example Pictures of the Skin

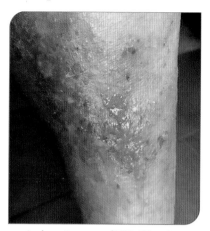

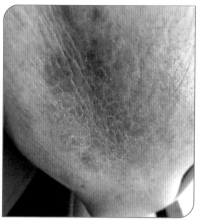

A chronic case of ND. The skin appears dark, scaly, cracks easily and occasionally damp exudate can be seen.

The same patient (chronic ND on the arm): The skin lesions appear dark in color and are scaling. This picture WAS taken during a stage where the skin didn't show damp exudate.

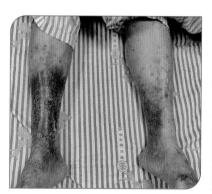

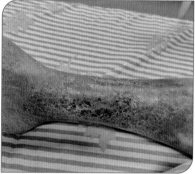

A chronic form of ND on a patient's lower legs. The skin appears very dark, is scaling, shows erosions and yellowish crusts due to damp exudate.

Suggestions for External Treatment

As already mentioned, this part is structured a little differently to the first part (on eczema). The difference in the suggestions for external treatment and examples for tailored herbal washes or wet compresses is that the recommendations are based on the appearance of the skin. Please keep in mind that all suggestions given below should serve as a practical orientation. Don't stick to the exact prescriptions, be flexible! Different formulas can be used for various skin appearances. The dosages and combinations can be adjusted, herbs can be replaced as required anytime. The choices are almost endless.

Erosive Lesions with Large Amount of Exudate

- *Huáng Bǎi Róng Yè* (Phellodendri Cortex Solution)

- *Qū Shī Sǎn* (Damp-Removing Medicinal Powder)

- *Sān Huáng Xǐ Jì* (Three Yellow Cleanser Formula)

- *Shé Chuáng Zǐ Tāng* (Cnidium Fruit Decoction)

- *Pí Shī Yī Hào Gāo* (Eczema Ointment No. 1)

Examples of individually tailored herbal formulas:

pú gōng yīng	Taraxaci, Herba	15 g
mǎ chǐ xiàn	Portulacae, Herba	15 g
yě jú huā	Chrysanthemi Indici, Flos	15 g

Boil with 350 ml water. Increase the doses of the herbs and the volume of water if the skin lesions are larger and more liquid is needed. Use as a cold compress on the affected skin area for 20–30 minutes each time, 2–3 times a day. If there is less exudate, this combination can be also used as an ointment. This also applies for all following combinations. Please see Appendix I for how to make ointments and pastes.

mǎ chǐ xiàn	Portulacae, Herba	30 g

Boil with 250 ml water and use as a cold compress on the affected skin area for 20–30 minutes each time, 2–3 times a day. Please note, *mǎ chǐ xiàn* compresses can be followed by the application of the formulas mentioned above, when required.

huáng bǎi	Phellodendri, Cortex	10 g
huáng qín	Scutellariae, Radix	10 g
dì fū zǐ	Kochiae Scopariae, Fructus	10 g
kǔ shēn	Sophorae Flavescentis, Radix	10 g
+/- *bái xiān pí*	Dictamni Radicis, Cortex	10 g

kǔ shēn	Sophorae Flavescentis, Radix	15 g
huáng bǎi	Phellodendri, Cortex	15 g
bái xiān pí	Dictamni Radicis, Cortex	15 g
cāng zhú	Atractylodis, Rhizoma	15 g
gān cǎo	Glycyrrhizae Uralensis, Radix	15 g

These combinations should be boiled with about 450 ml of water. If *bái xiān pí* is omitted from the first combination, use 350 ml water instead. Use as a cold compress on the affected skin area for 20–30 minutes each time, 2–3 times a day.

CLINICAL HINT: Whenever there are open skin lesions, advise your patients to avoid greasy creams. The skin must be able to breathe in order to heal, and the damp exudate has to have a chance to escape. If the skin is occluded, dampness moving transversely back will make the inflammation worse. Thus, patients can apply sesame oil as an emollient after using a wash or wet compress. This applies to each appearance of the skin no matter the TCM syndrome.

Erythema, Papules, Vesicles and Less Exudate

- *Huáng Lián Sǎn* (Coptis Rhizome Powder)[19]

- *Pí Fū Píng Ruǎn Gāo* (Skin Smoothing Ointment)[20]

- *Qīng Dài Sǎn* (Indigo Powder)[21]

- *Sān Huáng Xǐ Jì* (Three Yellow Cleanser Formula)

- *Zhǐ Yǎng Xǐ Jì* (Anti-Itch Wash)

Examples of individually tailored herbal formulas:

cāng ěr zǐ	Xanthii, Fructus	25 g
wáng bù liú xíng	Vaccariae, Semen	25 g
kǔ shēn	Sophorae Flavescentis, Radix	15 g
míng fán	Alumen	10 g

Boil with about 450 ml water. Use as cold compress on the affected skin area for about 15–30 minutes each time, twice a day.

huáng bǎi	Phellodendri, Cortex	10 g
huáng qín	Scutellariae, Radix	10 g
huáng lián	Coptidis, Rhizoma	5–10 g
gān cǎo	Glycyrrhizae Uralensis, Radix	10 g

This combination should be boiled with about 350 ml of water. Use as a cold compress on the affected skin area for about 15–30 minutes each time, usually twice a day. Please note that *yě jú huā, lián qiáo, jīn yín huā, pú gōng yīng,* or *tǔ fú líng* can be always added to increase the heat clearing action and reduce redness. It really depends what your patients need. Increase the amount of water accordingly, the more herbs you add. And as with any other combination, *yě jú huā* is particularly useful whenever the lesions are on the face.

jīn yín huā	Lonicerae Japonicae, Flos	15 g
lián qiáo	Forsythiae, Fructus	15 g
pú gōng yīng	Taraxaci, Herba	15 g
gān cǎo	Glycyrrhizae Uralensis, Radix	10 g
+/- *yě jú huā*	Chrysanthemi Indici, Flos	10–15 g

This combination is suitable for 450 ml of water, depending on how concentrated you want the wash to be. If you want to work more strongly, use less water and vice versa–if you want to work more mildly, use more water. Use as a cold compress on the affected skin area for about 15–30 minutes each time, twice a day. When using this combination without *yě jú huā*, just reduce the amount of water accordingly. This is a simple and visually appealing combination of fruits, flowers, and liquorice root. Never underestimate the visual effect of the herbs on healing. Patients often tell me how beautiful the herbs look, so they are not only effective, but also look beautiful and smell good when boiled, appealing to multiple senses. Applied topically, this combination can help with itching, heat, inflammation, papules, swellings, and healing of the skin.

yú xīng cǎo	Houttuynia Cordata Thunb., Herba	30 g

Boil with 250 ml water and use as a cold compress on the affected skin area for 20–30 minutes each time, 2–3 times a day. In China, I have often seen the use of *yú xīng cǎo* mixed with isotonic NACL solution (physiologic salt solution or isotonic sodium chloride solution). It is still used as a cold wet compress, just with a different base in this case. Either is possible and effective if the skin is intense red, burns, and is swollen.

A Word on Super-Infections

When secondary bacterial infections occur, with pain, swelling, and pustules on the affected areas of the skin, add herbs such as *mǎ chǐ xiàn*, *zǐ huā dì dīng*, and *pú gōng yīng* to the external applications. They clear heat and have a detoxifying effect. Furthermore, *yú xīng cǎo* is known for its anti-bacterial and anti-inflammatory effects.

Erosion, Pustules, and Crusting

- *Cāng Ěr Yāng Shuǐ Jì* (Cang Er Yang Wash)
- *Qīng Dài Sǎn* (Indigo Powder)[22]
- *Huáng Lián Sǎn* (Coptis Rhizome Powder)[23]

Examples of individually tailored herbal formulas:

In this case, similar herbs and combinations to those described above can be used. Remember that herbs can always be added or removed. It all depends on what the patient's skin looks like and needs. Be flexible!

Dry Skin, Scaly and Itchy Lesions

- *Guī Téng Xǐ Jì* (Gui Teng Wash)

- *Rùn Jī Gāo* (Flesh Moistening Ointment)

- *Yǎng Xuè Rùn Fū Yǐn* (Nourish the Blood and Moisten the Skin Drink)

Examples of individually tailored external herbal formulas:

dāng guī	Angelicae Sinensis, Radix	25 g
zhì gān cǎo	Glycyrrhizae Preparata, Radix	25 g

This is a very simple combination to moisten the skin and is usually given as an ointment or cream. For preparing as an ointment, sesame oil is the oil of choice.

dāng guī	Angelicae Sinensis, Radix	15 g
gǒu qǐ zǐ	Lycii, Fructus	15 g
sāng shèn	Mori, Fructus	15 g
dān shēn	Salviae Miltiorhizae, Radix	15 g

This combination is usually used as an ointment or cream. It nourishes the yīn, invigorates the blood, and moistens the skin. It is very effective in dry patterns of ND, as well as in chronic eczema with dark colored, dry and itchy skin. For using this combination as an ointment, the herbs can be mixed with sesame oil.

For my patients with dry skin and lesions located on the face and neck, I usually recommend my specially formulated TCM skincare products—CHINAMED COSMETICS®.

Lichenification and Scaling

- *Hēi Bù Yào Gāo* (Black Cloth Medicated Paste)[24]

- *Hēi Dòu Liú Yóu Ruǎn Gāo* (Black Soybean Distillate Ointment)

- *Zǐ Sè Xiāo Zhǒng Fěn* (Purple Powder to Reduce Swelling)[25]

Examples for individually tailored herbal formulas:

táo rén	Persicae, Semen	15 g
guā lóu rén	Trichosanthis, Semen	15 g

táo rén	Persicae, Semen	15 g
xìng rén	Armeniacae, Semen	15 g

Both combinations are essentially the same in function. They help moisturize and soften the skin, and help reduce the dark color of the skin. Grind the two herbs into a fine powder. Mix them with water or sesame oil and use as an ointment. This combination is also suitable for mixing into a natural base cream to use as a fine spreadable cream. It is very important to inform patients not to expose their skin to the sun after using this combination. We want to soften the skin and reduce the dark discoloration of the skin.

In order to strengthen the blood moving action of both combinations, herbs like *dāng guī* 15 g, *chuān xiōng* 15 g, *chì sháo* 15 g, or *dān shēn* 15 g can be added to soften the hard skin by tonifying and moving blood. Keep in mind, hard skin usually appears greyish or dark purplish in color, and herbs which treat blood stagnation are a perfect choice in this case. Two or three of these herbs are enough, and it goes without saying that the more herbs you add, the more water, oil, or cream is required.

Herbs like *dà huáng* and *zhāng nǎo* might be possible as stand-alone topical herbs to promote blood circulation, remove blood stasis and, thus, soften the skin. However, I prefer combinations for getting the most effective results for this pattern.

Clinical Hint for Treating Children

In children, or during severe inflammatory flare-ups, other natural substances can also be used externally besides Chinese herbs. Tannins,[26] such as black tea, used in cold wet compresses are good, for example. Because of their tolerability, tannin agents are often used in childhood for mild forms of ND or as a supportive measure in severe cases of the disease. They have an anti-inflammatory effect, soothe itching, and regulate the water balance of the skin. Green tea used as a cold wet compress can sometimes work miracles on the skin.

Aloe vera is another useful home remedy. It has a cooling effect, soothing the skin and relieving redness and itching due to inflammation. Aloe vera generally supports skin regeneration and has a moisturizing effect. Thus, it can also be used in mild cases and for general skin care when the skin is red and feels warm. When used as a gel, patients should be advised to store the product in the refrigerator because it is very sensitive to oxidation.

Please keep in mind, and this applies for all pictures throughout this book, that the pictures of the tongues and the skin should serve as examples for you. Remember that all your observations about the patient in front of you should complete the diagnosis.

Patient Education, Skincare, Dietary, and Lifestyle Advice for ND

Above, I have talked about the different treatment options with Chinese herbal medicine for patients with ND. This next section discusses tips for patients with ND exclusively; tips for patients with eczema in general will be covered later.

Patient Education

As I have said, treatment in TCM doesn't just involve giving Chinese herbs. It also involves educating patients–or their parents when treating children– on prevention, and proper diet and health education. This means sharing health-related knowledge, skills, and behavior in the context of a healthy diet, sufficient sleep, maintaining a good work-life balance, physical activity, skincare routines, and so forth. This is so important and is a great part of TCM therapy. What sense does it make for us to give herbs if the patient acts against the therapy again and again (i.e., they do not modify the behaviors or lifestyle factors that negatively affect their skin)? In the past I didn't highlight this enough to patients. However, since I keep observing the same mechanisms in my practice, I have started to communicate this very clearly. Always tell your patients that they are doing this for themselves, never for the therapist.

Most of the information given below might seem simple, but I find that patients are often not aware of it. So sometimes a gentle reminder really changes the patient's thinking.

Some background information you can share with your patients for clarity:

- In severe cases, the Western dermatologist will usually prescribe a cortisone ointment/cream to treat ND. Inform your patients that this only treats the symptoms, never the disease (in TCM: the root) itself. Make them aware that it is not a long-lasting or sustainable form of treatment like TCM. What I see in practice is that when cortisone is dropped, ND comes back. Always!

- Often, greasy and strong lipid-replenishing creams (containing petroleum jelly, such as Vaseline®[27]) are prescribed to soothe and hydrate the skin, but they do not work! Aside from the fact that petroleum jelly is a cheap and low-quality substance, the creams sit only on the surface and do not moisten the skin in any way. The truth is it is of no use to the patient.

- Inform your patients that they can use an oil or a thin and easily spreadable ointment after using Chinese herbs for external treatment. I often ask: Do you have something that you have had a good experience with? Something that does not irritate your skin? Then keep using a thin layer of this after using Chinese herbs as a wash or wet compress. Almond oil is a good choice if they don't have a preferred product.

Things that can irritate the skin and should be avoided:

- Hot showers and baths.

- Extreme sunbathing.

- Extreme climatic factors, as much as possible, e.g., extreme dryness, cold, humidity, and heat. In winter, for example, it is not only the cold that dries out the skin, but also the warm indoor air from heating. In summer, on the other hand, increased sweating can also worsen the symptoms of ND.

- Excessive hygiene. As mentioned earlier in this book, excessive hygiene is associated with a reduced microbial exposure in early life. The child cannot strengthen their immune system and develop a strong acquired immune defence. Normal hygiene and living standards are recommended.

- Perfume, essential oils, alcoholic additives in skincare products, such as shower gels, facial creams and body lotions–in general, anything that dries or irritates the skin.

- Chemicals—and this is important for particular professional groups such as painters, chemists, doctors, lab workers, nurses and so on—as they can severely irritate the skin.

- Environmental toxins, e.g., cigarette smoke, exhaust gases, air pollution.

- Potential allergens and/or triggers, such as grass, pollen, dust, pets, drugs, insect bites, and certain foods, just to name a few. First, they must be identified and then, of course, avoided.

- If possible, synthetic clothing, or clothing made of wool, which rubs on the skin and can also cause itching. Wearing clothing made of synthetic materials can encourage acute sweating and prevent the sweat from evaporating properly. The skin is softened and becomes a potential target for damage from external factors. Clothing made of cotton, which is breathable and has slight cooling properties, is more suitable for patients with ND.

- Colored clothes should be washed before wearing them for the very first time. The dyes are often very aggressive. This is particularly important for babies and infants because they are so sensitive.

- We all know that stress and psychological strain can increase the symptoms of ND. Thus, it is best to avoid those factors as much as possible. Yes, it is not always easy, especially in a professional environment. The pressure and mental stress in the workplace is obviously increasing, I hear this from my patients every day. But maybe it is possible to find better coping strategies, or different ways to cope, because the reality is that many can't just leave their jobs, right?

- Finally, be sure to avoid micro-bacterial super-infections. Warn your patients to always keep wounds and broken skin with fissures clean. A super-infection will absolutely worsen the symptoms due to serious inflammation of the skin. The skin burns and feels extremely painful in this case. It should always be ensured that the affected areas of skin are clean but also well-ventilated.

Patient Education in Children

Many children do not understand skin diseases in the same way that adults do and educating children with ND is, thus, different to educating adult patients. It can help to make sure children and their parents fully understand your advice and the benefits of your treatment. When working with young children, some kind of reward system might also help to encourage them to comply with your treatment plan even if they don't like it. Another possible strategy can be to encourage the child's involvement in tasks. This can be especially effective at times when scratching is most likely to occur, e.g., when learning, concentrating or feeling upset. It's a simple form of distraction not to scratch.

Best Skincare Routines When Dealing with ND

As I have said before, with ND it is very important to use mild products. Skincare products without any harming substances, such as alcohol, perfume, and even essential oils, are most beneficial.

When taking a bath or a shower, patients should avoid rubbing the lesions vigorously and scrubbing the affected skin area. As general advice, a bath or a shower should be lukewarm or warm rather than hot, and short. It is also not recommended to rub with a towel. They should gently press the skin with a towel to absorb moisture. Towels and washing-gloves should also be changed frequently to be as hygienic as possible. (This is very important with any skin condition, not just with ND.) After bathing or having a shower, an externally applied moisturizer—be it an ointment or any other natural lotion—can help maximize skin hydration.

I often hear that patients don't tolerate any skincare products on the face, especially during an outbreak of ND. Many natural products contain essential oils, although they claim to be mild and suitable for sensitive skin. Essential oils should not be used on the face. They can irritate the skin and especially the mucous membranes, most of all when they are used near the eyes. We are dealing with allergy sufferers here. Therefore, any products should be free of essential oils and other irritant substances. For my patients with dry skin, I usually recommend my TCM skincare products—CHINAMED COSMET-ICS®. The same applies to deodorants. It makes more sense to forgo them or to use irritant-free and non-alcoholic ones.

Diet and Food Advice for ND

In general, dietary changes are crucial to implement when treating eczema and ND. I will go into more detail about special nutritional advice later in the text, but while the development of ND has clearly been shown to be multifactorial, one area of research has focused on food allergies as an exacerbating factor. So, I want to mention advice that is particularly important for ND patients.

As mentioned earlier in this book, almost all ND patients have allergies to pollen, house dust (house dust mites), certain foods, and/or to additives in foods. It is well known that ND and food allergy are highly correlated.[28] From the TCM viewpoint, the root problem of allergies generally originates in the digestive system, namely the Spleen and Stomach. Consequently, first it is necessary to find out what specific food the patient is allergic to and then, logically, avoid it (as far as this is possible). If the patient is unsure whether a food is reactive, I advise to remove it from the diet for at least one week. Then reintroduce the food and observe any reactions in the digestive system and the skin. Allergy testing can also make sense, but this process is often just as reliable.

Dairy Products / Cow's Milk

- Dairy products, which in TCM terms create dampness and phlegm, should be avoided. Goat's or sheep's milk is definitely more digestible.

- For patients with severe sinus or nasal congestion, constant runny nose or thick phlegm expectoration from the Lungs, cow's milk should be avoided completely.

- Many of my patients think that soy milk is a good substitute, but in reality it is not. Soy milk is difficult to digest and can be gas-producing, and thus should be avoided.

Foods Known to Be Triggering for ND and Best Avoided

- Glutinous wheat, corn, eggs, tree nuts, peanuts, and, of course, peanut butter.

- Shellfish (shrimp, crab, lobster etc.).

- Spices and spicy food.

- Sugar, alcohol, and coffee.

- Fruit acid in oranges, lemons etc., or their juices.

Foods Considered Beneficial for Patients with ND According to TCM:

- Beans, such as mung beans and aduki beans. These can clear heat, reduce skin inflammation and thus, help with ND.

- Fruit such as watermelon, pears, persimmons, or bitter melon. These have cooling properties, can eliminate heat and calm symptoms of ND.

- Vegetables such as spinach, broccoli, Chinese cabbage, lentils, peas, celery, kelp, etc. They are considered to reduce inflammation in your body.

Stress and Emotions in Relation to ND

ND puts a strain on the psyche and ultimately leads to emotional stress. This stress can in turn trigger or worsen ND. On the other hand, stress and strain can trigger or worsen ND. Therefore, tell your patients that it is advisable to learn methods for coping with stress. Relaxation methods such as *tài jí, qì gōng*, meditation, yoga or autogenic training can help. In addition, stress can impair the immune system leading to an increased risk of susceptibility to infections, which in turn can cause an active flare-up of ND. It can help to inform your patients about these connections.

ND: Good Sleep and Prevention for Scratching

So far, I have described behavioral and psychological aspects to consider to improve ND. As ND symptoms such as scratching often worsen at night, they can interrupt or delay sleep. Besides, patients are more likely to scratch their skin while they sleep, which can in turn make itchiness worse again. Long-term sleep problems further worsen the skin through exhaustion and psychological stress. It is therefore very helpful to emphasize the importance of good sleep and how to maximize the chances of getting good sleep.

The following tips may help patients to reduce or prevent night-time flare-ups of ND:

- Any triggers that can disturb sleep must be avoided before bed, such as stressful events or stimulating exercise.

- Moisturizing the skin well before bed to keep the skin hydrated may be beneficial.

- Avoid sheets or pyjamas made from harsh fabrics that can irritate the skin, such as wool or polyester.

- It may help to avoid common allergens, including certain foods, drinks, pollen, or even pet cuddles, alas.

- Keeping the bedroom cool can help prevent sweating or feeling hot, which can make the skin feel itchier.

- Wearing gloves to bed makes it more difficult to scratch and can help control ND itching at night.

- Patients should keep their nails short. It is not just more hygienic, it also prevents scratching as well as bleeding and deep scratch marks when scratching during the night.

- Getting into a good sleep pattern is essential–it may be helpful to go to bed at the same time each night. The body loves rhythm in order to stay healthy.

TCM Insight

Why is good sleep so important from the TCM point of view? Healthcare (in Chinese *yǎng shēng*) is a very crucial part of TCM. *Yǎng shēng's* aim is always to "nourish life" and maintain and improve health. This also includes when is best to go to sleep, how many hours one sleeps, and the best time for sleeping. In my opinion, adults should sleep 7–8 hours, ideally eight hours, but at least six when seven hours are not possible for whatever reason. However, when discussing sleep and the ideal sleeping time, I like to explain the ancient Chinese way of measuring time and the term "*shí chén*" (时辰). In ancient China, people divided a day into 12 two-hour periods, and they called each two-hour period *shí chén*. According to TCM theory, qì and blood flow into a specific meridian (*zàng fǔ* organs) during each "*shí chén*."

So far so good, but what does that have to do with ND? In my opinion, building up the blood plays a very important role in TCM when treating ND, especially in the blood deficiency pattern where dryness and itching are predominant. If there is enough blood, the skin is nourished, moisturized, and looks good. There should be no basis for the development of a skin disease like ND, in theory. So let's focus now on the blood and sleep. I think there are two important aspects of time: First, sleep should begin before 11pm at night, because between 11pm and 1am is the time when the yáng qì begins to recover and regenerate. This is when qì and blood flow into the Gallbladder meridian. The *Huáng Dì Nèi Jīng* says: "The 11 *zàng* all hinge upon Gallbladder." This means that when the qì in the Gallbladder channel arises, only then will all the qì and blood in the body begin its resurgence.[29] Thus, getting into the habit of falling asleep before 11pm is most important. Secondly, according to Chinese medicine, another very important time slot is 1am to 3am, which belongs to the Liver. It is absolutely important to be asleep during this time, too. It is the "golden time" for resting and nurturing both the Liver and the blood. Keep in mind, according to TCM theory, the Liver stores the blood. By sleeping deep and well between 1am and 3am, the Liver and the blood will be nourished well. When there is enough blood, there will be neither deficiency nor stagnation. (Remember, blood deficiency can also lead to blood stagnation in the long term.) Consequently, skin health is maintained.

In conclusion: Sleep is important in every *shí chén* at night, best before 11pm and 5am in the morning. The night comes to an end and after 5am the energy of the day and activity begins. Waking up at 5am is considered to be normal. Interesting, isn't it? However, the advice I prefer to give to my patients is: Go to bed at 10pm and try to sleep until 6am.

Can Acupuncture Help with ND?

Even though I have written a book about treating ND with Chinese herbs, that doesn't mean I don't practice acupuncture. Of course I do! And I like to recommend acupuncture, especially for those patients who are stressed, feel tense, and have difficulty relaxing and calming down. This is why: Acupuncture proactively reduces stress by helping the qì flow smoothly. Moreover, never underestimate the time you spend with the patient. Time and understanding are very important aspects of the patient–therapist relationship. And another, very trivial, reason: Have you ever considered that an acupuncture treatment feels like a kind of vacation for the patient? Here, they don't have to do anything, just rest. The needles do their job. That's exactly what my patients keep telling me again and again.

If the patient can afford the treatment, decide whether to include acupuncture. Preferably once a week and five visits should be enough. Then you can decide if the patient needs more. I find it dubious to arrange 10 or 15 appointments straight away during the first consultation. As a TCM practitioner, you should be able to assess after five sessions whether treatment is helping and/or whether the patient still needs it. Never forget that, although we are there to help, any therapy, depending on the patient's background, may be a financial and practical obstacle for them. We are down to earth, so even those aspects must be kept in mind when explaining the therapy plan to your patient. At least this is how I work in my practice. However, if you really must decide—for whatever reason (time, costs, and so forth)—which treatment is best for skin conditions, I always recommend Chinese herbs before acupuncture.

Course and Prognosis of the Treatment of ND

ND patients in acute stages or with any other very serious skin conditions must be treated and monitored continuously, without breaks. At the very beginning, two weeks of taking the herbs twice (or three times) a day is recommended. If there is no improvement after two weeks, the prescription needs to be changed, assuming, of course, that the patient has complied with all instructions. If the treatment is followed too nonchalantly, the desired effect will not occur. It can be helpful to warn your patient about this, as they are always an essential part of the therapy. Later, the monitoring can be eased to every three weeks. Inform your patients that they should contact you sooner if they need you sooner. Patients are often reluctant to come forward for whatever reason.

Last but not least, it is crucial to inform your patient about the duration of treatment. Interestingly, many patients have an unrealistic expectation of what can happen with TCM. Again, ND is one of the most complex and difficult to treat skin diseases, even in TCM. Be sincere and tell your patient that. Trust is an equally important aspect in therapy. Almost all patients have received conventional drugs before, or they are still undergoing treatment, plus they have often tried one or several psychotherapies, before they finally consult a TCM doctor. So many challenges before they see us. Regardless, instant results cannot be expected. We, as TCM doctors, cannot work miracles in weeks and fulfil an expectation that conventional medicine with cortisone has not fulfilled in 15, 20, or even 30 years, as almost all adult patients have had ND their whole life. You need to confidently represent your standpoint, because this is the truth. A good and realistic benchmark you can promise to your patients is a minimum of six months of treatment with Chinese herbal medicine. I always say: I as a therapist like to see good results, and you as a patient do too. So let's do our best to fight the disease–me by giving you the best possible treatment plan and you by being compliant. If your patient trusts you, they will be patient and compliant over the course of treatment.

Endnotes

1 Bensky, D., Clavey, S., and Stöger, E. (2004) *Materia Medica* (3rd Ed.). Seattle, WA: Eastland Press, p.96.

2 Penetrating and Conception Vessel.

3 Bensky, D., Clavey, S., and Stöger, E. (2004) *Materia Medica* (3rd Ed.). Seattle, WA: Eastland Press, p.96.

4 Please note that some sources advise to cook gypsum for about 30 minutes before adding the other herbs, however I usually cook all the herbs together at once.

5 The original formula contained *mù tōng*. I have substituted this herb with *tōng cǎo* for safety reasons.

6 Please keep in mind, if the lesions are redder and a blood cooling aspect is needed, *shēng dì huáng* is better than *shú dì huáng*. If the lesions are paler and the patient needs more tonification, *shú dì huáng* may be used. You may also use both herbs in combination.

7 Repetition: Guiding herbs convey the formula to the corresponding affected area of the body. They send the formula / herbs to body regions that are far from the trunk, such as the extremities or the head.

8 Please note, some sources mention that this "sore" seems to be contagious.

9 Also called: five center heat, which is heat manifesting on the *yīn* surfaces of the body, such as the palms, bottom of the feet and the chest.

10 Scheid, V., Bensky, D., Ellis, A., and Barolet, R. (2009) *Formulas & Strategies* (2nd Ed.). Seattle, WA: Eastland Press, p.366.

11 Bensky, D., Clavey, S., and Stöger, E. (2004) *Materia Medica* (3rd Ed.). Seattle, WA: Eastland Press, p.579.

12 First reference of the formula: *Wēn Bìng Tiáo Biàn* (Systematic Differentiation of Warm Pathogen Diseases, 1798), Author: Wú Jū-Tōng (Wú Táng).

13 In China, *mài mén dōng* is usually just called *mài dōng*.

14 A detailed elaboration of the herb can be found in my 2013 article: "Jiao Gu Lan: The Herb of Immortality." *RCHM Journal (Register of Chinese Herbal Medicine) (UK)* 10, 2, 50–53.

15 Source: Shutterstock.

16 Source: Shutterstock.

17 Care should be taken not confuse this formula with another formula that has the same name, originating from the *Wài Kē Zhèng Zōng (True Lineage of External Medicine)* written by Chén Shí-Gōng, 1617. These are two completely different formulas with different ingredients.

18 People's Medical Publishing House (PMPH) Beijing, 1979.

19 Use as an ointment with sesame oil or as a wash, or wet compress.

20 Chinese herbal patent formula for topical use.

21 Use as a wash or wet compress to clear heat and dry dampness.

22 Use as an oil with sesame oil or as a wash, or wet compress.

23 Use as an oil with sesame oil or as a wash, or wet compress.

24 May contain herbs that are restricted or forbidden in some countries.

25 May contain restricted and/or unavailable herbs in some countries.

26 Tannins are widespread in nature and can be found, for example, in oak bark, roots, leaves, tea or fruit. They help to heal sore skin, have an anti-microbial, anti-inflammatory, and anti-pruritic effect.

27 Again, petroleum jelly is a byproduct of the oil industry, and not a high-quality solution. It is thick and poorly spreadable and it doesn't smell good.

28 Katta, R. and Schlichte, M. (2014) "Diet and dermatitis: Food triggers." *The Journal of Clinical and Aesthetic Dermatology 7*, 3, 30–36.

29 Li-Min, Q. (2015) Yang Sheng according to the time of day. *The Lantern 9*-3, 2–5.

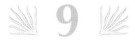

9

Modern Pharmacological Research

S O FAR, I have discussed the TCM formulas and their individual ingredients from the classic TCM point of view. This chapter provides an overview of the outcomes in experimental pharmacology, and clinical efficacy of pharmacologically active substances of herbs utilized in Traditional Chinese Medicine, applying modern scientific research methods.

Each herb has its own biochemical fingerprint, proven by analytical techniques and described in individual monographs. A monograph summarizes a report of the macroscopic descriptions, a list of all the main bioactive constituents of a drug, the pharmacological and biological activities of a single herbal drug, and their therapeutic application. Although I follow a classical approach, I find the meeting of traditional ways of thinking and modern biomedicine interesting. Not just for the medical insights, but it can also be very beneficial when talking to your patients. The concept of TCM is completely different from conventional medicine. Most of your patients probably aren't familiar with TCM terminology, so it can be helpful to explain the effect of a single herb as well as a complete prescription in a way that does not require in-depth TCM knowledge. Treatment itself should be regarded as a communicative process and patients need to be on board with it. If you explain mechanisms of action in a language they understand, it is very easy for them to follow your treatment suggestions. Using words like anti-inflammatory or anti-bacterial can sometimes be easier for the patient to understand than speaking of "toxins" or "damp-heat." However, this depends on the patient and their interest and educational background in TCM.

Below, I will discuss the pharmacological properties of the 15 most commonly used Chinese herbs in my practice in the treatment of eczema and ND. For the sake of simplicity, I have arranged the herbs in alphabetical order.

The left column names the most important active biochemical constituents, the right column their therapeutic effects in the treatment of eczema and neurodermatitis.

Bái Xiān Pí (白鲜皮–Dictamni Radicis, Cortex)

Main bioactive constituents	Useful therapeutic effects
limonoids[1], furoquinoline alkaloids, flavonoids, coumarins, sesquiterpene and sesquiterpene glycosides[2]	anti-inflammatory[3], anti-pruritic and anti-allergic[4], anti-bacterial, anti-fungal[5]

Dāng Guī (当归–Angelicae Sinensis, Radix)

Main bioactive constituents	Useful therapeutic effects
polysaccharides, Z-Ligustilide (3-butylidene-4,5-dihydrophthalide) and ferulic acid (4-hydroxy-3-methoxycinnamicacid)[6]	anti-oxidant, anti-inflammatory,[7] anti-pruritic[8]

Fáng Fēng (防风–Saposhnikoviae, Radix)

Main bioactive constituents	Useful therapeutic effects
chromones, coumarins, polyacetylenes, and acid esters[9]	anti-inflammatory, analgesic, immune-regulatory, anti-oxidative, and anti-proliferative[10]

Gān Cǎo (甘草–Glycyrrhizae Uralensis, Radix)

Main bioactive constituents	Useful therapeutic effects
glycyrrhizic acid, triterpene saponins, flavonoids, isoflavonoids, and chalcones[11]	anti-inflammatory, anti-viral, anti-microbial, anti-oxidative, immune-modulatory effects[12]

Huáng Qín (黄芩–Scutellariae, Radix)

Main bioactive constituents	Useful therapeutic effects
flavonoids: flavones (baicalein, wogonin, oroxylin A) and glycosides (baicalin, wogonoside, oroxylin A-7-glucuronide)[13]	anti-inflammatory,[14] anti-bacterial,[15] anti-oxidative and potential immunomodulatory activities,[16] anti-pyretic, analgesic, and anti-oxidant[17]

Jīng Jiè (荆芥–Schizonepetae, Herba)

Main bioactive constituents	Useful therapeutic effects
flavonoids, tannins[18], volatile oil, monoterpenes, sesquiterpenes, phenols, carboxylic acids[19]	anti-inflammatory, anti-oxidant, analgesic and immunomodulatory effects[20]

Jīn Yín Huā (金银花–Lonicerae Japonicae, Flos)

Main bioactive constituents	Useful therapeutic effects
phenolic carboxylic acids and esters, iridoid glycosides, flavones, triterpenoid saponins, essential oils[21]	anti-bacterial and anti-viral,[22] anti-inflammatory,[23] anti-pyretic[24] and detoxicant,[25] anti-exudative[26]

Lián Qiáo (连翘–Forsythiae, Fructus)

Main bioactive constituents	Useful therapeutic effects
phenolic glycosides, lignans, natural alcohols, triterpenes, flavon glycoside[27]	anti-bacterial, anti-inflammatory, supports immunity,[28] anti-viral,[29] analgesic[30] and anti-pyretic effects,[31] anti-oxidant[32]

Lóng Dǎn Cǎo (龙胆草–Gentianiae, Radix)

Main bioactive constituents	Useful therapeutic effects
secoiridoids, iridoids, xanthones, and xanthone glycosides[33]	anti-oxidant, anti-microbial, anti-bacterial, anti-fungal, wound-healing,[34] anti-inflammatory and immunological effects[35]

Mǔ Dān Pí (牡丹皮–Moutan, Cortex)

Main bioactive constituents	Useful therapeutic effects
monoterpenes, monoterpene glycosides, flavonoids, tannins, triterpenoids, phenols[36]	anti-oxidant and anti-inflammatory,[37] anti-allergic[38]

Pú Gōng Yīng (蒲公英–Taraxaci, Herba)

Main bioactive constituents	Useful therapeutic effects
cholin, inulin, pectin,[39] lactones, triterpenes and sterols (taraxasterol, taraxerol, cycloartenol, beta-sitosterol, stigmasterol),[40] vitamin A, B, and D[41]	anti-bacterial and anti-viral,[42] anti-oxidant and anti-inflammatory[43]

Shēng Dì Huáng (生地黄–Rehmanniae Glutinosae, Radix)

Main bioactive constituents	Useful therapeutic effects
iridoid and iridoid glycosides, ionones and ionone glycosides, phenylethanoid glycosides, lignans, phenylpropanoids, and sugars[44]	anti-bacterial, anti-inflammatory, and anti-oxidant[45]

Yě Jú Huā (野菊花–Chrysanthemi Indici, Flos)

Main bioactive constituents	Useful therapeutic effects
flavonoids, phenolic acids, and sesquiterpene[46]	anti-inflammatory, analgesic, anti-pyretic[47]

Yú Xīng Cǎo (鱼腥草–Houttuynia Cordata Thunb., Herba)

Main bioactive constituents	Useful therapeutic effects
volatile oils,[48] alkaloids, flavonoids, and other polyphenols[49]	anti-bacterial, anti-viral, anti-inflammatory,[50] anti-microbial, and anti-oxidative effects[51]

Zhī Zǐ (栀子–Gardeniae, Fructus)

Main bioactive constituents	Useful therapeutic effects
iridoids and crocetins, monocyclic monoterpenes, organic acids, and flavonoids[52]	anti-allergic and anti-inflammatory,[53] anti-phlogistic and anti-oxidant[54]

Endnotes

1 Chen, Y., Ruan, J., Sun, F., Wang, H., et al. (2020) "Anti-inflammatory limonoids from cortex dictamni." *Frontiers in Chemistry 8*, 73.

2 Jiang, S., Nakano, Y., Rahman, M.A., Yatsuzuka, R., and Kamei, C. (2008) "Effects of a Dictamnus dasycarpus T. Extract on allergic models in mice." *Bioscience, Biotechnology, and Biochemistry 72*, 3, 660–665.

3 Chen, Y., Ruan, J., Sun, F., Wang, H., et al. (2020) "Anti-inflammatory limonoids from cortex dictamni." *Frontiers in Chemistry 8*, 73.

4 Jiang, S., Nakano, Y., Rahman, M.A., Yatsuzuka, R., and Kamei, C. (2008) "Effects of a Dictamnus dasycarpus T. Extract on allergic models in mice." *Bioscience, Biotechnology, and Biochemistry 72*, 3, 660–665.

5 Yang, W., Liu, P., Chen, Y., Lv, Q., et al. (2022) "Dictamnine inhibits the adhesion to and invasion of Uropathogenic Escherichia Coli (UPEC) to urothelial cells." *Molecules 27*, 1, 272.

6 Wu, Y.C., and Hsieh, C.L. (2011) "Pharmacological effects of Radix Angelica Sinensis (Danggui) on cerebral infarction." *Chinese Medicine 6*, 32.

7 Wu, Y.C., and Hsieh, C.L. (2011) "Pharmacological effects of Radix Angelica Sinensis (Danggui) on cerebral infarction." *Chinese Medicine 6*, 32.

8 Lee, J., Choi, Y.Y., Kim, M.H., Han, J.M., et al. (2016) "Topical application of Angelica sinensis improves pruritus and skin inflammation in mice with atopic dermatitis-like symptoms." *Journal of Medicinal Food 19*, 1, 98–105.

9 Kreiner, J., Pang, E., Lenon, G.B., and Yang, A.W.H. (2017) "Saposhnikoviae divaricata: A phytochemical, pharmacological, and pharmacokinetic review." *Chinese Journal of Natural Medicines 15*, 4, 255–264.

10 Kreiner, J., Pang, E., Lenon, G.B., and Yang, A.W.H. (2017) "Saposhnikoviae divaricata: A phytochemical, pharmacological, and pharmacokinetic review." *Chinese Journal of Natural Medicines 15*, 4, 255–264.

11 Asl, M.N. and Hosseinzadeh, H. (2008) "Review of pharmacological effects of Glycyrrhiza sp. and its bioactive compounds." *Phytotherapy Research 22*, 6, 709–724.

12 Asl, M.N. and Hosseinzadeh, H. (2008) "Review of pharmacological effects of Glycyrrhiza sp. and its bioactive compounds." *Phytotherapy Research 22*, 6, 709–724.

13 Zhong, Z., Lin, G., and Li, C. (2011) "Pharmacological effects and pharmacokinetics properties of Radix Scutellariae and its bioactive flavones." *Biopharmaceutics and Drug Disposition*, Sep 19, 427–445.

14 Chi, Y., Lim, H., Park, H., and Kim, H.P. (2003) "Effects of wogonin, a plant flavone from Scutellaria radix, on skin inflammation: In vivo regulation of inflammation-associated gene expression." *Biochemical Pharmacology 66*, 7, 1271–1278.

15 Kowalczyk, E., Krzesiński, P., Kura, M., Niedworok, J., Kowalski, J., and Błaszczyk, J. (2006) "Pharmacological effects of flavonoids from Scutellaria baicalensis." *Przeglad Lekarski 63*, 2, 95–96.

16 Zhong, Z., Lin, G., and Li, C. (2011) "Pharmacological effects and pharmacokinetics properties of Radix Scutellariae and its bioactive flavones." *Biopharmaceutics and Drug Disposition*, Sep 19, 427–445.

17 Song, J.W., Long, J.Y., Xie, L., Zhang L.L., et al. (2020) "Applications, phytochemistry, pharmacological effects, pharmacokinetics, toxicity of Scutellaria baicalensis Georgi. and its probably potential therapeutic effects on COVID-19: A review." *Chinese Medicine 15*, 102.

18 Ding, X., Wang, H., Li, H., Wang, T., et al. (2023) "Optimization of the processing technology of schizonepeta herba carbonisata using response surface methodology and artificial neural network and comparing the chemical profiles between raw and charred schizonepetae herba by UPLC-Q-TOF-MS." *Heliyon 9*, 2.

19 Zhao, X., and Zhou, M. (2022) "Review on chemical constituents of Schizonepeta tenuifolia Briq. and their pharmacological effects." *Molecules 27*, 5249.

20 Ding, X., Wang, H., Li, H., Wang, T., et al. (2023) "Optimization of the processing technology of schizonepetae herba carbonisata using response surface methodology and artificial neural network and comparing the chemical profiles between raw and charred schizonepetae herba by UPLC-Q-TOF-MS." *Heliyon 9*, 2.

21 Wagner, H., Bauer, R., Peigen, X., Jianming, C., and Bächer, S. (2007) "Chinese drug monographs and analysis." *Verlag für Ganzheitliche Medizin 8*, 51.

22 Huang, K.C. (1993) *The Pharmacology of Chinese Herbs*. Boca Raton, FL: CRC Press, p.292.

23 Yoo, H.J., Kang, H.J., Song, Y.S., Park, E.H., and Lim, C.J. (2008) "Anti-angiogenic, antinociceptive and anti-inflammatory activities of Lonicera japonica extract." *Journal of Pharmacy and Pharmacology 60*, 6, 779–786.

24 A substance that reduces fever.

25 Wagner, H., Bauer, R., Peigen, X., Jianming, C., and Bächer, S. (2007) "Chinese drug monographs and analysis." *Verlag für Ganzheitliche Medizin 8*, 51.

26 Nadav Shraiborn, Sirbal Ltd., published June 30, 2015, patent citation US9066974 B1.

27 Wagner, H., Bauer, R., Peigen, X., Jianming, C., and Bächer, S. (2007) "Chinese drug monographs and analysis." *Verlag für Ganzheitliche Medizin 8*, 51.

28 Huang, K.C. (1993) *The Pharmacology of Chinese Herbs*. Boca Raton, FL: CRC Press, p.293.

29 Wang, Z., Xia, Q., Liu, X., et al. (2018) "Phytochemistry, pharmacology, quality control and future research of Forsythia suspensa (Thunb.) Vahl: A review." *Journal of Ethnopharmacology 210*, 318–339.

30 A substance that relieves pain.

31 Liu, C., Su, H., Wan, H., Qin, Q., Wu, X., Kong, X., and Lin, N. (2017) "Forsythoside A exerts antipyretic effect on yeast-induced pyrexia mice via inhibiting transient receptor potential vanilloid 1 function." *International Journal of Biological Sciences 13*, 1, 65–75.

32 Wagner, H., Bauer, R., Peigen, X., Jianming, C., and Bächer, S. (2007) "Chinese drug monographs and analysis." *Verlag für Ganzheitliche Medizin 8*, 51.

33 Gibitz-Eisath, N., Seger, C., Schwaiger, S., Sturm, S., and Stuppner, H. (2022) "Simultaneous quantitative analysis of the major bioactive compounds in Gentianae Radix and its beverages by UHPSFC–DAD." *Journal of Agricultural and Food Chemistry 70*, 24, 7586–7593.

34 Gibitz-Eisath, N., Seger, C., Schwaiger, S., Sturm, S., and Stuppner, H. (2022) "Simultaneous quantitative analysis of the major bioactive compounds in Gentianae Radix and its beverages by UHPSFC–DAD." *Journal of Agricultural and Food Chemistry 70*, 24, 7586–7593.

35 Singh, A. (2008) "Phytochemicals of Gentianaceae: A review of pharmacological properties." *International Journal of Pharmaceutical Sciences and Nanotechnology 1*, 1.

36 Wang, Z., He, C., Peng, Y., Chen, F., and Xiao, P. (2017) "Origins, phytochemistry, pharmacology, analytical methods and safety of cortex moutan (Paeonia suffruticosa Andrew): A systematic review." *Molecules 22*, 946.

37 Wu, M., and Gu, Z. (2009) "Screening of bioactive compounds from moutan cortex and their anti-inflammatory activities in rat synoviocytes." *Evidence-Based Complementary and Alternative Medicine: eCAM 6*, 1, 57–63.

38 Jiang, S., Nakano, Y., Yatsuzuka, R., Ono, R., and Kamei, C. (2007) "Inhibitory effects

of moutan cortex on immediate allergic reactions." *Biological and Pharmaceutical Bulletin 30*, 1707–1710.

39 Bensky, D., Clavey, S., and Stöger, E. (2004) *Materia Medica* (3rd Ed.). Seattle, WA: Eastland Press, p.164.

40 Kania-Dobrowolska, M., and Baraniak, J. (2022) "Dandelion (Taraxacum officinale L.) as a source of biologically active compounds supporting the therapy of co-existing diseases in metabolic syndrome." *Foods 11*, 2858.

41 Huang, K.C. (1993) *The Pharmacology of Chinese Herbs*. Boca Raton, FL: CRC Press, p.294.

42 Huang, K.C. (1993) *The Pharmacology of Chinese Herbs*. Boca Raton, FL: CRC Press, p.294.

43 Kania-Dobrowolska, M., and Baraniak, J. (2022) "Dandelion (Taraxacum officinale L.) as a source of biologically active compounds supporting the therapy of co-existing diseases in metabolic syndrome." *Foods 11*, 2858.

44 Li, M., Jiang, H., Hao, Y., Du, K., et al. (2022) "A systematic review on botany, processing, application, phytochemistry and pharmacological action of Radix Rehmnniae." *Journal of Ethnopharmacology 285*, 114820.

45 Kim, S.H., Yook, T.H., and Kim, J.U. (2017) "Rehmanniae Radix, an effective treatment for patients with various inflammatory and metabolic diseases: Results from a review of Korean publications." *Journal of Pharmacopuncture 20*, 2, 81–88.

46 Tian, D., Yang, Y., Yu, M., Han, Z.Z., et al. (2020) "Anti-inflammatory chemical constituents of Flos Chrysanthemi Indici determined by UPLC-MS/MS integrated with network pharmacology." *Food and Function 11*, 7, 6340–6351.

47 Wu, L.Y., Gao, H.Z., Wang, X.L., Ye, J.H., Lu, J.L., and Liang, Y.R. (2010) "Analysis of chemical composition of Chrysanthemum indicum flowers by GC/MS and HPLC." *Journal of Medicinal Plants Research 4*, 5, 421–426.

48 Yang, L., and Jian-Guo Jiang, J.-G. (2000) "Bioactive components and functional properties of Houttuynia cordata and its applications." *Pharmaceutical Biology 47*, 12, 1154–1161.

49 Fu, J., Dai, L., Lin, Z., and Lu, H. (2013) "Houttuynia cordata Thunb: A review of phytochemistry and pharmacology and quality control." *Chinese Medicine 4*, 3, 101–123.

50 Wagner, H., Bauer, R., Peigen, X., Jianming, C., and Bächer, S. (2007) "Chinese drug monographs and analysis." *Verlag für Ganzheitliche Medizin 8*, 51.

51 Wu, L.Y., Gao, H.Z., Wang, X.L., Ye, J.H., Lu, J.L., and Liang, Y.R. (2010) "Analysis of chemical composition of Chrysanthemum indicum flowers by GC/MS and HPLC." *Journal of Medicinal Plants Research 4*, 5, 421–426.

52 Zhou, J., Zhang, Y., Li, N., Zhao, D., Lu, Y., Wang, L., and Chen, X. (2020) "A systematic metabolic pathway identification of Common Gardenia Fruit (Gardeniae Fructus) in mouse bile, plasma, urine and feces by HPLC-Q-TOF-MS/MS." *Journal of Chromatography. B, Analytical Technologies in the Biomedical and Life Sciences 1145*, 122100.

53 Debnath, T., Lee, Y.M., Lim J.H., and Lim, B.O. (2018) "Anti-allergic and anti-atopic dermatitis effects of Gardenia Fructus extract." *Food and Agricultural Immunology 29*, 1, 665–674.

54 Wagner, H., Bauer, R., Peigen, X., Jianming, C., and Bächer, S. (2007) "Chinese drug monographs and analysis." *Verlag für Ganzheitliche Medizin 8*, 51.

10

Preventive Healthcare: Dietary, Lifestyle, and Skincare Advice; Patient Communication

WE LIVE IN a society that has changed a lot. Changed at least in the sense that it is different from what our parents and grandparents knew. Working environments have changed; personal computers, for example, didn't exist 50 years ago, not to mention mobile phones. Everyone has to be constantly available, and everything has to happen immediately. Furthermore, too much stress and too little sleep go hand in hand with stressful urban lifestyles. In my practice, it is clear to see that many people have lost the balance between activity (work, computer, thinking, and so on) and rest. In such a society, I observe that the idea of health prevention is unfortunately not on people's minds–prevention in the sense of maintaining health and avoiding disease. Many things seem to be prioritized over the well-being of one's own body, and alarm signals are all too often ignored. So let's take the time in our practices and do our job the best we can–which includes informing our patients how important preventive healthcare and self-care is. Patients need to know that there is a very deep connection between emotions, lifestyle, and work-life balance, and that it is not only their responsibility, but also their right to take care of themselves. And clearly it is our job as TCM and healthcare professionals to remind patients of this.

In this chapter I will discuss the general advice you can give your eczema / ND patients regarding diet, lifestyle, and skincare. At the very end of this chapter, I will touch on patient communication.

Let me describe the reality I observe with so many new skin patients in my practice: Many of them come to me, a TCM practitioner, for the very first time after years of visiting various Western practitioners and/or dermatologists. Yet, despite years of complaints, they have never been advised on nutrition, hygiene, or skincare. Strange, isn't it? Although it is so simple and so important, conventional medicine hardly ever takes the time to do it. Maybe it's the time factor that's missing, maybe it's just the ignorance of the positive effects of things like nutrition—or simply the lack of interest in thinking outside the box.

Diet

According to a Chinese proverb, "He that takes medicine and neglects diet, wastes the skills of the physician." I've already stressed this elsewhere in the book. I believe in the medicinal value of food and consider it crucial, especially for improving skin conditions. The Chinese idea of the importance of balance and harmony in every aspect of life, thus, applies to food, too. So, what we put into our bodies is so important. However, this does not mean that dietary changes alone will cure a complex skin disease. This also does not mean that when a person dislikes something, they have to eat it regardless just because they have been told "It is good for your health." No, absolutely not. Why? Because I really think that patients should still enjoy eating and like the food they eat.

ALWAYS KEEP THIS IN MIND: Patients have the ability to speed their skin's healing at home if we make them aware of their own responsibility in their healing process. Or—on the flip side—they may also contribute to the aggravation of their skin disease if they follow an inappropriate diet and lifestyle habits.

We know that the effects of a "bad" diet accumulate over time and should be seen in a long-term context. The issue is not just the quality of food but also the quantity, and irregular food consumption. The following section details information on eating habits, lists the foods that should be avoided, provides preferable alternatives, and offers other practical tips we can share with our patients.

General Guidelines

Certainly, doctors and health experts from different fields have different perspectives on food and thus different dietary recommendations. However, in TCM (and many other nutritional philosophies agree) the general guidelines for patients are:

- eat only when hungry

- stop before feeling completely full, the 80%[1] rule suits best here

- have three meals per day (warm food if possible)

- do not eat too late in the evening (ideally not after 6 pm).

When It Is Getting Tricky

I frequently hear the sentence "But I like it!" Show understanding, but know that it will likely prove worthwhile to educate the patient and explain that food they like is not necessarily what they need or what is good for them. The other sentence I regularly hear is "I can't do that!" We need to deconstruct such a statement for what it is: The patient might say they cannot do it, but they actually mean that they do not want to. We need to accept that change is difficult for many patients, but also tell them straight up that they shed their responsibility by claiming change is impossible. Many people are afraid of change, although nature—including our physical body—is in the process of constant change. To make it easier for patients, take the time and make suggestions that they can easily adopt without having to change their routines completely. Fortunately, modern society offers so many alternatives to products that we can usually find a solution for everything.

A good example is sugar. I have patients who tell me that they eat a bar of chocolate a day. Their world will fall apart if I tell them that this is not a good idea, and really it is the worst thing they can do for their skin. I always take my time in this case and ask what they particularly like, and search for alternatives. It can be fruit, or products from the organic market without refined sugar, for example sweetened with dates or cane sugar. All of this, of course, only in moderation. Apropos "moderation," as I have said earlier in this book, I often use the term "measure and middle" in practice, be it with a balanced diet or way of life. Less excess in life means a healthier one! Eating like a king or queen will definitely promote sickness. Interestingly, every patient will agree here. So, this can be a good time to change things.

Food and Drinks to Be Avoided, and Those Recommended

In this section I will mention food and drinks to be strictly avoided when dealing with eczema or ND. I will split my hints for you into acute/subacute and chronic conditions because it makes a difference in what to advise. My tips given below are easy to implement.

As mentioned above, when advising patients, it is helpful to not only list the individual products that need to be avoided, but also to give alternatives. In my experience, being too strict and dogmatic in our recommendations can be counterproductive. Moreover, complicated technical language and too much information at the beginning can be overwhelming, and sometimes even cause stress. Give every patient a simple but clear overview in a language that they can grasp.

ACUTE AND SUBACUTE PHASE OF ECZEMA AND/OR ND

The main principle during acute and subacute phases is to clear heat and drain dampness. Thus, any food and drinks which, from the TCM point of view, produce inner heat and dampness should strictly be avoided.

The following food and drinks are considered to be a potential source of heat:

- in general, oily, greasy, and fatty foods

- alcohol, spirits (the higher the alcohol content, the hotter the drink) and red wine in particular

- hot spices, such as chilli, curry, dried ginger, pepper, cumin

- garlic, spring onions, onions, leek

- hot (or warm) in nature meats, especially lamb and grilled beef

- shellfish (shrimp, crab, lobster etc.)

- sugar and coffee

- mustard and vinegar, if you're being particular.

The following foods and drinks are considered to be an ideal breeding ground for dampness, which transforms into heat later on:

- cow's milk and dairy products

- sugar and sweet foods, such as desserts, cakes, even sticky rice

- wheat flour products

- soft drinks like cola and lemonade

- alcohol.

For eczema and ND, as for any other skin condition, it is particularly important to stop—or at least heavily restrict—consumption of alcohol, cigarettes, and coffee, as well as oily and spicy food. Patients should preferably eat mildly spiced food and steam their food instead of roasting or frying in excess oil. It is also recommended to eat lighter meals, like vegetables and fresh fruits, and foods that cool heat, such as apple, watermelon, bamboo shoots, green tea, mint, radish, or mung beans. Foods that can resolve dampness can also be beneficial, such as coix seed (*yì yǐ rén*), Chinese yam (*shān yào*), adzuki bean (*chì xiǎo dòu*), cherries or kohlrabi etc.

> Let me share a case from my practice which illustrates the connection between food and skin: A young man in his early 40s came to my practice because of eczema on his legs. He had this for more than 10 years, a typical case of damp-heat from what I saw during our first appointment. With the use of Chinese herbs, applied internally and externally, we got a grip on it pretty quickly and his legs looked really good. The inflammation disappeared almost completely. I saw him again for a check-up at the beginning of the new week, a Monday or a Tuesday. He was very unhappy and said his skin had incredibly worsened again. The skin on his legs was inflamed again and was itching badly. He scratched so hard that he hurt some parts of the skin. I asked him what happened. He was almost too scared to admit that, the previous weekend, he had a barbecue with his family and friends. He said the weather was so nice and he did everything he hadn't done in a long time: he drank alcohol and ate hot, spicy, and grilled food (fish and beef). His skin looked good for so long, but that day he went beyond his limits, so the skin quickly worsened. Well, we improved his condition again with herbs, but this example clearly shows the tight connection between nutrition and skin—in this case, in a negative sense.

A Word on Dairy

Chinese medicine considers cow's milk cooling and damp-forming, especially if consumed in excess. It can be helpful when talking to patients to explain how the Spleen works according to Chinese medicine: dairy products slow down digestive and absorptive functions, resulting in excess fluids and phlegm that block the skin. Thus, cow's milk products should be strictly avoided by those who have any skin problems (not just eczema or ND) where dampness is involved.

The Western world consumes a large quantity of dairy products.[2] This trend seems to be expanding into the Asian world: I have observed that products from cow's milk, including milk, yoghurt, and cheese are now consumed more. Whatever the reason—global trends and advertising, or corporations seeking new markets—from a TCM point of view, this is a rather unfortunate development. Luckily, there are plenty of alternatives. Patients can substitute cow's milk cheese with sheep's or goat's milk cheese. According to TCM theory, both are easier to digest. Tell them about alternative options for milk: almond, rice, soy, or oat milk. Help your patients and make suggestions that they can easily adopt without having to change their routines completely.

Adult patients often tell me that they still drink a big glass of milk every day, despite the fact that milk is really not meant to be a beverage. Many people still believe that cow's milk contains a lot of calcium and that it is good for them. But if this is the case, why is the rate of osteoporosis in Asian people not significantly higher than in Caucasians? The truth is that most industrially advanced countries—like the US, Australia, New Zealand, and most Western European nations—have higher fracture rates, yet consume more dairy products than the rest of the world. Meanwhile, the people in much of Asia and Africa consume little or no milk (after weaning), few dairy products, and next to no calcium supplements, yet their fracture rates are 50 to 70% lower.[3] I usually tell patients that calcium as an essential mineral is important for good health, but bone health does not depend on calcium alone. Moreover, I show them a table with natural calcium sources and patients are usually surprised that cow's milk is not in the top spot. Many foods like vegetables (including kale, broccoli, fennel, spinach), algae or sardines contain the same, or even higher levels of calcium than cow's milk products. Debunk this myth for the benefit of your patients.

CHRONIC PHASE OF ECZEMA AND/OR ND:
During the chronic phase, it is preferable to nourish blood and moisturize the skin. The following foods might be considered here:

- dates (*dà zǎo*), goji berry (*gǒu qǐ zǐ*), longan fruit (*lóng yǎn ròu*)

- white fungus, lily root (*bǎi hé*)

- dark leafy greens, kelp, shiitake mushroom, spinach

- fruits, such as fig, pear, raspberries etc.

These are examples of foods that nourish blood in order to moisten the skin, just to name a few. As well as paying attention to diet, of course, advice given during an acute phase should be taken just as seriously.

Fā Wù 发物

Finally, when talking about nutrition in Chinese medicine, I like to explain the concept of *fā wù*. What does *fā wù* mean exactly? *Fā* means to emit, *wù* means a material or substance. In the context of food, *fā wù* usually describes a specific category of food in Chinese medicine that increases or exacerbates disease rather than preventing it. Simply put, *fā wù* food can be risky when eaten too much. In China, *fā wù* is usually applied in skin diseases, such as psoriasis, acne, urticaria, and eczema. During my studies in China, I often heard my Professor saying to her skin patients: Avoid *fā wù* foods.

These tips are similar to my previous advice, but I would like to describe everything in detail so that you know exactly what *fā wù* is when you hear it.

Foods Considered to Be *Fā Wù* and Their Six Mechanisms According to TCM[4]

- Food that generates heat and fire inside the body and injures fluids, e.g., ginger, lamb, stir-fried food.

- Food that generates wind, e.g., shrimps, crabs, chicken, eggs.

- Foods that generate dampness because they are considered to be sticky and greasy and cause stagnation, e.g., maltose, glutinous rice, rice wine. All these tend to impede the function of the Spleen and generate dampness.

- Food that generates cold inside the body, e.g., watermelon, pear, ice etc.

- Food that generates bleeding, e.g., pepper, wine, etc. They can damage and drive blood out of the blood vessels.

- Food that generates qì stagnation, e.g., lotus seed, Chinese yam, beans, and some fruits. They are difficult to digest and easily impede the flow of qì, thus making the qì stagnate.

Generally, if you are in good health you don't have to avoid *fā wù* food. The concept of "avoiding something" only applies when sick. A skin condition like eczema is a very good example of this. In the case of red skin lesions, as seen in acute eczema and ND, heat is already predominant. When *fā wù* food is consumed, it adds even more heat to the pre-existing heat, and thus makes the skin rash worse. Never add fuel to the flames! The following table provides an overview of foods considered as *fā wù* specifically in eczema, to be avoided.[5] Please note that I will not distinguish between eczema and ND in this table. These are general rules for the umbrella term "eczema."

Food to avoid	Pathogenic mechanisms that make eczema worse
sweet and greasy food (e.g., maltose, glutinous rice, rice wine)	produce internal dampness
sugary sweets (e.g., candy, cookies, other desserts)	produce internal dampness
dairy (e.g., milk, yoghurt, ice cream)	produce internal dampness
Acrid, spicy, and irritating food (e.g., green onion, lamb, pepper, lychee, mustard, aniseed)	warm/hot in nature with drying properties, tend to generate heat and fire inside the body
stir-fried, toasted, and smoked food	produce internal heat
wind-stirring food (e.g., mushroom, chicken, eggs, crabs, shrimps, coriander)	generate wind inside the body
seafood (e.g., crabs, shrimps, lobster)	trigger allergic reactions and aggravate the skin by increasing inflammation

This knowledge can also be helpful in other skin diseases, for example, psoriasis, acne, and urticaria.

Bowel Movement

Let's talk about elimination and how important it is that the bowels are able to flow freely. The bowels take in the good a person needs and easily release what the body no longer requires. When the body is able to release, it does not hold on to toxins, thereby also maintaining healthy skin. So far, so good– but in reality, many patients have no regular bowel movement. Constipation is an issue that needs to be addressed. If the stool is too dry or irregular, the heat within the body cannot escape, which makes the skin worse. Thus, regular bowel movement helps relieve eczema by expelling heat from the body. If the patient is constipated, it is recommended to treat the constipation first. After this has been successful, address the other aspects. The patient should understand how important this is, even if they have come to regard constipation as "normal."

PRACTICAL HINT: Regular bowel movement is essential–at least once a day.

Exercise

In general, the patient should maintain a stable mood, have enough rest and sleep, and avoid overexertion with exercise until the condition improves. The latter is also a myth we need to debunk: Exercise is good for our body, but physical strain is not. Our society (from PE at school to fitness culture) too often claims that we need to push ourselves to the point of overexertion. Yet, patients need to learn to listen to their bodies and know when they need rest, when they need light exercise, and when they are fit enough for more intense training. And by the way, one should practice a sport that is also fun. Don't do any sport just because it's trendy!

Vaccinations

Another point to consider is that it is necessary to postpone any planned vaccinations during an acute phase of eczema or ND, as these will bring more heat to already existing heat in the body. I think it is important to take this into account again when patients ask about this. It is our duty to advise and inform patients professionally as best we can.

Skincare

Having covered nutrition and lifestyle habits in detail, I now come to the topic of skincare. Part of any initial consultation with a patient is to fully educate them on the topic of proper skincare. Cleaning and care should be adapted to the patient's skin's individual needs. Take your time to discuss what they should include in their daily skincare regimen, but also what they should avoid as much as possible. Appearance affects the patients' daily lives. The aim of a TCM consultation, therefore, is also to teach individuals simple techniques to improve their skin condition at home, enabling them to feel better in their skin. Herbs will take care of the rest.

The information below applies to eczema in general. I will not differentiate between eczema and ND at this point. Detailed information on ND and skincare in particular can be found in Chapter 9. The following lists useful advice on skincare routine basics you can give to your patients:

- Whether acute or chronic eczema, it is necessary to avoid scratching to prevent the possibility of a secondary infection.

- Don't wash the infected skin areas with hot water. Use lukewarm water instead.

- Washing too frequently, especially excessive scrubbing, will aggravate the problem. Don't overdo it! Wash the skin gently.

- Do not wash skin lesions with soap as they can disrupt the skin barrier and clog the pores.

- Always use a clean towel, as even after a single use, the fabric will pick up many bacteria, which will then land on the skin if the towel is reused. Change towels and cloths very regularly, even daily in acute cases.

- Avoid contact with washing powder and softener.

- It is advisable to wear 100% cotton clothes, silk, or any other breezy clothing.

- Do not wear tight clothes during an acute phase. The material may attach to the wounds and cause serious damage to the skin when taking them off. Tight clothes can also rub on damaged skin.

- Do not wear new colored clothes because of potential irritating chemicals. It is advisable to wash clothes before wearing.

- Avoid using strong, irritant shower gels or body lotion.

- Whenever possible, use products without perfume, essential oils and alcohol. Mild products without irritating substances are absolutely preferable. pH-neutral products are best.

While one would assume that everyone knows this, practice shows that this is not the case.

Prevention in Skincare

The holistic approach of TCM also includes preventive aspects which, if considered, may prevent disease from occurring in the first place. In skin health, preventive measures are particularly suitable, as they can be applied quickly and easily. To keep the skin healthy, care should be taken to ensure that it receives sufficient moisture. This makes the skin not only soft, but also supple and thus less prone to cracking. The necessary acidity (pH value) remains more stable and protects the skin from bacterial diseases.

Regarding creams—keep in mind that Cortisone creams are usually not the best solution for eczema, although in Western dermatology they are given all the time and seen as the only treatment. Cortisone is not the most effective, and also not the most sustainable solution. In my experience, Chinese herbs are more effective and longer lasting! Represent your point of view. Clinical experience proves efficacy.

Patient Communication

Finally, I want to touch briefly on patient–practitioner communication. As with any sort of communication, that between patients and doctors is a two-way street and poor communication can definitely affect a patient's treatment. Many of us have a horror story to tell about a visit to a doctor at a certain time in our lives, be it long waiting times, insensitivity, or simply feeling rushed. Do not forget that patients often bring a sense of anxiety into the consultation room. This kind of anxiety can also make it difficult to mention essential information and/or retain what information is given. Make it easy for your patient to share all you need for your diagnosis, but also to follow your advice. Don't use technical language. The use of jargon is a very common barrier in patient–practitioner communication. Explain everything in a way the patient can understand and follow. Always treat a patient as you would like to be treated in this situation. Please also remember to explain to your patients exactly what we do: that we practice individualized medicine and write tailored prescriptions. The prescriptions are always adjusted, and what we do is high-quality work. Often patients do not realize this because they only see the result: a wonderfully personalized TCM formula. Therefore, it is always worthwhile to mention it again in the initial consultation. We practice wonderful medicine that many patients are looking for, a holistic medicine. This is the great advantage of TCM. Especially in the field of dermatology, we can help many, if not most, patients with complex skin conditions.

Endnotes

1 Stop eating when feeling 80% full.

2 www.ourworldindata.org: Per capita milk consumption, 2017. www.statistica.com: Annual consumption of fluid cow milk worldwide in 2019, by country.

3 Castleman, M. (2009) "The calcium myth." *Natural Solutions*, July–August, 57–62.

4 张湖德，张玉苹主编.餐桌上的发物与忌口[M].上海：上海科学技术出版社.

Hu-De, Z., and Yu-Ping, Z. (eds) (2007) *Fa Wu and Taboos at the Dinner Table* [M]. Shanghai: Shanghai Scientific and Technical Publishers.

5 Most of the information is taken from the book: 张湖德，张玉苹主编.餐桌上的发物与忌口[M].上海：上海科学技术出版社. Hu-De, Z., and Yu-Ping, Z. (eds) (2007) *Fa Wu and Taboos at the Dinner Table* [M]. Shanghai: Shanghai Scientific and Technical Publishers.

11

Useful Advice on the Practical Application of Chinese Herbs

WELCOME TO the practical part of this book. So far, I have explained the causes, the diagnostic process, and different TCM syndromes of eczema and ND, as well as their characteristics and treatment with Chinese herbal medicine in detail. In this chapter, I will discuss frequently asked questions about Chinese herbs, treatment course, and frequency of appointments. The chapter on diet, lifestyle, and skincare follows next.

Frequently Asked Questions on Taking Chinese Decoctions
Why the Focus on Raw Herbs?

As I have mentioned, in my clinical experience, decoctions, or teas, of raw herbs are the most effective form of treatment. Clinical experience proves that it is almost impossible to treat a difficult chronic skin disease without prescribing herbs. Despite the popular assumption, acupuncture is actually just a small part of TCM. The essential TCM method is Chinese herbal medicine and specifically, in my view, using raw herbs.

Many colleagues tell me that patients do not want to take raw herbs because the herbs taste bad or are hard to cook. Well, I have not found this to be the case. Overwhelmingly, I find that my patients wish to have access to the best possible treatment they can have, and will put in the time—and even their courage because of the adventurous taste of herbs—to get it. I always say: effectiveness comes before taste. Medicine doesn't have to taste good, it should work! And you know, every patient would agree. In a nutshell: When

I advise patients, I don't discuss. I recommend fresh herbs, nothing else. I don't give any other choice, so there is simply no basis for discussion. I think it all depends on how you present your point of view. I am the therapist and patients follow my advice, otherwise we are not the right fit for each other. I also say, when it is necessary: Effectiveness always comes first!

How to Deal with Allergy Sufferers

Almost all eczema and ND patients have allergies and if not, almost all of them are sensitive and can easily have an allergic reaction to various kinds of external influences. This is why it is always advisable to be careful and start with a mild approach when it comes to treatment with Chinese herbs, whether it is a case of internal or external treatment. I usually start with prescribing just one bag of herbs in this case and wait for their feedback. If everything works well, i.e., no irritating reaction occurs, I order more bags of the same prescription. Never underestimate the psychological factor here. Patients who have had allergic reactions in the past are often relieved when I tell them how I work. I always explain how important it is to me that they tolerate my treatment well, that I care, and that it is my job to make them feel better. This can be very important for some patients. Remember this!

Herbs During Pregnancy

During pregnancy you should work gently with Chinese herbs. Since we often have to take a harsh and clarifying/draining approach in acute cases, I normally advise starting the treatment with herbs after delivery, to avoid any risks. Advise your patients to wait for any strong treatment—in your patient's and the child's interest. You can, of course, work mildly without hesitation and without any harmful effects, by using various cooling herbs. But as I said, that's often not enough and you won't always achieve the desired success in the treatment of acute eczema and cases of ND.

What to Do When Drinking a Herbal Decoction Causes Bloating or Stomach Issues

Sometimes a patient's digestion is very sensitive. Especially in the beginning it can happen that they experience bloating or slight stomach pressure. As a rule, patients should drink their herbs before meals. In the case of digestive complaints, advise your patients that they should take the herbs after meals, waiting at least 30 minutes after the meal. The herbs and the food should not influence each other, or the effectiveness could be mitigated. If all this is not enough, advise them to also reduce the dose a little: for example, taking 90 ml instead of 120 ml. Usually the problems are solved very quickly. General advice: For those patients with weak digestion, drinking the herbs after meals may be best.

What to Do When Patients Catch a Cold, Flu, or Gastrointestinal Infection

Advise your patients that whenever a severe cold or flu with fever, or a gastrointestinal infection occurs, that they should not continue drinking the tea. Tell them to pause the herbs during the worst days and to resume only when feeling better. This also applies when taking antibiotics—I usually advise patients to stop drinking the herbs during this time.

Can the Skin's Appearance Worsen During Treatment?

Yes, sometimes it can. Patients must be aware of this fact but that it's not necessarily a bad sign. Sometimes there can be an aggravation before everything gets better. Fortunately, I rarely see this in my practice. However, if patients are not informed about this process, they may be worried and also think that the treatment is not helping, and even that their skin is getting worse. I have found that if this mechanism is well explained, patients understand and will go along with it. However, as with all treatment processes: the better informed patients are, the less they worry when things appear to get worse.

Rules of Thumb for the Treatment Course with Chinese Herbs

Eczema and ND patients in acute stages or with very serious skin conditions must be treated and monitored continuously, without breaks. Therefore, at first, two or three weeks of taking the herbs daily is recommended. If there is no improvement after that, the prescription needs to be changed, assuming, of course, that the patient has complied with all instructions. If your dietary advice is not followed strictly, treatment success will also be difficult to achieve. Patients should be disciplined with changes in diet, as it will definitely improve their results.

How Long Does the Patient Have to Drink Chinese Herbs For?

This always depends on the problem being treated and the severity. A good and realistic benchmark you can offer your patients is a minimum of three to four months of treatment with Chinese herbal medicine for chronic and stubborn eczema and ND. However, a time period of six months is realistic. It is crucial to inform your patient about the duration of treatment.

Again, chronic and stubborn skin diseases, especially ND, have evolved over many years; often they are present since birth. Thus, instant results cannot be expected, but small changes will occur as treatment progresses. As mentioned already, a good rule of thumb is one month of treatment for every one year of illness. For chronic and severe types of eczema and ND, this is a very realistic rule to give to your patient. Of course, skin can often improve faster, and yes, I often see more rapid successes, especially in patients with acute skin conditions that have not lasted very long. However, do not give any false hope, because there is much more going on in the patient's life that plays a role in improvement as well as aggravation, such as stress, emotions, environmental factors, etc. You need to confidently represent your position, because this is the truth. We, as TCM doctors, cannot work miracles in weeks and achieve an outcome that conventional medicine has not achieved in several years. Also, compared with the harsh drugs and permanent topical treatments with cortisone that patients may have already used over the years, a natural medicine like TCM works gently, may take a little longer, but is effective and, above all, sustainable.

Frequency of Appointments

Finally, inform your patients that herbal treatment requires regular appointments. Although less frequent than acupuncture appointments, for example, the initial one or two appointments may also be about two weeks (in some cases one week) apart, to check on initial responses to the herbs. Discuss this at the initial consultation. If your patient cannot come in at this frequency, the point of long-term therapy must be questioned. I am saying this because I see many patients who drive long distances to see me. These really very practical things should also be discussed. Often a therapist located closer to the patient can make more sense if frequent visits are not possible for whatever reason.

12

Clinical Case Studies of Eczema and Neurodermatitis

HAVING DISCUSSED the theory of eczema and ND in TCM in detail, we now leave the theoretical part and come to the practical part of this book. In this section, I will discuss a total of six clinical cases. Three of these will be different types of eczema, and three will be ND. These case studies will clearly demonstrate how to apply the classical formulas, discussed earlier in this book, to different cases of eczema and ND. This will also make it very clear that you can work well with classical formulas as a basis in many individual cases of TCM eczema. On top of this, you will learn:

- how to change treatment strategies if you find that the first approach was not 100% correct

- that classical formulas are not limited to one type of eczema, and that they can be used flexibly

- how to make a TCM diagnosis even when you have very little information, as may be the case with infants

- when to employ external applications with Chinese herbs

- what additional information should be given to the patient to improve their skin condition, and what the patient can do at home (e.g., through nutrition, lifestyle changes, and appropriate skincare).

All in all, this practical part should teach you how to apply the theoretical knowledge of the first part of the book in your practice.

PRACTICAL NOTE: The following dosages are meant for one herbal bag. One bag lasts patients an average of 3–4 days, depending on the number of ml per day. The more severe the skin lesions, the higher the ml dosage. For adults, I usually work with about 100–150 ml per dose. For children, I usually work with light dosages (no more than 100 ml per dose).

#1: Male Patient, 51 Years Old–Eczema (Western Diagnosis: Endogenous eczema)
First Visit

This was a complex case of eczema with many pre-existing conditions. I would like to use this case to illustrate that every bit of information is necessary to understand the process and the development of a skin disease; to show that you must change your treatment strategy when you realize that the initial prescription is not 100% suitable; and also that knowledge of conventional medicine is absolutely necessary in order to treat a serious skin disease adequately with TCM. This case also illustrates that, regardless of the severity and poor response to all Western medications, TCM can work miracles on the skin.

The middle-aged male patient's medical history noted that he had been suffering from hypertension, COPD and hepatitis C for many years. Eight months ago, he had a pulmonary infarction with cerebral hemorrhage and was placed in an induced coma. In addition to all the medications he was already taking for his pre-existing conditions, more and more Western drugs were added during his hospitalization. Crucially, after hospital discharge one month later, he continued taking the diuretic medication Torasemide, and it was at this time that all his skin problems began.

This patient came on the recommendation of another patient and presented in my clinic with medium sized, bright red, slightly scaly and very itchy eczema lesions all over his body. Especially noticeable were the open eczema lesions on his lower legs, on both sides. The sores were open, oozed with large amounts of damp exudate and yellowish crusts, and felt warm and even slightly burning to the patient. In addition, the skin on his neck was intensely red and peeling. Within the past four months, neither a Western dermatologist nor his treating physician had been able to help him. His ankles and feet were extremely swollen, with a mixed red and purplish hue to the skin. On his feet, spider veins could also be observed. All in all, this was a very serious case of eczema on a background of overall poor health. The pictures at the end of this case study illustrate how serious his skin initially appeared. In general, he was not living the healthiest lifestyle. Despite his pre-existing conditions, he smoked and drank large amounts of coffee, and occasionally alcohol. Accompanying symptoms included: trunk obesity, red face, spider veins on his face, swollen and painful joints, fatigue particularly starting in the afternoon, no appetite in the morning, soft stools 1–3 times a day, a feeling of fullness after meals, and heat at night with sweating.

Please note that the Western umbrella term "endogenous eczema" refers to eczema due to an inherent tendency to develop dermatitis on the skin. According to the definition, the cause of the eczema is not related to direct contact with an inciting agent. The most common example of endogenous eczema is neurodermatitis (atopic eczema). However, for me, this case was clearly medication induced. It is very interesting that the most obvious cause was overlooked and, unfortunately, the patient was not taken seriously.

His tongue was thick and purplish in color, with a thin yellow coating. While checking his tongue, purplish lips could also be observed. His pulse was slippery and slightly rough, with weak Kidney and Spleen positions.

TCM Diagnosis
Blood Stasis combined with Yīn Deficiency and Dampness (*Yū Xuè Yīn Xū Shī Shèng* 瘀血阴虚湿盛).

Treatment Principle
Promote blood circulation to remove blood stasis, nourish yīn, clear heat, remove dampness and moisten the skin (*huó xuè huà yū, zī yīn qīng rè, qū shī rùn fū* 活血化瘀，滋阴清热，祛湿润肤).

Formula

shēng dì huáng	Rehmanniae Glutinosae, Radix	15 g
chì sháo	Paeoniae Rubrae, Radix	10 g
(chǎo) mǔ dān pí	Moutan, Cortex (dry-fried)	12 g
jī xuè téng	Spatholobi, Caulis	15
(chǎo) huáng bǎi	Phellodendri, Cortex (dry-fried)	10 g
(chǎo) zhī mǔ	Anemarrhenae, Rhizoma (dry-fried)	6 g
dān shēn	Salviae Miltiorhizae, Radix	15 g
lián qiáo	Forsythiae, Fructus	10 g
gān cǎo	Glycyrrhizae Uralensis, Radix	6 g

Raw herbs to be taken as a decoction for 10 days, 130 ml twice a day.

Formula for External Treatment

kǔ shēn	Sophorae Flavescentis, Radix	10 g
dì fū zǐ	Kochiae Scopariae, Fructus	10 g
bái xiān pí	Dictamni Radicis, Cortex	10 g
huáng bǎi	Phellodendri, Cortex	10 g
huáng lián	Coptidis, Rhizoma	5 g

Used as cold compresses for both legs, 20–30 minutes each time, twice a day.

Advise your patients to always work cleanly when using external treatments, and to avoid contamination of the liquid in any case.

Case Analysis

First, let me explain the nature of Torasemide, because this medication seemed to me to be the primary trigger of his skin rash. Torasemide is a diuretic medication used to treat fluid retention (oedema) due to heart failure, kidney disease, and liver disease and hypertension. It works by causing the kidneys to get rid of unneeded water and salt from the body via urination. So far so good. When the patient told me his story of suffering and emphasized several times that the skin itching and the rash all started at the same time as he began taking Torasemide, my alarm bells rang. I had seen a similar case in the past, a male patient with Parkinson's disease and heart insufficiency who was prescribed diuretics after hospital discharge, in addition to all the other medications he was already taking. That patients' skin was also red and itchy all over his body. In this particular case, the patient stopped the medication on his own and his skin got better. A short note on this: I never advise my patients to stop conventional medicine without consulting their doctor, and abruptly discontinuing a medication that someone has taken long-term is never advisable. The body often cannot handle these rapid changes. Patients should always do this after consultation with their treating physician, and systemic medication should always be gradually phased out. This is very important for patients to know.

However, in this current case, I stressed the issue of his medication, interactions and possible side effects. Along with its desired effects, Torasemide may cause some unwanted effects which may require medical attention. Potential side effects of Torasemide are: swelling of the hands, ankles, feet, or lower legs, blistering, peeling, or loosening of the skin, dry mouth, increased thirst and diarrhea, red skin lesions and itching,[1] just to name a few. Interestingly, he had already read the package insert and suspected the same—that his skin complaints were closely related to this diuretic medication. He had even asked his conventional doctor about it; however, they rejected his opinion and said there couldn't be any relationship. I advised him to see a pharmacologist[2] and discuss potential side effects as well as interactions of all his medications; and to be a strong advocate for his own health and not be brushed off. I, too, was firmly convinced that his skin rash was triggered by Torasemide. This case reminded me that Western medical knowledge is also a must for us as practitioners so we can grasp all the factors at play. Furthermore, it also clearly demonstrates that the more patients you see, the faster you become at gathering the necessary information and drawing conclusions. For me, the connection was quite clear, due in part to having seen a similar case before, and also due to my training in Western medications, their uses but also their potential harms.

Let's now discuss the initial formula: This was a patient with multiple chronic long-term conditions, e.g. COPD, Hepatitis C, and a lot of signs of "wear and tear" can be seen, e.g. fatigue and joint pain. Yīn and blood were exhausted, blood stasis was obvious; dampness was present, too. In this case, a short but effective formula was used. In addition to the internal treatment with Chinese herbal decoctions as described below, external Chinese herbal treatment was added twice daily as a cold wet compress to clear heat and cool blood. External treatments often work wonders on the skin and speed up the skin healing process, and in a case like this I would never treat without them.

In regard to addressing the blood cooling and heat clearing as well as blood moving and transforming blood stasis aspects, *shēng dì huáng, chì sháo, dān shēn, mǔ dān pí* and *jī xuè téng* were used. These herbs amplify the heat/fire clearing effect of the formula, cool the blood, and also invigorate the blood in order to prevent stasis. All these actions are needed for this degree of inflammation of the skin. *Jī xuè téng* not only moves the blood, it also soothes the sinews, unlock channels and collaterals, and was also selected to address the patient's joint pain. The cool and bitter herbs *zhī mǔ* and *huáng bǎi* nourish Kidney yīn and clear heat, but also strongly drain fire, especially from the lower *jiāo*. *Huáng bǎi* in particular is very effective when heat and fire-generated oozing sores are located in the lower part of the body. Combined with *shēng dì huáng* and mǔ dān pí, *zhī mǔ*, and *huáng bǎi* are components of the formula *Zhī Bǎi Dì Huáng Wán*, which is very effective in clearing heat from the lower *jiāo* as well as nourishing yīn. This again clearly demonstrates that you can easily construct and modify classic formulas. Always take the components you need. Classic formulas serve as a base. *Lián qiáo* was used to clear heat and resolve toxicity, and a higher dosage was used to amplify this effect during the early stage of treatment. Later on, it should be reduced to 6–9 g, for example, because it is very bitter and can harm the digestive system. Moreover, to minimize the bitter and cold character of *mǔ dān pí, zhī mǔ,* and *huáng bǎi*, they were dry-fried (*chǎo*). Considering that he already had loose stools, it was important to make these herbs more tolerable for the patients' digestive system. Finally, *gān cǎo* clears heat and relieves fire toxicity but also harmonizes the prescription because it mediates any extreme properties of the other herbs. *Gān cǎo* also strengthens the Spleen and replenishes qì in order to support the Spleen's transportive and transformative function.

Considering that the patient had been suffering from multiple chronic conditions and abusing his body for many years by eating unhealthily, smoking, and drinking, simply taking herbs would not be enough in this case. Thus, it goes without saying that the patient was informed in great detail about which foods he should definitely avoid and which are good for him. Without changing his lifestyle, his skin won't get better! I would like to emphasize once again that in the case of skin diseases in particular, nutritional advice always forms part of any consultation, and the patient needs to understand that this is an essential part of the therapy. At a minimum the patient needs a list of what to avoid, so that they know which foods will make their condition worse.

Second Visit

The patient returned for his follow-up consultation 10 days later. He took the first formula consistently every day for 10 days, but unfortunately, the skin on his legs hadn't changed much. He complained of slightly cold hands and feet and that the itching was worst at night. Please note that he had not previously differentiated the nocturnal itching in this way. The only significant change was that his ankles and feet were not as swollen and didn't feel tense anymore. The color of his tongue also hadn't changed significantly, and was still purplish with a thin yellow coating. His pulse was slippery and slightly rough. His Kidney position had improved but the Spleen position was still weak.

Formula Modification

The formula was adjusted to focus more on the blood moving aspect while continuing to nourish yīn, clear heat and remove dampness.

táo rén	Persicae, Semen	9 g
dān shēn	Salviae Miltiorhizae, Radix	15 g
dāng guī	Angelicae Sinensis, Radix	9 g
chuān xiōng	Chuanxiong, Rhizoma	4.5 g
chì sháo	Paeoniae Rubrae, Radix	6 g
niú xī	Achyranthis, Radix	9 g
shēng dì huáng	Rehmanniae Glutinosae, Radix	12 g
tǔ fú líng	Smilacis Glabrae, Rhizoma	15 g
chái hú	Bupleuri, Radix	3 g
gān cǎo	Glycyrrhizae Uralensis, Radix	6 g
(chǎo) mǔ dān pí	Moutan, Cortex (dry-fried)	9 g
(chǎo) huáng bǎi	Phellodendri, Cortex (dry-fried)	9 g
lián qiáo	Forsythiae, Fructus	9 g

Raw herbs to be taken as a decoction for 21 days, twice a day.

This formula is a modification of *Xuè Fǔ Zhú Yū Tāng* (Drive Out Stasis in the Mansion of Blood Decoction).[3] The main effect of this formula is to stimulate blood circulation, remove blood stagnation, move qì and unblock the channels. *Tǔ fú líng* was added to enhance the heat clearing process, reduce redness and swelling.

Formula for External Treatment

kǔ shēn	Sophorae Flavescentis, Radix	10 g
dì fū zǐ	Kochiae Scopariae, Fructus	10 g
bái xiān pí	Dictamni Radicis, Cortex	10 g
huáng bǎi	Phellodendri, Cortex	10 g

Used as cold compresses for both legs, 20–30 minutes each time, twice a day.

Third Visit

The herbal adjustments took the patient in the right direction because, after another three weeks of taking the modified formula, his skin significantly improved. The skin looked markedly less red, the itching disappeared completely and there were no more open and oozing sores. This was a very good result considering the severity of his skin condition initially, and that no Western medication had been helpful. In general, he felt better and had more energy. His digestion was stable, and he was passing stools twice a day. However, he reported that the heat and sweating at night had returned and his ankles were thick and felt warm and painful again. While he had an upcoming appointment with a pharmacologist, he had independently discontinued the diuretic medication (Torasemide) after his previous appointment at my practice. The discontinuation in combination with Chinese herbs showed a massive positive impact on his skin. The color of his tongue improved and was only slightly purplish now. The thin yellow coating remained. His pulse improved too, and was only slightly slippery and no longer rough, with only slight weakness remaining in the Spleen position.

Formula Modification

He received a prescription of Chinese herbal medicine for internal usage for a further three weeks to continue working on both the blood stasis and clearing the heat and dampness. Both aspects were addressed in equal measure. As his skin was completely healed and there were no open and oozing lesions anymore, the patient was instructed to discontinue the external treatment and return in another three weeks for a follow-up.

shēng dì huáng	Rehmanniae Glutinosae, Radix	12 g
(chǎo) huáng qín	Scutellariae, Radix (dry-fried)	10 g
chē qián zǐ	Plantaginis, Semen	15 g
zé xiè	Alismatis, Rhizoma	15 g
(chǎo) mǔ dān pí	Moutan, Cortex (dry-fried)	12 g
(chǎo) huáng bǎi	Phellodendri, Cortex (dry-fried)	10 g
pú gōng yīng	Taraxaci, Herba	15 g
dān shēn	Salviae Miltiorhizae, Radix	15 g
zé lán	Lycopi, Herba	15 g
bái xiān pí	Dictamni Radicis, Cortex	10 g
gān cǎo	Glycyrrhizae Uralensis, Radix	6 g

Clinical Course

I saw the patient two more times after that, at three-weekly intervals. His skin continued to look better at each visit, healing completely and fading more and more, although this took time. The swelling and pain in his ankles also resolved. Since the patient came to me because of his skin and not because of his other numerous pre-existing conditions, my job as a TCM therapist was done in terms of his skin. That was his wish: to heal his skin and to get rid of the pain. Interestingly, the visit to the pharmacologist never took place. However, it was now also up to the patient to change his lifestyle and to take better care of himself; as well as to keep an eye on his other chronic diseases and to continue his Western medical care. There was obviously a lot of work to be done. While he struggled to change his lifestyle considering his unhealthy eating, smoking, and drinking, at least he understood the sense in it, and awareness is the first step to making better choices. During his last appointment, I reminded the patient that whenever he had skin problems again or simply wished to address his other health issues, he could contact me at any time. I will always do my best to help with TCM!

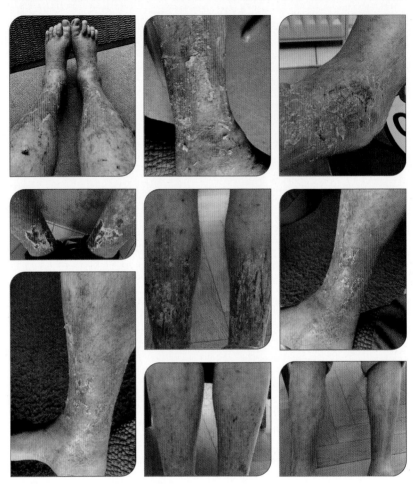

The progress of the patient's skin.

#2: Female patient, 23 Years Old–Eczema (Western Diagnosis: Seborrheic eczema)
First Visit

A young woman presented in the clinic with seborrheic eczema. She told me her skin had looked bad for several months and generally tended to worsen before her menstrual period. She had also noticed that, after eating seafood, her scalp started itching very badly, sometimes accompanied by pain or a burning sensation. This was new for her. The skin was not only itchy, it was also red, and not only on her scalp, but also her face. Her cheeks were slightly red, her throat felt dry, and she was a little thirsty. Besides slight bloating, breast distension, and mood changes before her period, no other symptoms were reported. The patient did appear somewhat stressed, however, and after asking her about her living circumstances, it became clear that she was under a lot of pressure at work.

The tongue was red (especially on the sides) with a thin yellow coating, which indicates internal heat. The pulse was thin, wiry, and rapid.

TCM Diagnosis

Liver Qì Stagnation with Excess Heat (*Gān Jīng Yù Rè Zhèng* 肝经郁热证).

Treatment Principle

Soothe the Liver, resolve constraint, clear excess heat, and expel wind (*shū gān jiě yù, qīng rè xī fēng* 疏肝解郁，清热熄风).

Formula
Modified *Dān Zhī Xiāo Yáo Sǎn*

chái hú	Bupleuri, Radix	9 g
bái sháo	Paeonia Albiflora, Radix	9 g
dāng guī	Angelicae Sinensis, Radix	9 g
bái zhú	Atractylodis Macrocephalae, Rhizoma	9 g
fú líng	Poriae Cocos, Sclerotium	9 g
gān cǎo	Glycyrrhizae Uralensis, Radix	6 g
mǔ dān pí	Moutan, Cortex	12 g
zhī zǐ	Gardeniae, Fructus	9 g
huáng qín	Scutellariae, Radix	9 g
bò hé	Menthae, Herba	5 g
shēng dì huáng	Rehmanniae Glutinosae, Radix	20 g
tiān mén dōng	Asparagi, Radix	10 g
bái jí lí	Tribuli Terrestris, Fructus	10 g
pú gōng yīng	Taraxaci, Herba	15 g

Raw herbs to be taken as a decoction, for 21 days, 120 ml twice a day.

Case Analysis

This case was relatively clear: the patient's tongue indicated heat, particularly in the Liver because the sides of the tongue were red and, according to TCM, the sides represent the Liver. Her wiry pulse, but also the tendency of her skin to get worse before her period, indicated Liver qì stagnation; and the rapidness of her pulse was a sign of excess heat. Considering that emotions and increased stress have been found to be negative factors which can trigger or worsen heat in the Liver, one can assume that seafood was not the only trigger here, but that the existing stress was the underlying main cause. The incident of eating seafood only came on top of that. Looking again at the TCM theory: the channels (meridians) serve physiologically as a pathway for transportation of qì and blood, but we know that, in pathological conditions, channels can also serve as a pathway for pathological factors like heat, or in more severe conditions, fire. Based on this theory, it makes complete sense that in this case, skin changes such as red skin can be seen along the pathway of the affected channel—the Liver channel—because if stress, overwork, or emotions are involved, the Liver channel is affected most often. Red skin lesions, sometimes warm, burning, and painful, accompanied by itching can be found especially in the upper regions—in this case on the head and face—because of the upward-rising nature of heat. Again, the red color, the warm (or hot) temperature, and burning all indicate excessive heat. Itching is due to internal wind, which is caused by dryness and blood deficiency, because excessive heat consumes the yīn fluids (body fluids) and exhausts qì. The blood becomes deficient, and the skin is no longer supplied with moisture.

In this case, *Dān Zhī Xiāo Yáo Sǎn* with modifications was used to soothe the Liver and clear excess heat, to ensure improvements to her skin condition. Always keep in mind, if a stronger approach is needed, one may use *Lóng Dǎn Xiè Gān Tāng* instead of *Dān Zhī Xiāo Yáo Sǎn*. However, in this case *Dān Zhī Xiāo Yáo Sǎn* was enough. The ingredients and detailed explanation of this formula can be found in Chapter 8, and will not be repeated again at this point. *Huáng qín* was added to increase the heat clearing function of the formula. *Shēng dì huáng* was added because the patient had a dry mouth and felt thirsty: *Shēng dì huáng* clears heat, cools blood and nourishes yīn. Remember that heat always tends to scorch and injure the yīn and body fluids as a consequence. Adding *tiān mén dōng* further increased the yīn and body fluids' nourishing function, in order to help moisten the skin. To reduce itching and calm the Liver, *bái jí lí* in a moderate dosage of 10 g was added. And finally, to maximize the heat clearing action, *pú gōng yīng* was added as well, in a relatively large dosage of 15 g. Considering the patient's current situation, I advised her to pay attention to balancing her emotions as much as possible. She should exercise if she likes in order to move her qì, and thus balance her emotions and reduce stress. I also reminded her to avoid hot and spicy foods. I want to stress that this has to be repeated in clinic again and again. Interestingly, patients often confirm that it is good for them to hear this again, even though they are aware of it deep inside. Sometimes this information is just too well hidden, buried deep because everything else seems to be more important.

Second Visit

The young woman returned to the clinic three weeks later. The eczema lesions had begun to decrease, and the redness on her scalp and face had receded. She reported that her skin wasn't as itchy or painful anymore. Her tongue was less red in color, and her pulse—although still slightly rapid—had begun to be less wiry. However, she said that with the herbs her stool was a little loose and that her bloating persisted.

Formula Modification

To protect the digestive system but continue to clear heat, *mǔ dān pí, zhī zǐ,* and *huáng qín* were used as dry-fried (*chǎo*). *Mǔ dān pí* was reduced to 9 g, *bò hé* to 3 g, and *shēng dì huáng* to 15 g. The patient was advised to continue taking the herbs for another three weeks.

Clinical Course

After another three weeks, her skin had significantly improved. The redness and the itching on her scalp were nearly gone. The skin on her face had completely faded back to its normal color. Her throat didn't feel dry anymore and she was no longer thirsty. She also reported feeling more relaxed than before. She had changed some things; for example, she started exercising again and doing things she liked but hadn't done for a long time. This all helped to improve her mood, but also her skin. Moreover, the bloating and breast distension were gone, and the stool was more normal than before.

The following herbs were taken out: *bái jí lí, tiān mén dōng,* and *pú gōng yīng. Jú huā* was added instead with a dosage of 9 g in order to cool and calm the Liver and protect the face against recurring inflammation.

I advised the patient to take the herbs for another month and to return to the clinic if her skin got worse again—or with any other new complaints.

#3: Female patient, 51 Years Old–Eczema
First Visit

A 51-year-old female patient presented to the practice with eczema on her legs. The skin lesions appeared dark red, were slightly swollen, felt warm and itchy. The patient was in her pre-menopausal phase: in the last six months her periods had become irregular, and when the period did come it was very short with only a little blood. She further reported feeling slightly nervous, experiencing heat sensations (especially at night), but also increasing hot flushes during the day, and stool that was a little dry. She said that her bowel movements were regular, but often dry and it was hard for her to defecate. Looking at her face and her hands, chloasma could be noticed. (Chloasma is often called "age marks" because it frequently appears on women's skin during menopause, when hormonal changes increase the formation of melanin. Strong sun exposure can also trigger chloasma. It is harmless and not clinically relevant, but its presence on the face can impact self-image.) Moreover, her hands were swollen and felt warm, and she told me that her ankles were also occasionally swollen and warm, and taut and painful. Other symptoms were a dry mouth with normal thirst.

The tongue was red and slightly purplish, and showed some cracks. The pulse was thready (thin) and rapid.

TCM Diagnosis

Kidney yīn deficiency with interior heat, combined with blood stasis (*shèn yīn xū nèi rè, yū xuè nèi zǔ* 肾阴虚内热，瘀血内阻).

Treatment Principle

Nourish Kidney yīn, clear heat, invigorate the blood, and remove blood stasis (*zī shèn yīn qīng rè, huó xuè qū yū* 滋肾阴清热，活血祛瘀).

Formula

Modified *Zhī Bǎi Dì Huáng Wán*

shēng dì huáng	Rehmanniae Glutinosae, Radix	30 g
zhī mǔ	Anemarrhenae, Rhizoma	3 g
huáng bǎi	Phellodendri, Cortex	9 g
(chǎo) huáng qín	Scutellariae, Radix (dry-fried)	9 g
mǔ dān pí	Moutan, Cortex	10 g
shān yào	Dioscorea, Rhizome	15 g
zé xiè	Alismatis, Rhizoma	10 g
chē qián zǐ	Plantaginis, Semen	15 g
mǎ chǐ xiàn	Portulacae, Herba	15 g
gān cǎo	Glycyrrhizae Uralensis, Radix	6 g
bái xiān pí	Dictamni Radicis, Cortex	10 g
xú cháng qīng	Cynanchi Paniculati, Radix	12 g
(chǎo) zhī zǐ	Gardeniae, Fructus (dry-fried)	6 g
yě jú huā	Chrysanthemi Indici, Flos	9 g
dì gǔ pí	Lycii, Cortex	15 g

Raw herbs to be taken as a decoction for two-and-a-half weeks, twice a day.

Case Analysis

This 51-year-old female patient was at the typical age when menopause usually begins, if it hasn't already begun. Please keep in mind: although the age of menopause around the world varies, global studies put the age-range of menopause at a mean average of 51 years.[4] However, from the TCM point of view, women's physiology is related to the seven-year cycles, and menopause usually occurs at 49 (7x7). This is very important to remember when talking about women and menopause. According to the classics, all menopausal symptoms are due to the physiological decline of *tiān guǐ* 天癸[5] (heavenly or celestial water of women, as the menstrual period is also called). As *tiān guǐ* derives from the Kidney *jīng*, that means that during the menopause, there is a gradual decline of Kidney *jīng*. Of course, there are always deviations but they will not be discussed here. Finally, due to the decline of Kidney *jīng*, the yīn and yáng of the Kidney becomes unbalanced. Usually, this is accompanied by heat, because the Kidney yīn decreases and yáng is overflowing.

So much for theory! Coming back to our patient and looking at her skin, considering the accompanying symptoms, her tongue and pulse condition, Kidney yīn with internal heat can be concluded. The cracks on her tongue indicate that yīn deficiency was already chronic, i.e., has been present for a long time, and that heat had already consumed yīn and blood, which will always eventually lead to blood stasis. That yīn deficiency had evolved to blood stasis was indicated by the color of her tongue, which was purplish–a clear sign. In order to nourish Kidney yīn and clear heat, the herbal prescription given to this patient was based on the formula *Zhī Bǎi Dì Huáng Wán*. Considering that the eczema was predominantly located on her legs, this formula was a perfect choice as a base because it effectively clears heat mainly located in the lower *jiāo*. Please see Chapter 8 for detailed analysis of this formula.

As *Zhī Bǎi Dì Huáng Wán* was certainly not enough to invigorate the blood and remove blood stasis, the following modifications were given: *huáng qín* (dry-fried) was added to enhance the heat clearing effect. It was used as dry-fried (*chǎo*) in order to reduce its cold properties and make it more tolerable for the digestive system. *Chē qián zǐ* eliminates dampness and drains heat from the lower *jiāo* by promoting urination. It is frequently given with *zé xiè* as a herbal pair for these functions. *Mǎ chǐ xiàn* is a very strong-acting herb, invigorating the blood and dispersing blood stasis, while at the same time it can facilitate urination and thus, resolve oedema. It is said that *mǎ chǐ xiàn* is particularly useful in "breaking up blood stasis…, facilitating dampness… and mainly treating lower body patterns."[6] Thus, it is very useful to treat the eczema on the patient's legs. *Gān cǎo* clears heat, relieves toxicity, and moderates and harmonizes the properties of the other herbs in the formula, which are extremely cooling. *Bái xiān pí* is very often seen in the treatment of eczema and I used it in the treatment of this patient, too, because it is very effective in clearing heat, resolving toxicity, expelling wind, and drying dampness, but also stopping itching. Please keep in mind, it should be used with caution if used for longer periods of time. *Xú cháng qīng* was used in this prescription because it resolves toxicity, dispels wind, and can thus alleviate itching. It is frequently used for this purpose in combination with *bái xiān pí*. *Xú cháng qīng* is, by the way, also very useful in invigorating the blood and reducing oedema, and is–considering all of its powerful actions–often seen in the treatment of stubborn and difficult to treat skin conditions, like chronic eczema or urticaria–imagine a picture of skin with deep red rashes, with itching and pain. *Zhī zǐ* was added in a very low dosage. It drains fire and relieves toxicity, as well as cooling the blood. It was given in its prepared form *chǎo* (dry-fried) to protect the digestive system while still being effective at clearing heat. As you can see, this formula already contains many cold and heat draining herbs, so a dosage at 6 g was enough in this case, and can be given to the patient for a longer period of time, if required. *Zhī zǐ* is also frequently given if the patient tends to feel irritated and nervous, as in this case. *Yě jú huā* increases the heat clearing action of the formula and reduces redness, but it is also good to give *yě jú huā* because of the hot flushes, which tend to make the patient feel warm (hot) on the face. And finally, *dì gǔ pí* was added to the formula in a relatively high dosage (15 g) to tonify yīn, cool blood and clear heat. *Dì gǔ pí* can be frequently seen in combination with *mǔ dān pí* and *shēng dì huáng*. However, using this herb in light dosage would almost certainly not suffice. As there were no oozing lesions, no additional external treatment with Chinese herbs was necessary.

Second Visit

The patient took the first formula daily without a break for two-and-a-half weeks. When I saw her again, the skin on her legs had become less red, warm, and itchy. Her ankles were also less swollen, and consequently didn't feel as painful and tense. The stool was less dry than before, and the heat sensation, both during night and day, began to decline. The swelling on her hands had also reduced, compared to the initial visit just two-and-a-half weeks ago. There were no real changes in her nervousness or chloasma spots, but change was not to be expected after such a short time. In my clinical experience, the treatment of chloasma takes a very long time. As this was not her main complaint, the patient didn't pay much attention to this. She was happy to see that TCM could work on her eczema and improve the pain in her legs and ankles, and also relieve the heat. Her tongue was less purplish in color. The pulse was still thready and rapid, however.

Formula Modification

The dosage of *shēng dì huáng* was reduced to 24 g, *chē qián zǐ* to 12 g, *mǎ chǐ xiàn* to 10 g, and *dì gǔ pí* to 9 g. I told the patient to continue with the herbs for another three weeks, twice a day.

Clinical Course

After taking the herbs for another three weeks, there was another obvious improvement to the eczema on her legs. There was practically no redness, swelling, pain, or itching anymore. Her heat sensations (night and day) markedly improved, presenting mildly from time to time but she said that this was absolutely tolerable for her. Her stool was normal (daily and not dry anymore), and her hands didn't feel swollen or painful. Her dry mouth and thirst also improved, as well as her mood. Finally, her tongue was less red and not purplish anymore. The pulse was still thready and slightly rapid.

The patient was discharged with this prescription:

shēng dì huáng	Rehmanniae Glutinosae, Radix	15 g
zhī mǔ	Anemarrhenae, Rhizoma	3 g
huáng bǎi	Phellodendri, Cortex	3 g
(chǎo) huáng qín	Scutellariae, Radix (dry-fried)	9 g
(chǎo) mǔ dān pí	Moutan, Cortex (dry-fried)	9 g
shān yào	Dioscorea, Rhizome	12 g
zé xiè	Alismatis, Rhizoma	9 g
chē qián zǐ	Plantaginis, Semen	9 g
gān cǎo	Glycyrrhizae Uralensis, Radix	6 g
xú cháng qīng	Cynanchi Paniculati, Radix	9 g
(chǎo) zhī zǐ	Gardeniae, Fructus (dry-fried)	6 g
yě jú huā	Chrysanthemi Indici, Flos	9 g
dì gǔ pí	Lycii, Cortex	6 g
dān shēn	Salviae Miltiorhizae, Radix	12 g

Mǎ chǐ xiàn and *bái xiān pí* were removed, *mǔ dān pí* was changed to *chǎo* (dry-fried) because this is always advisable when taking this herb for a longer period of time; dosages of the other herbs were reduced and *dān shēn* 12 g was added to improve her chloasma spots. I advised her to continue with the herbs for another four weeks, or for longer if her skin showed any discomfort again. She was reminded about the importance of reducing her intake of hot and spicy food, and to go to bed early to protect her yīn. You may have noticed that each patient gets nutritional and lifestyle advice from me, because this is something which they can easily implement at home to support their healing process. Never let a patient go home without reminding them about this!

A final word: although one might assume that the treatment in this case would be difficult, I have to say that such cases are very treatable with TCM. Without exception, I have had good results with women going through menopause, no matter their unique combination of symptoms. So you see, TCM helps the skin, but can also support women during this often challenging time.

#4: Child, Female Patient, Six Years Old–Neurodermatitis (ND)
First Visit

A six-year-old girl presented in the clinic with ND, accompanied by her mother. As I have mentioned before, working with children requires sensitivity as their systems are more delicate–so we must always tread carefully. The ND in her case manifested as a very red, dry, and swollen rash with many cracks on the skin, especially on her arms in the elbow flexures and the wrists. Her main complaint was very severe itching of the skin, especially at night. Moreover, her skin felt very warm and painful. The child could not sleep well, was a little restless during the night (due to both heat in the Heart and the itching), and felt thirsty. She was quite a lively girl during the day too–she could hardly sit still during the consultation. They didn't report any digestive issues, nor a history of common cold. A very important detail for later TCM diagnosis: the first visit took place end of March (Spring).

The tongue body was slightly thick, and showed little red spots on the tip, which was also red. The pulse was slippery and a little rapid.

TCM Diagnosis

Heat Accumulation in the Lung and Heart (*Xīn Fèi Jī Rè* 心肺积热).

Treatment Principle

Clear heat from the Lung and Heart, tonify the Spleen, remove dampness and reduce itching (*qīng xīn fèi zhī rè, jiàn pí, qū shī zhǐ yǎng* 清心肺之热, 健脾, 祛湿止痒).

Formula

huáng qín	Scutellariae, Radix	9 g
jīn yín huā	Lonicerae Japonicae, Flos	9 g
lián qiáo	Forsythiae, Fructus	9 g
(chǎo) huáng bǎi	Phellodendri, Cortex (dry-fried)	6 g
dà qīng yè	Isatidis, Folium	9 g

shēng dì huáng	Rehmanniae Glutinosae, Radix	12 g
lián zǐ	Nelumbinis, Semen	3 g
dì gǔ pí	Lycii, Cortex	9 g
bái sháo	Paeonia Albiflora, Radix	9 g
tiān má	Gastrodiae Elatae, Rhizoma	6 g
gōu téng	Uncariae, Ramulus Cum Uncis	6 g
dēng xīn cǎo	Junci, Medulla	3 g
shān yào	Dioscorea, Rhizome	12 g
jú huā	Chrysanthemi, Flos	10 g
(chǎo) mǔ dān pí	Moutan, Cortex (dry-fried)	6 g

Raw herbs to be taken as a decoction, taken for 14 days, 80–90 ml twice a day.

Case Analysis

First, it has to be said that when working with infants, it's not always easy to get all the information you need. You often have to rely on the parents for help, but sometimes this requires all your professionalism and sensitivity. Fortunately, in this case, the girl's tongue and pulse, combined with the skin's appearance, was sufficient to make a precise diagnosis. A good practitioner has to be able to accurately assess just a few key signs in order to design a beneficial treatment strategy. In those cases—either for severe skin conditions, or when the initial consultation was complex due to insufficient information—it is always recommended to arrange a quick follow-up appointment to check whether your treatment strategy was exact, and which modifications the patient's initial prescription might need.

Following the four main diagnostic methods according to TCM, I drew the following conclusions: the girl's tip of the tongue was red, which showed heat in the Heart but also heat in the Lungs, because the redness reached out into the Lungs' area (the immediate inner area behind the Heart area) as well. Thus, heat had to be cleared from both areas. Considering that the worsening of the skin happened in Spring, it was most likely that wind-heat was involved too. As I have explained earlier in this text, ND flare-ups occur more frequently or get worse in the Spring months. In this case, because this patient's flareup took place in Spring, this led me to suspect an underlying weakness of the Lungs. Another important fact is that, according to the principles of TCM, in children yáng is abundant.

In TCM it is said that "children are the body of pure yáng," with yáng here referring to the vigorous vitality of children's physiology. This means that in children, diseases tend to manifest as a quick, strong response to external pathogens, and they also tend to recover quickly. If wind-heat attacks the Lungs during Spring, the already existing heat in the Heart is stirred up, yáng (heat) becomes even more abundant, and skin rashes appear. (Note: remember, lesions on the arms are called "four bends of wind," after the lesions typical to ND in the arm flexure.) Examining the girl's pulse, I noticed dampness which, on the one hand, has to be drained and, on the other, can also be addressed by strengthening the Spleen.

The formula given to this child was based on Sān Xīn Dǎo Chì Yǐn with modifications, which has already been discussed in Chapter 6. The analysis of the basic formula will not be repeated at this point. In addition, jīn yín huā was included to clear heat from the Lungs and resolve toxicity. Jú huā was used to further boost the heat-clearing and toxicity-relieving effect, but also to subdue rising heat. Both light herbs are very suitable for children because they look nice while being very effective. Huáng bǎi, cool and bitter in nature, clears heat, drains fire, and directs it downward. Because the skin lesions on the arms were markedly fresh red, dà qīng yè was used. This herb is useful to clear heat, cool and regulate blood, and reduce inflammatory responses. Dà qīng yè is, by the way, often used in cases of severe heat with inflammation, for example, sore throat, mouth ulcers, erysipelas, and other skin eruptions. But be careful: don't use this herb for too long and in too large dosages, especially in children, because dà qīng yè is bitter and very cold. It is sometimes too harsh for children's digestive systems, but even in adults it should be used with care when the Spleen and Stomach are weakened. As soon as it isn't needed anymore, reduce the dosage or take it out. Dì gǔ pí clears heat and cools the Lungs. It is sweet and bland in taste and, thus, relatively tolerable even for small children. Bái sháo nourishes the (Liver) blood and has astringent properties for the yīn. Keep in mind, when blood is deficient due to reduced blood storage in the Liver, other important "blood organs" can be affected.[7] As the child in this case was irritable and restless at night, it was most suitable to nourish and calm the Heart by building up the Liver blood. Moreover, don't forget that wind-heat may injure the Lung yīn, thus, nourishing and restraining the yīn helps to prevent disharmonies due to yīn deficiency. For insomnia, disturbed and restless sleep, tiān má and gōu téng were added in order to sedate yáng. This herbal combination is able to calm the Liver and extinguish wind, which should help to reduce the itching at night, too. To strengthen the Spleen, *shān yào* was given. When the Spleen is working properly, dampness can be transformed and transported adequately. Finally, for the red skin rash with extreme pruritus, *mŭ dān pí* was added. It cools blood and clears heat as well as moving blood and transforming stasis. Don't forget that extreme heat exhausts yīn and blood, which leads to blood stasis in the long term. Thus, preventing blood stasis is an aspect that should never be forgotten.

You may have noticed that the dosages are relatively light because, as mentioned earlier in this book, this is the recommended approach for children and infants. When working with adults, increase the dosages accordingly. The herbs *huáng băi* and *mŭ dān pí* were used as *chăo* (dry-fried), which will make them more tolerable for the digestive system. When treating adults, I would have also recommended using *huáng lián*, but in children, it is most likely too bitter. Thus, herbs like *lián zĭ* are more suitable for cooling. *Lián zĭ* can cool the heart and quiet the spirit but also tastes very nice.

Second Visit

The family returned to the practice about two weeks later. The child's skin had improved slightly. It was no longer so intensely red, and the itching was somewhat reduced, but the girl was still very restless. The mother reported that it was somewhat difficult for the child to drink the decoction: she didn't enjoy the taste, so it was hard to get her to take it regularly. So, an external application with Chinese herbs was added to speed up the healing process of the skin. Some would think that granules are the better choice in this case, but I don't think so: the taste is equally bad, but the effectiveness is reduced. Therefore, the mother was instructed to use the external treatment either as a cold wet compress, or to dab the skin with a soaked cotton ball several times a day. (Please see earlier in the book for instructions for this process.) I told her that she should continue to give the herbal decoctions to the child as often as possible. She was asked to continue with the herbs for another two weeks, and then come back to see me. Now it was time to see how the girl's skin continued to react with the additional application of the herbs from the outside.

Formula Modification

Huáng qín was changed to *chăo* (dry-fried), (*chăo*) *mŭ dān pí* was increased to 9 g, and *gān căo* 3 g and (*chăo*) *zhī zĭ* 9 g were added.

As external treatment, the following combination was prescribed: jīn yín huā 10 g, *pú gōng yīng* 10 g, *lián qiáo* 10 g, *yě jú huā* 10 g, to be boiled with about 350 ml water and used as a wet compress once or twice a day, depending on the frequency the child tolerates. If this was not feasible, the parents were instructed to repeatedly dab the areas, let them dry and dab them again, using gauze or cotton balls. This could make wet compresses more tolerable.

Clinical Course

The child returned to the practice after another two weeks. The skin on her arms had improved significantly. There was hardly any redness visible and the itching was significantly reduced too. The child was sleeping better and did not wake up due to itching as frequently. She was no longer so restless. I once again talked to the parents about proper skin care, and which foods to avoid or consume. Please see earlier in this book for detailed information on dietary advice. The child was provided with herbs for another two-and-a-half weeks. *Dà qīng yè, tiān má,* and *gōu téng* were removed from the prescription. The external application was also to be continued until the skin had healed completely. The same external herbal combination was prescribed for another two weeks and I asked them to come in or give me a call when they needed more herbs for preparing the external application—or should the child need an additional follow-up.

#5: Female Patient, 20 Years Old– Neurodermatitis (ND)

First Visit

A young woman, aged 20, presented at my practice for treatment of her ND–a typical case. Her skin was very dry, slightly red, and very itchy, which was her main burden. She said that the itching was present both day and night, but most severe at night. The itching would often wake her at night and, therefore, she was also feeling a little tired. Signs of ND were present on her face, around the mouth and neck. Her mouth and lips were very dry, the latter also chapped. Because the mouth felt so dry, she also felt thirsty, constantly wanting to moisten the mouth. This young woman had experienced a lot of allergies since infancy. She reported house dust allergies, hay fever, and many allergies/intolerances to certain foods. She had a sallow complexion, was very slim and, due to the many intolerances, she couldn't eat everything she wanted to. While all her friends could eat out at restaurants, she has always had to be careful. Her stool was regular but a little dry. She was taking the contraceptive pill and reported very light menstruation, with regular but short bleeding: just three days, using two to three tampons maximum a day, which is far too little for a young woman of her age. Please keep in mind that while being on the pill, women usually have just a "withdrawal bleed" during the time when the active hormonal pill is paused. In my experience, the period becomes fuller when off the pill. However, in addition, she reported having dry and brittle fingernails, very dry skin over the entire body, and also very dry hair. Looking at her, she seemed very calm on the outside, however she complained about often feeling nervous and restless. Furthermore, she said that she could not sleep well, waking up often during the night due to the itching. Generally, it must be said that she seemed a rather sensitive patient and very fragile; the kind of person who is sensitive on a physical but also on an emotional level. For example, if she used paper towels or napkins, she would very quickly get skin rashes and the skin would itch. These products often contain a lot of chemicals, which the patient is often not aware of. I informed her that it was always best to use cotton as a towel, handkerchief, or napkin. Regarding her emotional sensitivity, she described herself as someone who thinks about everything, and cannot take anything lightly.

Her tongue was pale with a normal coating and the pulse was thin.

TCM Diagnosis
Blood Deficiency and Wind Dryness (*Xuè Xū Fēng Zào* 血虚风燥).

Treatment Principle
Nourish blood and yīn, calm down wind, stop itching and moisten the skin (*zī yīn yǎng xuè ān shén, zhǐ yǎng rùn fū* 滋阴养血安神，止痒润肤).

Formula

shēng dì huáng	Rehmanniae Glutinosae, Radix	15 g
gān cǎo	Glycyrrhizae Uralensis, Radix	9 g
xià kū cǎo	Spica Prunellae Vulgaris	9 g
shí gāo	Gypsum Fibrosum	15 g
xuán shēn	Scrophulariae Ningpoensis, Radix	9 g
tiān mén dōng	Asparagi, Radix	9 g

shān yào	Dioscorea, Rhizome	15 g
dà zǎo	Jujubae, Fructus	12 g
bò hé	Menthae, Herba	3 g
dì gǔ pí	Lycii, Cortex	15 g
dāng guī	Angelicae Sinensis, Radix	10 g
yù zhú	Polygonati Odorati, Rhizoma	9 g

Raw herbs to be taken as a decoction for 14 days, 110–120 ml twice a day.

Case Analysis

This was a classic case of ND, one often seen in practice. This young woman was not in an acute phase at the time, which was evident from the fact that the skin was not bright and intense red. However, she said that she gets short flare-ups with red and warm skin developing, especially on the face and neck, when she is stressed or upset. Otherwise, she presented with the usual symptoms of blood deficiency with dryness according to TCM: dry and itchy skin, dry hair, dry mouth, thirst, dry and brittle fingernails, sallow complexion, and scanty periods, just to name a few. Combined with her tongue and pulse condition, it was relatively easy to diagnose this TCM pattern: blood deficiency and wind dryness. Keep in mind that blood nourishes and moistens the skin, and blood deficiency can be at the root of many skin diseases. In this context, as already explained, when blood is deficient it often gives rise to "wind" (and dryness) and its manifestations are itching, and dry and scaly skin lesions, which become tight and easily crack. Why? Because the skin is no longer adequately nourished and dries out.

Another aspect I saw as detrimental for this young woman was her being on the contraceptive pill. Besides the fact that the pill is not a lifestyle drug, I explained to this young woman that from a TCM point of view we are looking at the health of the whole body. First, according to TCM the Liver is the main organ system responsible for the menstrual cycle. TCM recognizes the negative impact of hormones on the Liver function to be huge, as they suppress its functions over time. Secondly, the same applies for the blood. The longer a woman takes the pill, the more the blood will stagnate. As this young woman had been diagnosed with blood deficiency already, blood stagnation is even more likely, which would certainly make her skin worsen over time. It's kind of a vicious cycle. If there is little blood, it can easily stagnate. And conversely, if blood stagnation is already present, blood is being used up more and more. I advised her that she should think twice about continuing on the pill for the benefit of her skin, but also for the future, when she might want to have children (which she said she wanted–not now, but most certainly later).

In this case, a modified herbal prescription was given in which several basic formulas were combined: components of *Xiāo Fēng Sǎn, Sì Wù Xiāo Fēng Yǐn,* and *Zēng Yè Tāng* were used, aiming to nourish blood and yīn, calm down wind to stop itching, and to nurture and moisten the skin. Please see earlier in this book for detailed information about the ingredients of these formulas and exact formula analysis. In addition to these, *xià kū cǎo* was added to cool and disperse; useful here because the young patient had complained about nervousness, restlessness, and sleeplessness, but its yīn and blood nourishing functions were also beneficial in this case. Although opinions differ on these latter functions of *xià kū cǎo*, according to Zhū Dān-Xī, it nourishes the yīn and blood of the Liver.[8] When the Liver is deficient, yáng (heat) can rise and make the skin worse. From my clinical point of view, *xià kū cǎo* has shown very good results. If you recall that I mentioned earlier in this book that the neck represents the Liver area, the usage of this herb makes a lot of sense when the skin looks red. Remember, this young woman was mainly affected by ND on her face, around the mouth and neck. Let's move forward to *tiān mén dōng* in this prescription. Sweet and cold in nature, it enriches the yīn, clears heat, generates fluids, and thus moistens. Combined with *shēng dì huáng* and *xuán shēn* it acts to strongly tonify yīn. Together with *dāng guī*, it's beneficial for the patient's deficient blood, as well as improving her dry stools. Taking all the herbs together, the dryness on her skin, mouth and lips would certainly improve, and her stools would be moistened. Nearly the same actions apply for *yù zhú. Yù zhú,* sweet and slightly cold, is also able to nourish yīn and moisten dryness. In clinic, it is often used in combination with *shēng dì huáng* for this purpose. Although *shān yào* has a wide range of benefits, it was used in this particular prescription to improve the function of the Spleen. In order to produce blood, the Spleen must function properly. Keep in mind: the Spleen is responsible for making the blood, and the Spleen qì keeps the blood within the vessels. It is so important when talking about blood and the skin, but also, in this case, the young woman's menstruation (short periods with only a scanty amount of blood). *Shān yào* would certainly also help with this. Considering that this was a young woman with a somewhat weak constitution and many allergies and intolerances to foods, it was even more appropriate to strengthen her Spleen. Remember: The Spleen is responsible for producing the person's power, the qì. As the source of "post-heavenly" qì, it plays an important role in a person's acquired constitution and can also be considered as the person's immune system– looking at it from the Western medicine point of view. Thus, boosting this young woman was certainly a good idea for many of her complaints–her skin, her constitution, and gynaecological aspects, for instance. Finally, dì gǔ pí was added to the prescription in a relatively high dosage (15 g) to tonify yīn and clear heat due to deficient blood.

Second Visit

The young woman returned to the clinic two weeks later. The ND lesions had begun to decrease, and the redness on her face and neck had receded. She reported that her skin wasn't as itchy anymore, and that the thirst wasn't as obvious. Her sleep was slightly improved because her skin was less itchy. Thus, she also felt slightly stronger in her energy and was able to manage her day better. Despite this improvement, she still wanted me to work on her sleep and consolidate, as she felt so much better when sleeping more soundly.

She had one incident to report: some stress with her boyfriend, after which she felt a worsening of the skin on her face for a few days, becoming red and feeling very warm. This had dissolved again, but she wanted to report it because she saw the clear connection herself. Her tongue was only slightly pale and looked healthier. The pulse was still thin.

Formula Modification

To improve her sleep but also build up the blood, thus also working on reducing the itchiness and scaling of her skin, yè jiāo téng 20 g was added. As mentioned earlier in this book, it can calm the spirit and reduce itching due to dryness and blood deficiency, especially at night. When patients don't scratch as much, sleep is bound to improve. Shí gāo was removed, and jú huā 9 g was added to reduce redness on her face due to emotional stress, which also tends to make the patient feel warmth on the face. She was advised to continue taking the herbs for another three weeks.

Clinical Course

After taking the herbs for another three weeks, the young woman's skin condition continued to stabilize. As reported before, she was having difficulties and arguments with her boyfriend from time to time. Thus, I made the following adjustments to the next prescription: *shēng dì huáng* was reduced to 12 g, *gān cǎo* to 6 g, *xià kū cǎo* to 6 g, *dì gǔ pí* was removed, and *chái hú* 6 g was added. The patient was advised to take the herbs for another month. Please note, this would be a typical case where I would have given acupuncture in addition to the herbs; however, since the patient was in training and couldn't afford additional acupuncture, costs and benefits had to be weighed in the patient's interest. And since herbs were the most important and effective part of her therapy, I stuck to this treatment course. Importantly, these kinds of decisions also help build patient trust.

I treated this young woman with Chinese herbs for another six months. I had told her from the beginning that the treatment would take longer because she had had ND since childhood. Such diseases always take longer to treat—therefore what we achieved during this short period was remarkable. Because of her sensitivity to so many substances, I gave her my CHINAMED COSMETICS® face cream, created with Chinese herbs and based on the principles of TCM, so that she could create a daily skincare routine that was right for her skin type. She had previously complained that she had spent so much time and money on expensive cosmetic products, but couldn't tolerate any of them, often developing allergic reactions. You would be surprised how many of my patients bring a bag full of creams and other products to their first consultation and ask for my advice on which ones to use. It is clearly an essential part of any good TCM dermatology consultation to advise patients on what products are good for their skin. And how wonderful is this? We can help patients with Chinese herbs from the inside and outside! Now, this young patient comes back to my practice whenever her skin gets worse, or with any other new complaints.

#6: Female patient, 49 Years Old– Neurodermatitis (ND)

First Visit

A 49-year-old woman with ND presented in my practice, complaining about chronic ND lesions on her neck and elbows. The skin lesions were dark in color because they had been there for a very long time. In general, the skin was itchy and, due to scratching, the skin had become very thick and leathery. The skin on her face was very dry and felt taut, with some slightly red areas. The patient reported that, due to having suffered from

ND for so many years and experiencing bad reactions from cosmetic products, she only showered once a week, otherwise only practicing light hygiene with pure water without any products on her body and face. In my opinion, her skin was too dry and tight. I explained to her that moisturizing her face would be beneficial: The skin has to be well nourished and moisturized, otherwise it has a tendency to tear or crack. Nevertheless, it is completely understandable why this woman was so careful with showering and using products, especially after so many bad experiences and aggravations due to certain cosmetics. For me, it was important to allay her fear and worries, but also to inform her in detail on how to best practice skin hygiene, including pros and cons of a good skincare routine with light products on her face.

Appropriate skin hygiene in such a case of ND: Don't shower too often, and don't have showers that are too hot and too long. Use only lukewarm water to wash, and if the lesions are on the face and neck, avoid these areas as much as possible. Moisten them with water only briefly. Patients can also wash their hair upside down. (Strangely enough, many people have forgotten that they could do this.) Use only mild and natural skincare products without aggressive agents and alcohol—but use something to moisten the skin!

Interestingly, this woman had ND lesions on her earlobes too. Both earlobes appeared slightly red, swollen, and felt warm. The lesions were thick and crusted because they often oozed with a yellowish liquid; and, of course, they felt painful. I noticed that, even during our conversation, she kept touching her earlobes frequently and scratching them. The patient reported that her earlobes had been affected for several years, and that nothing had helped until now. Of course, she had almost always been prescribed cortisone ointments by conventional medicine dermatologists. Everything only helped for a short time, and after a certain period it did not help at all. The patient had come to the point where she no longer wanted to use cortisone ointment because her skin was becoming more and more irritated, more and more sensitive, and also very thin. She had the feeling that it was time for her to go in a different direction and look for a natural medicine that works gently but effectively.

Other symptoms included: Occasional heat sensations on her head/face, restlessness occurring now and then, a dry mouth and dry lips, and occasional thirst but not significant. Her bowel movements were relatively regular and only sometimes dry; her periods were regular but short with no significant discomfort. It is worth mentioning that the patient appeared very calm on the outside, but when asked–which I always do to assess the patients' living situation–she told me that she was experiencing a lot of stress at work, and even making appointments outside of work hours was not always easy for her. She constantly had the feeling that there was not enough time. Furthermore, she complained about increased fatigue recently, despite relatively normal sleeping patterns.

Her tongue was thick and swollen, red/purplish with a slightly thick, yellow coating at the root of the tongue. The pulse was deep and wiry.

TCM Diagnosis
Damp-Heat attacks the Skin (*shī rè yùn fū* 湿热蕴肤).

Treatment Principle
Clear Heat, drain dampness, and stop itching (*qīng rè lì shī zhǐ yǎng* 清热利湿止痒).

Formula

shí chāng pú	Acori Tatarinowii, Rhizoma	9 g
fú líng	Poriae Cocos, Sclerotium	12 g
zé xiè	Alismatis, Rhizoma	12
bái máo gēn	Imperatae, Rhizoma	15 g
dì fū zǐ	Kochiae Scopariae, Fructus	15 g
huáng bǎi	Phellodendri, Cortex	9 g
cāng zhú	Atractylodis, Rhizoma	9 g
bái xiān pí	Dictamni Radicis, Cortex	12 g
bái jí lí	Tribuli Terristris, Fructus	12 g
yì yǐ rén	Coices, Semen	15 g
Liù Yī Sǎn	Six-to-One Powder	15 g
tǔ fú líng	Smilacis Glabrae, Rhizoma	30 g

Raw herbs to be taken as a decoction for 14 days, 120 ml twice a day.

Case Analysis

This was long-term ND. The woman had been suffering from the skin disease all her life, showing in the thick and leathery structure of her skin. This is usually the result of constant scratching or rubbing over the years. Let's analyze this case step by step: The redness and oozing of her skin showed heat combined with dampness. There were occasional heat sensations on her head/face, restlessness occurring now and then, a dry mouth and dry lips because of the heat, yet the woman had no increased thirst or desire to drink because of the existing dampness. Her bowels were sometimes dry, again from the heat. Her tongue was thick and swollen, which indicated Spleen deficiency and dampness, with a slightly thick, yellow coating at the root of the tongue, which indicated dampness and internal heat (mainly in the lower *jiāo*, which is represented by the root of the tongue in TCM). Her pulse could only be felt at the deep level and felt wiry, which means that dampness was obstructing the channels and impairing the flow of qì and blood. When qì and blood cannot circulate properly, the pulse feels wiry (tense). All in all, considering her tongue and pulse condition, in combination with the skin appearance and other symptoms, damp-heat was diagnosed. The thickness of the tongue coating showed that heat was predominant. The redness of the tongue's body indicated heat, too, but the color was already turning purplish, which proved that yīn and/or blood had started to be consumed and blood stasis was already present. In this case, this most probably happened because damp, if stored in the body for a long period and left untreated, transforms into damp-heat, the resulting heat (fire) damages fluids and later on, blood stagnates. It takes a long time, but this process is very common in such a case. Please note, the transition between these patterns or stages is fluid. Thus, the treatment strategy is not just clearing heat and eliminating dampness, but also strengthening the Spleen, which is responsible for transforming, transporting and eliminating dampness (always consider the Spleen when treating dampness), and moving blood to prevent blood stagnation. And finally, the itching, which this patient had been suffering from for so long, had to be stopped.

The herbal combination was based on *Chú Shī Wèi Líng Tāng*. Please see pages 108–11 for a detailed list of ingredients and formula analysis. Only five herbs from this formula were used: *fú líng, zé xiè, cāng zhú,* and *Liù Yī Sǎn,* comprising *huá shí* and *gān cǎo* in a ratio of 6:1 and 15 g of the powder in total. *Shí chāng pú* was added to transform dampness and strengthen the Spleen. As it also moves qì and blood, it can work to reduce the obstruction in the channels and improve circulation. *Bái máo gēn* was added to clear heat and cool the blood, and as previously mentioned, it cools without any risk that it might injure the yīn or cause accumulation or stagnation. Because the patient's skin was very itchy, *dì fū zǐ* and *bái xiān pí* were added. Both herbs are very effective in clearing damp-heat and stopping itching. *Huáng bǎi* clears heat but also strongly drains fire and directs it downward. As I have already mentioned, it is particularly good when heat is located in the lower *jiāo*. You have probably seen *bái jí lí* quite frequently in this text and in the treatment of eczema and ND–this herb is used to reduce itching. *Yì yǐ rén* is frequently used to strengthen the Spleen, promote urination, and leach out dampness. It also clears heat and damp-heat, often used in combination with *huáng bǎi*, as seen in the formula Bì Xiè Shèn Shī Tāng. (By the way, when taking a closer look at our current herbal combination, five herbs of *Bì Xiè Shèn Shī Tāng* can also be identified: *huáng bǎi, yì yǐ rén, fú líng, zé xiè*, and *huá shí*. Interesting, isn't it?) Finally, *tǔ fú líng* was added to increase the heat-clearing action and reduce redness, but also to reduce exudation on her earlobes.

The patient was informed to stop–or at least heavily restrict–consumption of coffee, as well as oily and spicy food. She should preferably eat mildly spiced food, and steam food instead of roasting or frying in excess oil. I didn't need to warn her about alcohol and cigarettes, because this woman did not drink or smoke. I advised her to come back to my practice after two weeks.

Second Visit

The patient returned to my practice two weeks later. The ND lesions on her neck had begun to decrease, the color of the skin on her neck had started to fade to normal and the skin wasn't as itchy anymore. The lesions on her elbows also started to improve, but the most striking result was the improvement of her earlobes. After all these years of suffering, they began to heal and were not so painful anymore. For the first visit after drinking herbal decoctions for only two weeks, this was a very good result. Her tongue looked nearly the same as before, but the coating was slightly thinner. The pulse was still deep and tense.

Formula Modification

As the skin condition had lasted for so long, and as the color of her tongue had not improved significantly after two weeks, we continued to focus on healing her skin, but also started to work more on the blood aspect. *Shēng dì huáng* 12 g, *mǔ dān pí* 9 g, and *dān shēn* 9 g were added. The former clears heat, cools blood, and nourishes yīn. *Mǔ dān pí* and *dān shēn* cool and invigorate the blood. To reduce the thick and leathery skin lesions, the blood must also be moved. If you decide to just use one of the herbs, use either *mǔ dān pí* or *dān shēn* with a dosage of 12–15 g. The dosages of *bái máo gēn* and *dì fū zǐ* were reduced to 12 g. The patient was advised to take the herbs for another three weeks and then come back to see me.

Third Visit

After taking the herbs for another three weeks, the woman's skin condition continued to stabilize. The elbows looked really good, and her neck showed significant improvement. Her earlobes also looked better than three weeks before, and I was convinced that they could heal completely if she were to take the herbs regularly. I made the following adjustments to the next prescription: *shí chāng pú* was decreased to 6 g, *gān cǎo* was increased to 6 g, and *huá shí* was taken out; bái máo gēn and *dì fū zǐ* were reduced to 9 g, *bái jí lí* to 9 g. *Bái xiān pí* was taken out and *tǔ fú líng* was reduced to 15 g. *Mǔ dān pí* was changed to *chǎo* (dry-fried) because this was intended for longer term use. *Xuán shēn* 9 g was mainly added to soften hardness, which is useful because her skin was hardened after long-term disease. As she repeatedly shared that she had a lot of stress at work, *chái hú* 3 g was added to move qì. *Jú huā* was included to continue working on her facial skin. The patient was advised to take the herbs for another month.

Clinical Course

After one more month, her elbows and neck appeared nearly normal and the good news: Her earlobes looked very good, too. Her tongue was not as red and purple anymore; and her pulse was not as deep and tense as before. I prescribed another herbal combination for another month with the following modifications: *shí chāng pú, bái máo gēn, dì fū zǐ, bái jí lí,* and *yì yǐ rén* were taken out. *Huáng bǎi* and *cāng zhú* were reduced to 6 g, *fú líng* and *zé xiè* to 9 g. *Dāng guī* 9 g was added to help tonify and invigorate the blood. *Shān yào* 12 g was added to strengthen the Spleen.

I treated this woman with Chinese herbs for about one year. I saw her every six weeks, and prescribed her new herbal prescriptions as required. No matter the taste, she was happy to take them, because she was so happy to discontinue the cortisone treatments (which she did, by the way, from the beginning of our TCM treatment). There were no more oozing and painful earlobes, and her overall skin condition was very stable. Like the previous young female patient, I gave her my CHINAMED COSMETICS® face cream and she is now using it as her daily skincare to moisturize her face and neck. I advised her to return to my practice whenever her skin got worse, or whenever she felt she wanted to see me.

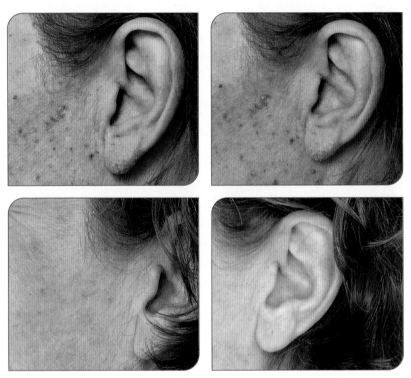

The improvement of the patient's skin on the earlobes.

Endnotes

1   www.drugs.com/sfx/torsemide-side-effects.html

2   Pharmacology is a medical discipline that deals with the interactions between exogenous substances and the body. Among other things, it deals with the nature of drug effects on the body, i.e. the biochemical and physiological effects on the organism, but it also advises on toxicology, which means it diagnoses and treats poisoning and carries out toxicological consultations.

3   *Xuè Fǔ Zhú Yū Tāng: táo rén, hóng huā, dāng guī, chuān xiōng, chì sháo, niú xī, chái hú, jié gěng, zhǐ ké, shēng dì huáng, gān cǎo.*

4   Vatankhah, H., Khalili, P., Vatanparast, M., et al. (2023) "Prevalence of early and late menopause and its determinants in Rafsanjan cohort study." *Scientific Reports* 13, 1847.

5 The classics say: *tiān guǐ* arrives when the girl is 14 (7×2) and it dries up when the woman is 49 (7×7).

6 Bensky, D., Clavey, S., and Stöger, E. (2004) *Materia Medica* (3rd Ed.). Seattle, WA: Eastland Press, p.192.

7 Bensky, D., Clavey, S., and Stöger, E. (2004) *Materia Medica* (3rd Ed.). Seattle, WA: Eastland Press, pp.753–754.

8 Bensky, D., Clavey, S., and Stöger, E. (2004) *Materia Medica* (3rd Ed.). Seattle, WA: Eastland Press, p.102.

Afterword

IN THIS BOOK, I have shared with you my many years of experience in treating patients with eczema and ND with Chinese herbal medicine. My hope is that you will bring the book's knowledge to life and apply it in your daily practice. That, indeed, would be a great gift, for that is why I have written it. I hope it enables you to help even the most challenging skin patients and to share the wisdom of TCM ever more widely in the world. And believe me, every patient will drink Chinese herbal decoctions if they really want to heal. If a patient refuses the treatment, then their disease is not severe enough. Always remember: medicine doesn't have to taste good, it has to work. Wishing you all the best on your path.

Sabine Schmitz
June 2023

Appendix I: The External Treatment of Eczema with Chinese Herbal Medicine

Welcome to Appendix I. This section provides you with a brief outline of TCM external treatment options for eczema and ND. While these external treatments are referred to throughout the book according to TCM syndrome in eczema, and skin appearance for ND, for the sake of simplicity the formulas are listed alphabetically here. I will describe to you in detail how to prepare them yourself, and this can also serve as useful background information to share with your patients if they are preparing them for themselves, or with collaborating TCM pharmacies, assuming all the herbs are available.

At this point it is important to mention that all suggestions given in this appendix serve as a practical orientation. Don't stick to the exact prescriptions, be flexible! Different formulas can be used for various TCM patterns. The dosages and combinations can always be adjusted, and multiple forms of treatment can be applied in the same session. Everything is described in a comprehensive and in a practical way. I'm sure you will find this easy to do yourself.

Bài Jiàng Cǎo Gāo (White Flower Patrinia Ointment)

bài jiàng cǎo	Patriniae, Herba	100 g

Overview and Functions

This formula has been mentioned in the *Zhào Bǐng-Nán Lín Chuáng Jīng Yàn Jí* (Zhào Bǐng-Nán's Clinical Experience Set, Vol. 2),[1] written by Zhào Bǐng-Nán.[2] Prof. Zhào worked extensively on creating new treatment options for many patients with various skin conditions, including, but not limited to, eczema and ND. The work of Prof. Zhào has greatly benefited Chinese dermatology. *Bài Jiàng Cǎo Gāo* is particularly useful for wounds that are slow to heal. It detoxifies, clears heat, expels pus, dries dampness, and reduces swelling. When inflammation is reduced, the skin can heal faster and the skin's appearance improves. Please note that the original text mentions ancient Chinese units of measurement and uses different amounts and boiling times, as well as using a paste mixed with honey. The method mentioned immediately below is the preparation method I would use to treat eczema.

Preparation

For application, soak 100–150 g washed *bài jiàng cǎo* in 1 litre of water for about 30 minutes. If you want to work with a more concentrated liquid, use less water and vice versa, if you want to work more mildly, use more water. After soaking, bring the herb to a boil over mild heat for approximately 20–30 minutes, filter off the herb-infused water and allow to cool. Apply as a (cold) wet compress or wash to the affected area two times a day, for about 15–30 minutes each time.

Please note: When using a wet compress or wash, the liquid should not be used for more than a week because after that it is no longer fresh. The effectiveness is certainly reduced and the risk of contamination increases. Patients should work cleanly and with care, avoiding touching the rim of the bottle while storing the liquid and only use liquids once, pouring out the daily "dose" and discarding after use on the skin. Concentrates can be diluted a little and should be stored in the refrigerator, of course.

Bái Zhú Gāo (White Atractylodis Ointment)

| *bái zhú* | Atractylodis Macrocephalae, Rhizoma | 100 g |

Overview and Functions

Yet another simple formula that has been mentioned by Zhào Bǐng-Nán in his *Zhào Bǐng-Nán Lín Chuáng Jīng Yàn Jí: Bái Zhú Gāo*. It consists of only one herb: *bái zhú* with the function of strengthening the Spleen and removing dampness. This formula treats eczema with stubborn dampness, but also chronic ulcers in the lower extremities (the original text mentions knee sores in particular), and blisters on hands and feet–just to name a few cases in which it can be used. In this case too, while the original text mentions ancient Chinese units of measurement and different amounts, using a paste mixed with honey, I have listed the amounts I would use in the treatment of eczema.

Preparation

Soak *bái zhú* 100 g in 1 litre of water for 20 minutes. Simmer slowly for approximately 6–7 hours to condense the liquid, filter off and mix with honey to form a thick ointment, and then let it cool for topical application. Apply the ointment twice a day to the affected areas. The original text asks for honey, but I tend to use it with sesame oil as a wash or wet compress when the skin oozes and becomes encrusted. When making an oil-based ointment, grind *bái zhú* 10 g to a fine powder and soak it in 100–150 ml of sesame oil for at least 24 hours. Bring to a boil over mild heat to dissolve the ingredients, filter off the herb-infused sesame oil, and then allow to cool. Apply the ointment once or twice a day to the affected areas of the skin. The instructions are for 100 ml oil, but all proportions can be changed as needed. If a thicker consistency is required, just melt a very small amount of beeswax (no more than a teaspoonful) into the prepared ointment. To prepare a herbal wash or wet compress, soak the ingredients in 850 ml of water for 20 minutes. Simmer slowly for approximately 20 minutes, strain the liquid and let it cool. Wash the affected area with the herbal liquid or apply a wet compress to the skin lesions twice a day, for about 15–30 minutes each time.

Cāng Ěr Yāng Shuǐ Jì (Cang Er Yang Wash)

cāng ěr yāng	Xanthii, Germen	50 g
kǔ shēn	Sophorae Flavescentis, Radix	50 g
mǎ chǐ xiàn	Portulacae, Herba	50 g
bài jiàng cǎo	Patriniae, Herba	25 g
chǔ táo yè	Morus Papyrifera, Folium	50 g

Overview and Functions

This formula originated from the book *Zhāng Zhì-Lǐ Pí Fū Bìng Yī Àn Xuǎn Cuì* (A Collection of Zhang Zhì-Lǐ's Medical Experience in Dermatology), written by the famous Chinese TCM dermatologist Zhāng Zhì-Lǐ. It clears heat, reduces swelling, stops itching, and astringes. Zhāng Zhì-Lǐ and Zhào Bǐng-Nán frequently mention this formula in the treatment of ND.

Let me first explain in detail the herbs *cāng ěr yāng* and *chǔ táo yè* which are listed in the original formula. Some of you might have never heard of either of these herbs before. While *cāng ěr zǐ* is the fruit of the plant (cocklebur), *cāng ěr yāng* means seedlings or stems and leaves according to the literal meaning. Based on my research, it is more likely to be the vine of the plant, which is clearly different from *cāng ěr zǐ*. It is bitter, slightly cold, and slightly toxic. It dispels wind, clears heat, detoxifies, and was mainly used for the treatment of rheumatism, paralysis, and pain in the extremities and other syndromes, but also for itching skin. However, the *yāng* part is not used anymore and is unavailable in TCM pharmacies. I suggest using *cāng ěr cǎo* instead, as it fulfils similar functions. While some might think it is the same herb or part of the plant, it is not. *Cāng ěr cǎo* is the entire plant, is acrid, bitter, slightly cold, and toxic. It dispels wind, clears heat, resolves toxins, and kills parasites. Let's come to the other rarely heard of herb: *chǔ táo yè*. My research has revealed that *chǔ táo yè* are the leaves of the paper mulberry (Broussonetia Papyrifera, syn. Morus Papyrifera L.), one species of the family Moraceae.[3] The leaves may be lobed or unlobed, but they are usually tri-lobed and have toothed edges. The upper part is dark green, covered with coarse hair, and the lower part is grey-green, densely covered with hair. Compared to the leaves of Morus alba, which are heart-shaped, the shape of the leaves is completely different, but the fruits of the paper mulberry are also entirely different in character. These are red or orange in color and are round, rather than oval. Based on their appearance, you can't confuse the fruits and leaves of the paper white mulberry with the mulberry tree, which most of us know and use nowadays in TCM. The following functions are attributed to *chǔ táo yè*: clear heat, resolve toxicity, kill insects, dispel wind, and relieve itching. These leaves are also not available in TCM pharmacies nowadays. As a substitute, *sāng yè*, the leaves of the white mulberry tree, would certainly not be enough. I suggest either increasing the dosages of the other ingredients or adding herbs such as *pú gōng yīng* and/or *yě jú huā* instead. This is an example that shows that you can work with ancient formulas even if some ingredients are unavailable and/or no longer in use.

Preparation

For a herbal wash or wet compress, soak the ingredients in 1.5 liters of water for 20 minutes. Simmer slowly for approximately 20 minutes, strain the liquid and let it cool for topical application. Wash the affected area or apply a wet compress to the skin lesions two to three times a day for about 15–30 minutes each time. This combination can also be used as an oil-based ointment. I suggest using sesame oil. Grind the ingredients to a fine powder and mix them thoroughly. Soak the herbs in a proportion of about 1:4 in sesame oil for about 24–48 hours, bring it to a boil over mild heat, filter off the herb-infused sesame oil and allow to gel. It can be mixed with a small amount of beeswax before applying to the skin to make a thicker ointment, but this is not essential. Apply the ointment once or twice a day to the affected areas of the skin. Proportions and doses can be varied to get the best effect, and herbs can be soaked for a longer time. In my experience, soaking the herbs for longer increases the potency of the liquid. We have also found in practice that crushing the herbs increases their surface area, which also increases the potency of the liquid. Experiment with variations in order to get the best effect and be flexible!

Cāng Zhú Gāo (Black Atractylodis Ointment)

| *cāng zhú* | Atractylodis, Rhizoma | 100 g |

Overview and Functions

Another formula originating from Zhào Bǐng-Nán's *Zhào Bǐng-Nán Lín Chuáng Jīng Yàn Jí*, consisting of only one herb: *cāng zhú*. It invigorates the Spleen, dries dampness, and neutralizes the middle. Similar to *Bái Zhú Gāo*, mentioned above, this formula treats eczema with stubborn dampness, and also chronic lower extremity ulcers (knee sores), and blisters on hands and feet, but with a slightly stronger effect on drying dampness. However, the name "Black Atractylodis Ointment" originates from the fact that *cāng* refers to the appearance of the outer skin of the rhizome, which is dark grey-black in color (as opposed to *Bái Zhú Gāo*, where *bái* refers to the white color when looking at the sliced rhizome).

Preparation

The method of preparation is identical to that of *Bái Zhú Gāo*. Please see above for detailed information. Here, I also prefer to use an oil-based ointment instead of honey, or a herbal wash or wet compress. Always feel free to adjust preparations according to the individual's needs.

Guī Téng Xǐ Jì (Gui Teng Wash)

jī xuè téng	Spatholobi, Caulis	30 g
yè jiāo téng	Polygoni Multiflori, Caulis	30 g
bái jí lí	Tribuli Terristris, Fructus	15 g
tòu gǔ cǎo[4]	Tuberculate Speranskia, Herba	30 g
bái xiān pí	Dictamni Radicis, Cortex	30 g
tǔ fú líng	Smilacis Glabrae, Rhizoma	30 g
zào jiǎo[5]	Gleditsiae, Fructus	30 g
chǔ táo yè[6]	Morus Papyrifera, Folium	30 g
ài yè	Artemisiae Argyi, Folium	15 g
dāng guī	Angelicae Sinensis, Radix	30 g

Overview and Functions

According to my research, this herbal combination seems to originate from the Běijīng Chinese Medicine Hospital.[7] First of all, please note that *tòu gǔ cǎo* is considered to be toxic and is not available everywhere; in Germany, for example, it is not. It clears heat, eliminates toxins, removes blood stasis, and improves blood circulation. It is known for its ability to relieve inflammation, pain and swelling. However, if it is not available, just leave it out. As discussed above, *chǔ táo yè* are the leaves from the paper mulberry. They are usually not available in TCM pharmacies, not even in China nowadays. Use the formula without this herb. For the sake of completeness, I have listed both herbs, but the formula is still potent enough without them. Its functions are to nourish blood, moisten the skin, and stop itching, and it is frequently mentioned in Zhào Bǐng-Nán's notes for chronic hypertrophic skin diseases, such as psoriasis, eczema, and neurodermatitis.

Preparation

Soak the ingredients in 2 liters of water for 20–30 minutes. Bring them to a boil, then reduce the heat to a low flame, allowing the herbs to simmer slowly for approximately 20 minutes, then strain the liquid. For application, wash the affected area or apply as a wet herbal compress two or three times a day, for about 15–20 minutes each time. *Guī Téng Xǐ Jì* can also be applied with a cotton ball, up to four times a day. This actually applies for all herbal washes and wet compresses, but this is up to you and the individual needs of your patient. For children, for example, I do recommend using cotton balls because they usually don't stay still for that long.

Hēi Bù Yào Gāo (Black Cloth Medicated Paste)[8]

lǎo hēi cù	Atrum Vetum, Acetum	2500 ml
wǔ bèi zǐ	Rhois Chinensis, Galla	840 g
wú gong	Scolopendra	10 pieces
bīng piàn	Borneolum	3 g
fēng mì	Mel	180 g

Overview and Functions

This formula was invented by Professor Zhào Bǐng-Nán. He mentions it in his *Zhào Bǐng-Nán Lín Chuáng Jīng Yàn Jí* (Zhào Bǐng-Nán's Clinical Experience Set). *Hēi Bù Yào Gāo* clears heat, resolves toxicity, and cools the blood. Although some of the ingredients may be restricted or banned in some countries, I am mentioning it because of its effectiveness in speeding up the healing process and improving the appearance of skin prone to lichenification and scaling. It reduces inflammation, and helps soften and smooth the skin, while reducing its dark color and improving its appearance.

Preparation

Grind each herb separately to a fine powder. Boil the black vinegar for about 30 minutes, add the honey and boil again for about a minute. After that, gradually add the fine herbal powder of *wǔ bèi zǐ* and let it cook over mild heat. Stir constantly, always in the same direction until the texture is thick. Now, add *wú gong* and *bīng piàn*. The result should be a black, shiny, and soft paste. Pour the paste into a glass or porcelain container. No metal container should be used. Apply a thin layer over the affected areas of the skin and allow to dry fully once or twice a day. A black film will form, which should be gently washed off with warm water before re-applying the paste the next time. The frequency can be increased up to 3–5 times daily, depending on individual needs.

Hēi Dòu Liú Yóu Ruăn Gāo (Black Soybean Distillate Ointment)

hēi dòu yóu	5 % Black Soybean Oil	5 g
	15 % Zinc oxide	5 g
	Vaseline®	90 g

Overview and Functions

This is another formula invented by the famous Chinese dermatology professor, Professor Zhào Bĭng-Nán, again mentioned in his *Zhào Bĭng-Nán Lín Chuáng Jīng Yàn Jí* (Zhào Bĭng-Nán's Clinical Experience Set). *Hēi Dòu Liú Yóu Ruăn Gāo* is used for long-lasting lesions in chronic skin conditions, which are painful, fissured, and/or show intense itching, such as those seen in chronic eczema and ND, but also in psoriasis. The formula softens hardness, smooths the skin, and relieves itching.

Preparation

These quantities will produce an ointment of 100 ml. The original text mentions the ointment with Vaseline®. The pros and cons of Vaseline® are described earlier in this book in Chapter 3. For the skin to heal, it must be able to breathe; a thick and barely spreadable substance like Vaseline® prevents this and an inflammatory process could certainly worsen this way. Some practitioners may like to use it for making this ointment. In Chinese dermatology, however, it is recommended to use pure, natural, environmentally friendly options instead. You can either use Vaseline® or any other organic base, such as paraffin-free Vaseline (paraffin-free petroleum jelly). While the name is misleading, the latter contains purely natural ingredients based on vegetable fat instead of petroleum components. Alternatives are sesame oil, beeswax, or shea butter. To prepare this formula as an ointment, mix all substances thoroughly, and apply topically two to three times a day to the skin lesions.

Huà Dú Sàn (Toxicity Transforming Powder) and *Huà Dú Sàn Gāo* (Toxicity Transforming Powder Paste)

huáng lián	Coptidis, Rhizoma	60 g
rŭ xiāng	Olibanum, Gummi	60 g
mò yào	Myrrha	60 g
chuān bèi mŭ	Fritillariae Cirrhosae, Bulbus	60 g
tiān huā fĕn	Trichosanthis, Radix	120 g
dà huáng	Rhei, Radix et Rhizoma	120 g
chì sháo	Paeoniae Rubrae, Radix	120 g
xióng huáng	Realgar	60 g
gān căo	Glycyrrhizae Uralensis, Radix	45 g
niú huáng	Bovis Calculus	12 g
bīng piàn	Borneolum	15 g

Overview and Functions

Two more formulas by Zhào Bĭng-Nán, which were written down in the *Zhào Bĭng-Nán Lín Chuáng Jīng Yàn Jí*. The herbal composition, mentioned above, is called *Huà Dú Sàn* (Toxicity Transforming Powder). Please note that two substances in the formula are not available outside of China, namely *xióng huáng* and *niú huáng*. *Xióng huáng* might be substituted with *liú huáng* as both substances can resolve toxicity. The prescription can, however, be used without *xióng huáng* and *niú huáng*, and would still be strong enough to clear heat, remove toxins, promote blood circulation, and resolve swelling. It is recommended for use in cases of eczema and ND where the skin lesions appear swollen and bright red in color, often accompanied by vesicles or pustules, erosions, oozing, and the formation of yellowish crusts. In this case, the skin generally feels very painful, warm/hot, and itchy, and the patient often has a burning sensation on the skin.

Preparation

Huà Dú Sàn can be used as an ointment with sesame oil, or as a wash or wet compress. To use it as an oil-based ointment, grind the ingredients of *Huà Dú Sàn* to a fine powder and mix them thoroughly. Soak the herbs in a proportion of 1:4 in sesame oil for about 24 hours. The next day, bring it to a boil over mild heat, filter off the herb-infused sesame oil and allow to gel. It can be mixed with a small amount of beeswax before applying to the skin to make a thicker ointment, but this is not essential. Apply the ointment once or twice a day to the affected areas of the skin. For a herbal wash or wet compress, simply boil the herbs in 1.5–2 liters of water for a maximum of 20 minutes, strain, and use two or three times a day.

For *Huà Dú Sàn Gāo,* while the original prescription recommends Vaseline® as a carrier, the use of natural substances is always preferable. Let me describe how to make it as an oil-based paste without the use of Vaseline®. Grind the ingredients of *Huà Dú Sàn* to a fine powder and mix them thoroughly. For *Huà Dú Sàn Gāo*, about 50 g of the powder should be sufficient for use on the face or wrists, for example. Mix it well with 150 ml of sesame oil (or any other organic base). If the lesions are larger, use more herbs and more sesame oil. Apply the paste once or twice a day to the affected areas of the skin. Please don't forget: all pastes can be prepared with oil or with water. When preparing a paste with water, just use boiled water instead of sesame oil. Simple as that! Although it is not advised in classic books, I am sure that high-quality green tea as a base would also work.

Huáng Băi Róng Yè (Phellodendri Cortex Solution)

huáng băi	Phellodendri, Cortex	100 g

Overview and Functions

This formula is simply *huáng băi* distilled in water and used as a herbal wash or cold wet compress. I have mentioned it several times in this book before, but I am explaining it in more detail at this point in combination with the formula name for completeness. It is an empirical formula and very frequently seen in clinic. *Huáng Băi Róng Yè* clears heat, removes toxins and dead tissue, and alleviates pain.

Preparation
In my practice I prepare this by soaking 100 g *huáng bǎi* in 800 ml–1 liter of water for 20 minutes. It really depends how concentrated you want the liquid to be and/or how large the skin lesions are. For large skin areas, increase the quantity of water and herbs. Remember, it is advisable to crush a herb like *huáng bǎi* because it is a bark (cortex). In my opinion, the biochemical components dissolve better this way. Bring to a boil, reduce the heat to a low flame allowing it to simmer slowly for approximately 20 minutes, then strain the liquid. For application, wash the affected area or apply a wet compress to the skin lesions two to three times a day for about 15–30 minutes each time. The more severe the lesions, the longer and the more often the solution should be used.

Huáng Lián Sǎn (Coptis Rhizome Powder) and Huáng Lián Gāo (Coptis Rhizome Ointment)

huáng qín	Scutellariae, Radix	12 g
huáng lián	Coptidis, Rhizoma	10 g
jiāng huáng	Curcumae Longae, Rhizoma	10 g
dāng guī	Angelicae Sinensis, Radix	15 g
shēng dì huáng	Rehmanniae Glutinosae, Radix	15 g

Overview and Functions
Huáng Lián Gāo initially appeared in the *Yī Zōng Jīn Jiàn* (The Golden Mirror of Medical Tradition, 1742), written by Wú Qiān et al. It is *Huáng Lián Sǎn* prepared as an ointment (*gāo*). It is highly effective in clearing heat, dispelling toxins, relieving inflammation, and stopping any itching. In my clinical experience, *huáng lián* seems to have very strong effects and can be used as a standalone herb in ointments. You do not need to add all herbs mentioned in the formula to reach the desired effect.

Preparation
Like *Huà Dú Sàn, Huáng Lián Sǎn* can be used as an ointment with sesame oil (this is *Huáng Lián Gāo*), or as a wash or wet compress. For using it as *Huáng Lián Gāo*, grind the ingredients to a fine powder and soak them in

500 ml of sesame oil for 24 hours. Cook over mild heat until the ingredients have a dark yellow color. Filter off the sesame oil, allow to gel and apply the ointment twice a day to the affected areas of the skin. For *Huáng Lián Sǎn,* simply boil the herbs in 550–650 ml of water for a maximum of 20 minutes, strain, and use as a wash, or a wet compress for about 15–30 minutes, two or three times a day.

Jiě Dú Xǐ Yào (Detoxifying Lotion)

pú gōng yīng	Taraxaci, Herba	30 g
kǔ shēn	Sophorae Flavescentis, Radix	12 g
huáng bǎi	Phellodendri, Cortex	12 g
lián qiáo	Forsythiae, Fructus	12 g
mù biē zǐ[9]	Momordicae, Semen	12 g
jīn yín huā	Lonicerae Japonicae, Flos	10 g
bái zhǐ	Angelica Dahuricae, Radix	10 g
chì sháo	Paeoniae Rubrae, Radix	10 g
mǔ dān pí	Moutan, Cortex	10 g
gān cǎo	Glycyrrhizae Uralensis, Radix	10 g

Overview and Functions

The sources for this formula vary, but it seems that the original formula comes from the Shāndōng University of Traditional Chinese Medicine, Jǐnán, China. Please note that some sources mention this formula with *mù biē zǐ,* some with *ér chá* (Catechu) instead and some may even mention it without either of these substances. As neither are available in every country, it is absolutely fine and still very effective when prepared without these two herbs. This herbal combination strongly clears heat, resolves toxicity, invigorates the blood, reduces swelling, and eliminates exudate. It is quite effective for eczema that is accompanied by severe inflammation, exudation and where the skin feels warm/hot, painful, and extremely itchy.

Preparation

As with most of the other external herbal applications, *Jiě Dú Xǐ Yào* can be used in many ways: either as a wash or a wet compress, but also as a paste.

To prepare a wash or a wet compress, soak the ingredients in 1.5 liters of water for 20 minutes. Bring them to a boil, and then reduce the heat to a low flame allowing the herbs to simmer slowly for approximately 20 minutes, then strain the liquid. Wash the affected area or apply a wet compress to the skin lesions two to three times a day for about 15–30 minutes[10] each time. To prepare an oil-based paste, grind the ingredients to a fine powder and mix thoroughly with sesame oil. To prepare a water-based paste, replace the oil with boiled water or green tea.

Pí Fū Píng Ruǎn Gāo (Skin Smoothing Ointment)

fáng fēng	Saposhnikoviae, Radix	10 g
kǔ shēn	Sophorae Flavescentis, Radix	10 g
bái xiān pí	Dictamni Radicis, Cortex	10 g
cāng zhú	Atractylodis, Rhizoma	10 g
huáng qín	Scutellariae, Radix	10 g

Overview and Functions

Pí Fū Píng Ruǎn Gāo is a Chinese patent formula for topical treatment. I am using this example to demonstrate that you can make nearly all patent formulas yourself or order them from TCM pharmacies, as long as the ingredients are known and, of course, available. In China, I have often seen patients in TCM hospitals being prescribed formulas for external but also for internal use. These prescriptions are mainly based on the experience of the local TCM doctors, or modifications of classical formulas. One doesn't usually find them outside the hospital–even the ingredients are often kept a secret. However, in this particular case, *Pí Fū Píng Ruǎn Gāo* seems to be available in many countries via TCM shops. As the original patent product is ready-made with stearic acid, glycerol stearate, and glycerine, I thought this a good opportunity to demonstrate how to make it entirely with natural ingredients. It can be prepared as a wash, wet compress, ointment, or cream–depending on the skin of your patient. The main ingredients are effective in clearing heat, reducing inflammation and exudation, and stopping itching. This formula has a curative effect on skin eruptions and can be used in eczema, ND but also urticaria and psoriasis, for example.

Preparation

Please note that the dosages mentioned above are the ones that I recommend. To prepare *Pí Fū Píng Ruǎn Gāo* as a herbal wash or wet compress, simply boil the herbs in 500 ml of water for a maximum of 20 minutes, strain, and use two or three times a day. If you want to work with a more concentrated substance, use more water and vice versa. To prepare it as an ointment, grind the ingredients to a fine powder and mix them thoroughly. Soak the herbs in a proportion of about 1:4 in sesame oil for about 24–48 hours, then bring to a boil over mild heat, filter off the herb-infused sesame oil, and allow to gel. As usual, it can be mixed with a small amount of beeswax before applying to the skin to make a thicker ointment. Apply twice a day to the affected areas.

When applying as a cream, soak the herbs in about 300 ml of sesame oil for two or three days. Then cook over mild heat until the herbs turn dark.[11] Strain to remove the herbal residues, add beeswax and a little bit of shea butter if you prefer a softer (and more spreadable) consistency, and melt in the hot oil. Allow the oil to cool and stir constantly until the texture is thick. (Please note that the oil can also be mixed with any other natural cream base, or paraffin-free petroleum jelly.) Apply the cream once or twice a day to the affected areas of the skin. Finally, if in addition to the other functions, a cooling effect is desired, a small amount of *bò hé* 3–5 g, *bīng piàn* 1.5–3 g, or *zhāng nǎo* (camphor) 3 g can be added to the formula. One of these is sufficient, depending on your patient's needs.

Caution: *zhāng nǎo* is suitable for external applications only. Patients should be informed that if taken internally, it is toxic! It should also be used very carefully by people with skin allergies.

Pí Shī Yī Hào Gāo (Eczema Ointment No. 1)

(duàn) shí gāo	(calcinated) Gypsum Fibrosum	93 g
dì yú (fěn)[12]	Sanguisorbae, Radix (powder)	93 g
(duàn) bái fán[13]	Alumen (calcinated)	3 g
	Vaseline®	31 g

Overview and Functions

Pí Shī Yī Hào Gāo originates from the *Zhōng Yī Pí Fū Bìng Xué Jiǎn Biān* (Compendium of TCM Dermatology, 1979), in which Chéng Yùn-Qián summarized his experiences in Chinese dermatology. However, to be precise it seems that the original formula called *Pí Shī Yī Gāo* (Pus Absorbing Ointment),[14] comes from Zhū Rén-Kāng's *Zhū Rén-Kāng Lín Chuáng Jīng Yàn Jí*, also published in 1979. Its function is to clear heat, absorb discharge (pus) and relieve itching. It is suitable for any form of eczema in which red, thick, oedematous, inflamed, and very painful skin lesions are seen; or any other skin condition with toxic swollen sores.

Preparation

The original text suggests preparing the powder with Vaseline®. However, when discharge absorbing action is needed, I would always suggest preparing a formula as a wash, wet compress or an ointment instead. A thick and hardly spreadable cream would not be advisable as the discharge has to be drained, not occluded. As already explained, a thick substance like Vaseline® would prevent this and keep inside what should be discharged. An inflammatory process could certainly worsen this way. Therefore, to prepare this formula as an ointment, grind all substances to a fine powder. Mix them thoroughly with a liquid such as sesame oil and apply two to three times a day to the affected skin lesions. Alternatively, bring the ground herbs to a gentle boil in about 1–1.5 liters of water until they dissolve, then strain and use the liquid as a topical wash. Reduce the quantities of herbs and water if only small areas of skin are affected. You might also use this formula as a wet compress, gently applied to the affected skin areas.

Qīng Dài Sǎn (Indigo Powder)

qīng dài	Indigo Naturalis	60 g
huáng bǎi	Phellodendri, Cortex	60 g
huá shí	Talcum	120 g
shí gāo	Gypsum Fibrosum	120 g

Overview and Functions

Qīng Dài Săn is a popular, modern formula and is widely used amongst TCM practitioners. It is an empirical formula and different compositions of the powder are available—I am describing the classical version here. *Qīng Dài Săn* has a broad application and delivers effective results by relieving inflammation, stopping itching, clearing heat, dispelling toxins, absorbing fluids, and, thus, reducing swelling. It is widely used to treat a broad range of skin conditions, such as eczema, ND, urticaria, and psoriasis.

Preparation

The ingredients mentioned above are *Qīng Dài Săn* (Indigo Powder), not to be confused with powdered *qīng dài*. I am highlighting this because in Chinese, *săn* always means powder. This formula can be used in many different ways. For application as an ointment, grind the ingredients (except *qīng dài*) to a fine powder and soak them in 500 ml of sesame oil for 24 hours. Cook over mild heat until the ingredients have a dark yellow color. Filter off the sesame oil and, finally, add *qīng dài* to the medicated oil and mix well. Allow to gel and apply once or twice a day to the affected areas of the skin. For a herbal wash or wet compress, soak the herbs in 1–1.5 liters of water for about 30 minutes. As with all washes and wet compresses, the amount of water varies, depending on how concentrated you want it to be. Bring the herbs to a boil, and then reduce the heat to a low flame allowing them to simmer gently for approximately 20 minutes, and finally strain the liquid. For application, wash the affected area or apply a wet compress to the affected skin lesions two to three times a day for about 15–30 minutes each time.

Qīng Liáng Gāo (Clearing and Cooling Ointment)

Weathered Lime	500 g
(clear) Water	1 l

Overview and Functions

The sources, but also the ingredients, here vary. It seems that the original formula comes from the *Yī Zōng Jīn Jiàn*. This is the original version, a very simple and easy to prepare combination. It clears heat and moistens the skin, and is best used when the skin appears red, with or without blisters.

Preparation

The original text mentions the use of weathered lime. Nowadays, I suggest using a fresh lime you can get in any fruit market. Take 500 g of fresh lime and cut it into small pieces. Mix with 1 liter of water, boil for a very short time over mild heat, strain the liquid, and keep the clear water. Then, mix it with sesame oil thoroughly and apply to the affected skin areas twice a day. Don't forget to shake the ointment before each use because the oil and water might separate.

To give a complete picture let me describe two other versions of *Qīng Liáng Gāo* I have found in medical textbooks. The latter one is mentioned by Zhào Bǐng-Nán in his *Zhào Bǐng-Nán Lín Chuáng Jīng Yàn Jí*, for example. Both versions are prepared with sesame oil and beeswax to form an ointment.

qīng dài	Indigo Naturalis	25 g
huáng bǎi	Phellodendri, Cortex	25 g
tiān huā fěn	Trichosanthis, Radix	25 g
yì yǐ rén	Coices, Semen	25 g

This formula cools the blood, dries dampness and clears toxins from the skin. In eczema, it is helpful whenever the skin is red, swollen, feels warm, burning, and painful. Contact eczema is a good example in this context.

dāng guī	Angelicae Sinensis, Radix	30 g
zǐ cǎo	Arnebiae seu Lithospermi, Radix	6 g
dà huáng	Rhei, Radix et Rhizoma	3 g

This combination clears away heat and detoxifies, cools blood and relieves pain; and is recommended for when eczema or ND appears as inflammation with red, dry, and scaly skin. Select the option that is the best fit for your patient's skin.

Qū Shī Sǎn (Damp-Removing Medicinal Powder)

dà huáng	Rhei, Radix et Rhizoma	30 g
huáng qín	Scutellariae, Radix	30 g
hán shuǐ shí	Calcitum	30 g
qīng dài	Indigo Naturalis	3 g

Overview and Functions

This formula comes from the book *Zhū Rén-Kāng Lín Chuáng Jīng Yàn Jí* (A Collection of Zhu Renkang's Clinical Experiences, 1979), written by Zhū Rén-Kāng. It clears heat, detoxifies and dispels dampness, and it is quite effective in eczema and ND showing erosive inflamed skin lesions with large amounts of exudation.

Preparation

Grind the ingredients into a fine powder called *Qū Shī Sǎn*. This can be used in many different ways; in this book, I will mention the two most popular methods. The first one is: Mix with vegetable oil to form a paste or sprinkle the powder directly onto the lesion. Apply twice or three times daily, for about 20 minutes each time. The second one[15] is: Boil *mǎ chǐ xiàn*[16] in 2 liters of water for approximately 20 minutes, filter off and allow to cool. When the decoction is cool, use it as a cold wet compress and apply to the affected skin areas for 20 minutes each time. Directly after finishing this, dust *Qū Shī Sǎn* directly onto the affected skin areas and leave to dry.

Interestingly, there is another herbal combination called *Qū Shī Sǎn*, mentioned by Zhào Bǐng-Nán in his *Zhào Bǐng-Nán Lín Chuáng Jīng Yàn Jí* (Vol. 2), consisting of *huáng lián, huáng qín, huáng bǎi*, and *bīng láng*. If you find this combination works better for you, the method of preparation is quite similar to that described above. It can be used with vegetable oil as an ointment, sprayed directly onto the affected skin area, and also mixed together with fresh aloe vera.

Rùn Jī Gāo (Flesh Moistening Ointment)

dāng guī	Angelicae Sinensis, Radix	15 g
zǐ cǎo	Arnebiae seu Lithospermi, Radix	3 g
fēng là	Beeswax	15 g
zhī má yóu	Sesame Oil	120 ml

Overview and Functions

This formula first appeared in the *Wài Kē Zhèng Zōng* (Orthodox Lineage of External Medicine,[17] 1617) by Chén Shí-Gōng. It nourishes, moistens the skin, alleviates itching and invigorates the blood while clearing heat. It is an ideal choice in the treatment of eczema and ND when the skin is dry, thickened, scaly and itchy; but is also often used in the treatment of psoriasis. Unfortunately, *zǐ cǎo* is not available everywhere. In Germany, for example, it is not.

Preparation

Soak *dāng guī* and *zǐ cǎo* in 120 ml of sesame oil for two or three days. Then cook over mild heat until the herbs turn a dark yellow. Remove the herbal residues, mix the oil with *fēng là* (beeswax) and allow to cool before applying to the affected skin areas twice a day. If the skin lesions are larger, increase all dosages proportionally, of course.

Sān Huáng Xǐ Jì (Three Yellow Cleanser Formula)

dà huáng	Rhei, Radix et Rhizoma	10 g
huáng bǎi	Phellodendri, Cortex	10 g
huáng qín	Scutellariae, Radix	10 g
kǔ shēn	Sophorae Flavescentis, Radix	10 g

Overview and Functions

Sān Huáng Xǐ Jì is an empirical formula from China, which clears heat, relieves inflammation, and stops secretion and itching. In clinic, this manifests as eczema or ND with red, hot, and burning skin lesions, sometimes accompanied by pain and/or itching. If there are erupted skin lesions, add *pú gōng yīng* to the formula.

Preparation

Soak the ingredients in 500 ml of water for 20–30 minutes. Bring them to a boil, then reduce the heat to a low flame allowing the herbs to simmer slowly for approximately 20 minutes and at the end, strain the liquid. For application, wash the affected area or apply as a wet compress two or three times a day, for about 15–30 minutes each time. *Sān Huáng Xǐ Jì* can also be applied with a cotton ball, up to four times a day, depending on the severity of the skin lesions. The more severe, the more often it should be applied.

Shé Chuáng Zǐ Tāng (Cnidium Fruit Decoction)

shé chuáng zǐ	Cnidii, Fructus	15 g
dāng guī	Angelicae Sinensis, Radix	15 g
wēi líng xiān	Clematidis, Radix	15 g
shā rén	Amomi, Fructus	9 g
dà huáng	Rhei, Radix et Rhizoma	15 g
kǔ shēn	Sophorae Flavescentis, Radix	15 g
cōng bái	Allii Fislulosi, Bulbus	7 pieces

Overview and Functions

As mentioned earlier in this book, *Shé Chuáng Zǐ Tāng* originates from the *Yī Zōng Jīn Jiàn* (The Golden Mirror of Ancestral Medicine, 1742) by Wú Qiān. Functions include clearing away heat and dampness, expelling wind and relieving itching, and it is frequently used as external application for the genital area, in particular for scrotum eczema with oozing and itching.

Preparation

To prepare a wash or a wet compress, soak the ingredients in about 1000 ml of water for 20 minutes. Bring them to a boil, then reduce the heat to a low flame allowing the herbs to simmer slowly for approximately 20 minutes, then strain the liquid. For application, wash the affected area or apply a wet compress to the skin lesions two to three times a day for about 15–30 minutes each time. If used in the genital area, it can be useful to tell your patient to lie down when applying wet compresses. I normally say, "Just listen to the news or to nice music, or just close your eyes and relax for a while. This time will also give you a little 'me-time' within your day in which you do something good just for you!"

Shī Zhěn Sǎn (Eczema Powder)

shé chuáng zǐ	Cnidii, Fructus	300 g
mǎ chǐ xiàn	Portulacae, Herba	300 g
cè bǎi yè	Platycladi Cacumen	325 g
fú róng yè	Hibsci, Folium	325 g

lú gān shí	Calamina	150 g
fú xiǎo mài (fěn)	Tritici Levis, Fructus (powder)	300 g
(duàn) zhēn zhū mǔ	Margaritaferae, Concha	150 g
dà huáng	Rhei, Radix et Rhizoma	300 g
gān cǎo	Glycyrrhizae Uralensis, Radix	160 g
huáng bǎi	Phellodendri, Cortex	300 g
bīng piàn	Borneolum	150 g
(duàn) bái fán[18]	Alumen (calcinated)	150 g
kǔ shēn	Sophorae Flavescentis, Radix	350 g

Overview and Functions

This formula seems to originate from the *Zhōng Huá Rén Mín Gòng Hé Guó Wèi Shēng Bù Yào Pǐn Biāo Zhǔn Zhōng Yào Chéng Fāng Zhì Jì Dì Wǔ Cè* (Drug Standards for Traditional Chinese Medicine Prescriptions Volume V), which most likely was published in 1992 by the Pharmacopoeia Committee of the Ministry of Health of the People's Republic of China, but the publishing year differs depending on the source, as well as the ingredients. The ingredients mentioned above are, however, those listed in the original text. This formula clears heat, dispels dampness, and stops itching.

Preparation

Grind the ingredients into a fine powder. Mix them with vegetable oil to form a paste or sprinkle the powder directly onto the affected skin lesions. Apply once or twice daily. Please note, *lú gān shí* and other herbs in this formula are for external use only. Do not apply this formulation to children's faces, as they can easily lick the skin around their mouths. For use with children, be sure to ask the parents to work with care.

Sì Huáng Sǎn (Four Yellow Powder) and Sì Huáng Gāo (Four Yellow Cream)

huáng qín	Scutellariae, Radix	30 g
huáng lián	Coptidis, Rhizoma	30 g
huáng bǎi	Phellodendri, Cortex	10 g

dà huáng	Rhei, Radix et Rhizoma	30 g
zé lán	Lycopi, Herba	30 g
huáng là	Yellow Wax (Beeswax)	125g
zhī má yóu	Sesame Oil	250 ml

Overview and Functions

This formula originated from the book *Zhū Rén-Kāng Lín Chuáng Jīng Yàn Jí*, written by Zhū Rénkāng. The ingredients mentioned above form *Sì Huáng Sǎn* (Four Yellow Powder). The name "*Sì Huáng*" is given because the first four of the Chinese names of its ingredients contain the word *huáng*, which means yellow. "*Sì*" is the Chinese word for the number four. All these herbs are bitter in flavour and cold in nature. They clear heat and drain fire. This powder is used to make the cream called *Sì Huáng Gāo*, which can be effectively used for the treatment of hot toxic skin lesions, in particular eczema lesions that show severe inflammation, are oozing or itching. Due to the presence of *zé lán*, it can also be used to relieve painful skin lesions and swelling, because this herb invigorates the blood and dispels stasis.

Preparation

Melt the yellow wax (beeswax) and the sesame oil over moderate heat. Grind all other ingredients to a fine powder and stir into the oil (after removing the pot from the heat) to form a paste. Allow to cool, and gently apply the paste twice a day to the affected areas of the skin. The paste should be left on for about 20–30 minutes, then gently washed off with clean water. Always work gently as the patient's skin tends to be very sensitive and inflamed, and usually feels very painful.

In the case of eczema, however, I recommend using it as a herbal wash or wet compress. Simply omit *huáng là* (beeswax) and *zhī má yóu* (sesame oil) and boil the ingredients for about 20 minutes with 1 liter of water and apply as a wash or wet compress twice a day to the affected areas of the skin. The principle is always the same: water is used to make a herbal wash or wet compress; while with oil (and beeswax) it is an ointment.

Wǔ Huáng Gāo (Five Huang Cream)[19]

dà huáng	Rhei, Radix et Rhizoma	15 g
huáng qín	Scutellariae, Radix	15 g
huáng bǎi	Phellodendri, Cortex	15 g
huáng lián	Coptidis, Rhizoma	15 g
jiāng huáng	Curcumae Longae, Rhizoma	15 g

Overview and Functions

Pǔ Jì Fāng (Prescriptions of Universal Relief). This book is the most extensive collection of prescriptions and methods of treatment in TCM in Chinese history, containing over 61,739 prescriptions in 168 volumes. Compiled by Zhū Sù et al., this book was published in 1406 under the leadership of Emperor Zhū Dì, the third emperor of China's Míng Dynasty.[20]

Preparation

For application in eczema, I recommend using the herbal combination as a wash or a wet compress. Soak the ingredients in about 750 ml of water for 20 minutes. Bring them to a boil, then reduce to a low flame allowing the herbs to simmer slowly for approximately 20 minutes and at the end, strain the liquid. Wash the affected area or apply a wet compress to the affected skin lesions two to three times a day for about 15–30 minutes each time. The original book mentions using equal parts of all the ingredients. Here I have described it with 15 g of each component for smaller skin lesions. If your patient has larger lesions, simply increase the dosages and the amount of water proportionally. The same applies for varying the concentration, as with previous formulas. And if you prefer to use it as an oil-based ointment, use the same preparation methods as described previously.

Xīn Sān Miào Sǎn (New Three Marvels Powder)

huáng bǎi	Phellodendri, Cortex	100 g
hán shuǐ shí	Calcitum	250 g
qīng dài	Indigo Naturalis	50 g

Overview and Functions

Xīn Sān Miào Săn was first mentioned by Zhào Bǐng-Nán in his *Zhào Bǐng-Nán Lín Chuáng Jīng Yàn Jí* (Vol. 2). It dries dampness and clears away heat, detoxifies, and relieves itching; and is frequently seen in the treatment of acute eczema, infantile eczema, and allergic contact eczema whenever the skin is severely inflamed, oozes, feels hot, painful, and itchy.

Preparation

Spread the powder directly onto the affected skin lesions or mix it with fresh aloe vera; alternatively, make a paste with vegetable oil for external use, two or three times a day, for about 15–30 minutes each time. The frequency and application time depends on the severity of the condition.

Zào Shī Xǐ Gāo (Damp-Heat Eliminating Ointment)

bái xiān pí	Dictamni Radicis, Cortex	10g
mǎ chǐ xiàn	Portulacae, Herba	10 g
kǔ shēn	Sophorae Flavescentis, Radix	10 g
huáng bǎi	Phellodendri, Cortex	10 g
cāng zhú	Atractylodis, Rhizoma	10 g

Overview and Functions

This formula is mentioned in Xú Xiàngcái.[21] It clears heat and thus relieves irritation, dispels wind and thus eases itching, dries dampness and thus improves swelling. It is frequently used not just for eczema, but also for acne, urticaria etc.

Preparation

Grind the ingredients to a fine powder. Soak them in 300 ml of sesame oil for two or three days, then cook over mild heat for a short time. Filter off the herbal residues and allow the oil to cool before applying to the skin. Apply the ointment two or three times a day to the affected areas. Please note that the ointment can be mixed with beeswax to get a thicker consistency before application.

It can also be prepared as a wash or a wet compress and this is how it was described in Xú Xiàngcái's book: Soak the ingredients in about 500 ml of water for 30 minutes.[22] Bring them to a boil, then reduce to a low flame allowing the herbs to simmer slowly for approximately 20 minutes, and at the end, strain the liquid. Wash the affected area or apply a wet compress to the affected skin lesions two to three times a day for about 15–30 minutes each time. In the interval of this process, dust the powder of *Huáng Bǎi Sǎn* onto the affected skin, consisting of *huáng bǎi, huáng lián,* aloe vera, *sōng xiāng,*[23] *huá shí, bīng piàn,* and *cāng zhú. Huáng Bǎi Sǎn* can, by the way, be mixed with vegetable oil to form a paste to make it stick to the skin more easily.

Zhǐ Yǎng Xǐ Jì (Anti-Itch Wash)[24]

chuān jiāo	Xanthaxyli, Semen	15–30 g
xì xīn	Asari, Radix	4–10 g
chuān jǐn pí	Hibisci, Cortex	20–30 g
kǔ shēn	Sophorae Flavescentis, Radix	20–30 g
shè gān	Belamcandae, Rhizoma	15 g
huáng bǎi	Phellodendri, Cortex	15 g
lián qiáo	Forsythiae, Fructus	15 g
wǔ bèi zǐ	Rhois Chinensis, Galla	15 g
cāng zhú	Atractylodis, Rhizoma	15 g
bái xiān pí	Dictamni Radicis, Cortex	15 g
bǎi bù	Stemonae, Radix	30 g
shé chuáng zǐ	Cnidii, Fructus	30 g
dì fū zǐ	Kochiae Scopariae, Fructus	30 g
bǎn lán gēn	Isatidis, Radix	30 g
dà qīng yè	Isatidis, Folium	30 g
pú gōng yīng	Taraxaci, Herba	30 g
cāng ěr zǐ	Xanthii, Fructus	30 g
ài yè	Artemisiae Argyi, Folium	30 g
(duàn) bái fán	Alumen (calcinated)	30 g
jú huā	Chrysanthemi, Flos	30 g
mǎ chǐ xiàn	Portulacae, Herba	30 g
jīn yín huā	Lonicerae Japonicae, Flos	50 g

ér chá	Catechu	12 g
bái jí lí	Tribuli Terristris, Fructus	12 g
bái zhǐ	Angelica Dahuricae, Radix	10 g
hǎi zǎo	Sargassum	20 g
dà huáng	Rhei, Radix et Rhizoma	20 g
shí chāng pú	Acori Tatarinowii, Rhizoma	9 g
zǎo xiū	Paridis, Rhizoma	15–20 g

Overview and Functions

This extensive herbal formula comes from an article by Dīng Wén-Fēng.[25] It seems to be an empirical formula and clears heat, drains dampness, relieves inflammation, and stops itching.

Preparation

Most of the ingredients mentioned above are available in most countries. The original version is a very long formula and the careful reader would have noticed that it contains useful combinations that can be taken individually without using the whole formula. However, when working according to the original text, I suggest reducing the dosages proportionally by a third. When doing this, the amount of water for boiling the herbs would be approximately 1500 ml. The preparation method is as usual: Soak the herbs in the water for about 20 minutes. Bring them to a boil, reduce the heat to a low flame allowing the herbs to simmer slowly for approximately 20 minutes, and then strain the liquid. For application, wash the affected area or apply a wet compress to the affected skin lesions two to three times a day for about 15–30 minutes each time.

Zǐ Sè Xiāo Zhǒng Fěn (Purple Powder to Reduce Swelling)[26]

zǐ cǎo	Arnebiae seu Lithospermi, Radix	25 g
chì sháo	Paeoniae Rubrae, Radix	50 g
dāng guī	Angelicae Sinensis, Radix	100 g
guàn zhòng	Cyrtomii, Rhizoma	10 g

shēng má	Cimicifugae, Rhizoma	50 g
bái zhǐ	Angelica Dahuricae, Radix	100 g
jīng jiè	Schizonepetae, Herba	250 g
zǐ jīng pí	Kadsurae Radicis, Cortex	25 g
hóng huā	Carthami, Flos	25 g
ér chá	Catechu	25 g
hóng qǔ[27]	Monascus	25 g
qiāng huó	Notopterygii, Rhizoma Seu Radix	25 g
fáng fēng	Saposhnikoviae, Radix	25 g

Overview and Functions

This formula is mentioned by Zhào Bǐng-Nán in his *Zhào Bǐng-Nán Lín Chuáng Jīng Yàn Jí* (Vol. 2). It disperses wind, activates blood circulation, removes blood stasis, and reduces swelling and is, thus, useful for chronic conditions of eczema and ND with dark colored, dry, thick, and itchy skin. Precaution: Do not use for boils and carbuncles presenting with severe heat and toxicity at the beginning.

Preparation

Please note that not all ingredients of this powder are available everywhere. For application, grind the ingredients into a fine powder. This can be used in many ways: alone or mixed with other medicinal powders. The original text suggests using it with honey, or decocted in water with lotus leaves (*hé yè*) for external use as a wash or wet compress. As *hé yè* can clear heat, it makes sense to decoct the powder with the leaves whenever the skin lesions appear reddish and, thus, a slight heat clearing effect is also wanted. Otherwise, leave it out. For dry, thick, and itchy skin, as seen in chronic eczema and ND, I recommend using it as an oil-based ointment though. Sesame oil is best for this, but any other vegetable oil works too. As preparation has been described previously, this will not be repeated at this point.

Please note that the formulas mentioned in this Appendix on external treatments are just a selection of the enormous range of options. This just serves as a basis, and a good starting point for you to explore.

Endnotes

1 Volume 2, published by People's Medical Publishing House Beijing, 2006.

2 Professor Zhào Bǐng-Nán (Chinese: 赵炳南, 1899–1984).

3 The mulberry tree belongs to the mulberry family (Moraceae). There are about ten species of mulberry trees native to Asia, Europe and North America. The best-known mulberry tree is the white mulberry (Morus alba), which is mainly found in Asia. Other species include: black mulberry (Morus nigra), native to Europe; red mulberry (Morus rubra), native to North America; but also Himalayan mulberry tree (Morus serrata), Japanese mulberry (Morus bombycis), Texas mulberry (Morus microphylla), Pakistan mulberry (Morus macroura), African mulberry (Morus mesozygia), and Korean mulberry (Morus australis).

4 This herb is toxic and not available everywhere. In Germany, for example, it is not.

5 Please note that the original source text mentioned: dà zào jiǎo 大皂角, which is actually the same herb.

6 Not available.

7 Cannot be verified with 100% certainty.

8 May contain herbs that are restricted or banned in some countries.

9 If available.

10 The application time can vary.

11 This process can be very fast. Ten minutes can often be enough, so be careful and observe the cooking process. Otherwise, the oil turns too dark and is too smelly.

12 If available.

13 Also known as kū fán 枯矾.

14 Chin: 皮湿一膏.

15 Xiàngcái, X. (1998) Complete External Therapies of Chinese Drugs. Beijing: Foreign Languages Press.

16 Please note that the original text does not mention the amount of mǎ chǐ xiàn. I would either use 200 g of the herb, or reduce the amount of water and use 30 g mǎ chǐ xiàn, boiled in 300 ml of water.

17 Also known as "True Lineage of External Medicine."

18 Also known as kū fán 枯矾.

19 Don't confuse this formula with Wǔ Huáng Gāo (Five Huang Cream) from the book Liú Juān Zǐ Guǐ Yí Fāng, (Liu Juan-Zi's Ghost-Bequeathed Formulas) by Liú Juān-Zǐ, which is used for ulcers. It has the same name but totally different ingredients.

20 Míng Dynasty (1368–1644 AD).

21 Xiàngcái, X. (1998) Complete External Therapies of Chinese Drugs. Beijing: Foreign Languages Press. Also: Xú Xiàng-Cái.

22 The original text mentions higher dosages with a larger amount of water and one hour of soaking time.

23 Might not be available everywhere.

24 May contain herbs which are not available everywhere.

25 Wén-Fēng, D. (1984) "Observation of 100 cases of pruritus skin diseases treated with traditional Chinese medicine antipruritic lotion." Journal of Integrated Traditional Chinese and Western Medicine 7, 436–437.

26 May contain restricted and/or unavailable herbs in some countries.

27 Also known as red yeast rice, this is rice that has been fermented with the yeast monascus purpureus. The fermentation process changes the color of the rice from white to red, thereby giving it its name. It invigorates blood circulation and eliminates blood stasis.

Appendix II: *Pīnyīn*-Chinese-English Herb Cross Reference

Pīnyīn	Chinese	Pharmaceutical
ài yè	艾叶	Artemisiae Argyi, Folium
bái biǎn dòu	白扁豆	Lablab Album, Semen
bǎi bù	百部	Stemonae, Radix
bái fán	白矾	Alumen
bǎi hé	百合	Lilii, Bulbus
bái huā shé shé cǎo	白花蛇舌草	Hedyotis Diffusae, Herba
bái jí lí	白蒺藜	Tribuli Terristris, Fructus
bài jiàng cǎo	败酱草	Patriniae, Herba
bái máo gēn	白茅根	Imperatae, Rhizoma
bái sháo	白芍	Paeonia Albiflora, Radix
bái xiān pí	白鲜皮	Dictamni Radicis, Cortex
bái zhǐ	白芷	Angelica Dahuricae, Radix
bái zhú	白术	Atractylodis Macrocephalae, Rhizoma
bǎn lán gēn	板蓝根	Isatidis, Radix
bì xiè	萆薢	Dioscoreae, Rhizoma
bīng láng	槟榔	Arecae, Semen
bīng piàn	冰片	Borneolum
bò hé	薄荷	Menthae, Herba
cāng ěr cǎo	苍耳草	Xanthii, Herba
cāng ěr yāng	苍耳秧	Xanthii, Germen
cāng ěr zǐ	苍耳子	Xanthii, Fructus
cāng zhú	苍术	Atractylodis, Rhizoma
cè bǎi yè	侧柏叶	Platycladi Cacumen
chái hú	柴胡	Bupleuri, Radix
chán tuì	蝉蜕	Cicadae, Periostracum
chē qián cǎo	车前草	Plantaginis, Herba

Pīnyīn	Chinese	Pharmaceutical
chē qián zǐ	车前子	Plantaginis, Semen
chén pí	陈皮	Citri Reticulatae, Pericarpium
chì sháo	赤芍	Paeoniae Rubrae, Radix
chì xiǎo dòu	赤小豆	Phaseoli, Semen
chǔ táo yè	楮桃叶	Morus Papyrifera, Folium
chuān jǐn pí	川槿皮	Hibisci, Cortex
chuān jiāo	川椒	Xanthaxyli, Semen
chuān xiōng	川芎	Chuanxiong, Rhizoma
cì jí lí	刺蒺藜	Tribuli, Fructus
cōng bái	葱白	Allii Fislulosi, Bulbus
dà huáng	大黄	Rhei, Radix et Rhizoma
dà qīng yè	大青叶	Isatidis, Folium
dà zǎo	大枣	Jujubae, Fructus
dàn dòu chǐ	淡豆豉	Sojae Praeparata, Semen
dān shēn	丹参	Salviae Miltiorhizae, Radix
dàn zhú yè	淡竹叶	Lophatheri, Herba
dāng guī	当归	Angelicae Sinensis, Radix
dāng guī wěi	当归尾	Angelicae Sinensis, Radicis Cauda
dǎng shēn	党参	Codonopsis, Radix
dēng xīn cǎo	灯心草	Junci, Medulla
dì fū zǐ	地肤子	Kochiae Scopariae, Fructus
dì gǔ pí	地骨皮	Lycii, Cortex
dì yú	地榆	Sanguisorbae, Radix
dōng guā pí	冬瓜皮	Benincasae, Exocarpium
dú huó	独活	Angelicae Pubescentis, Radix
é zhú	莪术	Curcumae, Rhizoma
ér chá	儿茶	Catechu
fáng fēng	防风	Saposhnikoviae, Radix
fēng mì	蜂蜜	Mel
fú líng	茯苓	Poriae Cocos, Sclerotium
fú píng	浮萍	Spirodelae, Herba
fú róng yè	芙蓉叶	Hibsci, Folium
fú xiǎo mài	浮小麦	Tritici Levis, Fructus
gān cǎo	甘草	Glycyrrhizae Uralensis, Radix
gé gēn	葛根	Puerariae, Radix

Pīnyīn	Chinese	Pharmaceutical
gǒu qǐ zǐ	枸杞子	Lycii, Fructus
gōu téng	钩藤	Uncariae, Ramulus Cum Uncis
gǔ yá	谷芽	Oryzae Germinatus, Fructus
guā lóu rén	瓜蒌仁	Trichosanthis, Semen
guàn zhòng	贯众	Cyrtomii, Rhizoma
hǎi zǎo	海藻	Sargassum
hán shuǐ shí	寒水石	Calcitum
hé shǒu wū	何首乌	Polygoni Multiflori, Radix
hé yè	荷叶	Nelumbinis, Folium
hēi zhī má	黑芝麻	Sesami Nigrum, Semen
hóng qǔ	红曲	Monascus
hóng huā	红花	Carthami, Flos
hòu pò	厚朴	Magnoliae Officinalis, Cortex
hòu pò huā	厚朴花	Magnoliae Officinalis, Flos
hú má rén	胡麻仁	Sesami Indici, Semen
huá shí	滑石	Talcum
huáng bǎi	黄柏	Phellodendri, Cortex
huáng dān	黄丹	Minium
huáng jīng	黄精	Polygonati, Rhizoma
huáng là	黄蜡	Yellow Wax (Beeswax)
huáng lián	黄连	Coptidis, Rhizoma
huáng qí	黄芪	Astragali, Radix
huáng qín	黄芩	Scutellariae, Radix
huǒ má rén	火麻仁	Cannabis, Semen
huò xiāng	藿香	Agastachis, Herba
jī xuè téng	鸡血藤	Spatholobi, Caulis
jiāng cán	僵蚕	Bombyx Batryticatus
jiāng huáng	姜黄	Curcumae Longae, Rhizoma
jiǎo gǔ lán	绞股蓝	Gynostemma Pentaphyllum, Herba
jié gěng	桔梗	Platycodi, Radix
jīn yín huā	金银花	Lonicerae Japonicae, Flos
jīng jiè	荆芥	Schizonepetae, Herba
jīng mǐ	粳米	Oryzae, Semen
jú hóng	桔红	Citri Reticulatae Rubrum, Exocarpium
jú huā	菊花	Chrysanthemi, Flos

Pīnyīn	Chinese	Pharmaceutical
kǔ shēn	苦参	Sophorae Flavescentis, Radix
lǎo hēi cù	老黑醋	Atrum Vetum, Acetum
lián qiáo	连翘	Forsythiae, Fructus
lián zǐ	莲子	Nelumbinis, Semen
líng xiāo huā	凌霄花	Campsis, Flos
lóng chǐ	龙齿	Draconis, Dentium
lóng dǎn cǎo	龙胆草	Gentianiae, Radix
lóng gǔ	龙骨	Calcinated Draconis, Os
lóng yǎn ròu	龙眼肉	Longan, Arillus
lú gān shí	炉甘石	Calamina
lú gēn	芦根	Phragmitis, Rhizoma
mǎ bó	马勃	Lasiosphaera/Calvatia
mǎ chǐ xiàn	马齿苋	Portulacae, Herba
mài mén dōng	麦门冬	Ophiopogonis Japonici, Tuber
mài yá	麦芽	Hordei Germantus, Fructus
méi guī huā	玫瑰花	Rosae Rugosae, Flos
míng fán	明矾	Alumen
mǔ dān pí	牡丹皮	Moutan, Cortex
mù guā	木瓜	Cydonium Sineuse
mù tōng	木通	Akebiae, Caulis
niú bàng zǐ	牛蒡子	Arctii Lappae, Fructus
niú xī	牛膝	Achyranthis, Radix
nǚ zhēn zǐ	女贞子	Ligustri Lucidi, Fructus
pú gōng yīng	蒲公英	Taraxaci, Herba
qiān dān	铅丹	Minium
qiān niú zǐ	牵牛子	Pharbitidis, Semen
qiāng huó	羌活	Notopterygii, Rhizoma Seu Radix
qīng dài	青黛	Indigo Naturalis
qīng fěn	轻粉	Calomelas
quán xiē	全蝎	Scorpio
rén shēn	人参	Ginseng, Radix
rén zhōng huáng	人中黄	Glycyrrhizae Extractionis Sedilis, Rulvis
ròu guì	肉桂	Cinnamomi, Cortex
sān léng	三棱	Sparganii, Rhizoma
sāng shèn	桑椹	Mori, Fructus

Pīnyīn	Chinese	Pharmaceutical
sāng yè	桑叶	Mori Albae, Folium
sāng zhī	桑枝	Mori, Ramulus
shā rén	砂仁	Amomi, Fructus
shā shēn	沙参	Adenophonrae seu Glehniae, Radix
shān yào	山药	Dioscorea, Rhizome
shān zhā	山楂	Crataegi, Fructus
shān zhū yú	山茱萸	Corni, Fructus
shé chuáng zī	蛇床子	Cnidii, Fructus
shè gān	射干	Belamcandae, Rhizoma
shén qǔ	神曲	Massa Medica Fermentata
shēng dì huáng	生地黄	Rehmanniae Glutinosae, Radix
shēng má	升麻	Cimicifugae, Rhizoma
shí chāng pú	石菖蒲	Acori Tatarinowii, Rhizoma
shí gāo	石膏	Gypsum Fibrosum
shú dì huáng	熟地黄	Rehmanniae Preparata, Radix
shuǐ niú jiǎo	水牛角	Bubali, Cornu
sōng xiāng	松香	Colophonium
tài zǐ shēn	太子参	Pseudostellaria, Radix
táo rén	桃仁	Persicae, Semen
tiān huā fěn	天花粉	Trichosanthis, Radix
tiān má	天麻	Gastrodiae Elatae, Rhizoma
tiān mén dōng	天门冬	Asparagi, Radix
tōng cǎo	通草	Tetrapanacis, Medulla
tòu gǔ cǎo	透骨草	Tuberculate Speranskia, Herba
tǔ fú líng	土茯苓	Smilacis Glabrae, Rhizoma
wáng bù liú xíng	王不留行	Vaccariae, Semen
wēi líng xiān	威灵仙	Clematidis, Radix
wǔ bèi zǐ	五倍子	Rhois Chinensis, Galla
wú gōng	蜈蚣	Scolopendra
wū shāo shé	乌梢蛇	Zaocys
xì xīn	细辛	Asari, Radix
xià kū cǎo	夏枯草	Prunellae Vulgaris, Spica
xiāng fù	香附	Cyperi, Rhizoma
xīn yí huā	辛夷花	Magnoliae, Flos
xìng rén	杏仁	Armeniacae, Semen

Pīnyīn	Chinese	Pharmaceutical
xú cháng qīng	徐长卿	Cynanchi Paniculati, Radix
xù duàn	续断	Dipsaci, Radix
xuán shēn	玄参	Scrophulariae Ningpoensis, Radix
yè jiāo téng	夜交藤	Polygoni Multiflori, Caulis
yě jú huā	野菊花	Chrysanthemi Indici, Flos
yì mǔ cǎo	益母草	Leonuri, Herba
yì yǐ rén	薏苡仁	Coices, Semen
yù jīn	郁金	Curcumae Radix
yú xīng cǎo	鱼腥草	Houttuynia Cordata Thunb., Herba
yù zhú	玉竹	Polygonati Odorati, Rhizoma
zào jiǎo	皂角	Gleditsiae, Fructus
zǎo xiū	蚤休	Paridis, Rhizoma
zé lán	泽兰	Lycopi, Herba
zé xiè	泽泻	Alismatis, Rhizoma
zhāng nǎo	樟脑	Camphora
zhēn zhū mǔ	珍珠母	Margaritaferae, Concha
zhì gān cǎo	炙甘草	Glycyrrhizae Preparata, Radix
zhǐ ké (zhǐ qiào)	枳壳	Citri Aurantii, Fructus
zhī má yóu	芝麻油	Sesame Oil
zhī mǔ	知母	Anemarrhenae, Rhizoma
zhǐ shí	枳实	Immaturus Citri Aurantii, Fructus
zhī zǐ	栀子	Gardeniae, Fructus
zhū líng	猪苓	Polyporus
zǐ cǎo	紫草	Arnebiae Seu Lithospermi, Radix
zǐ huā dì dīng	紫花地丁	Violae, Herba
zǐ jīng pí	紫荆皮	Kadsurae Radicis, Cortex

Appendix III: *Pīnyīn*-Chinese-English Formula Cross Reference

Pīnyīn	Chinese	English
Bái Hǔ Tāng	白虎汤	White Tiger Decoction
Bài Jiàng Cǎo Gāo	败酱草膏	White Flower Patrinia Ointment
Bái Zhú Gāo	白术膏	Dark Atractylodis Ointment
Bì Xiè Shèn Shī Tāng	萆薢渗湿汤	Dioscorea Decoction to Leach Out Dampness
Cāng Ěr Yāng Shuǐ Jì	苍耳秧水剂	Cang Er Yang Wash
Cāng Ěr Zǐ Sǎn	苍耳子散	Xanthium Powder
Cāng Zhú Gāo	苍术膏	Black Atractylodis Ointment
Chú Shī Wèi Líng Tāng	除湿胃苓汤	Eliminate Dampness Decoction by Combining Calm the Stomach with Five Ingredient Powder with Poria
Dān Zhī Xiāo Yáo Sǎn	丹栀逍遥散	Moutan and Gardenia Rambling Powder
Dāng Guī Yǐn Zǐ	当归饮子	Chinese Angelica Drink
Dǎo Chì Sǎn	导赤散	Guide Out the Red Powder
Èr Miào Sǎn	二妙散	Two-Marvel Powder
Guī Téng Xǐ Jì	归藤洗剂	Gui Teng Wash
Hēi Bù Yào Gāo	黑布药膏	Black Cloth Medicated Paste
Hēi Dòu Liú Yóu Ruǎn Gāo	黑豆馏油软膏	Black Soybean Distillate Ointment
Huà Bān Jiě Dú Tāng	化斑解毒汤	Maculae Transforming and Toxicity Removing Decoction
Huà Bān Tāng	化斑汤	Transform Maculae Decoction
Huà Dú Sǎn	化毒散	Toxicity Transforming Powder
Huà Dú Sǎn Gāo	化毒散膏	Toxicity Transforming Powder Paste
Huáng Bǎi Róng Yè	黄柏溶液	Phellodendri Cortex Solution
Huáng Bǎi Sǎn	黄柏散	Phellodendron Bark Powder

Pīnyīn	Chinese	English
Huáng Lián Gāo	黄连膏	Coptis Rhizome Ointment
Huáng Lián Jiě Dú Tāng	黄连解毒汤	Coptis Decoction to Relieve Toxicity
Huáng Lián Sǎn	黄连散	Coptis Rhizome Powder
Jiě Dú Xǐ Yào	解毒洗药	Detoxifying Lotion
Liù Wèi Dì Huáng Wán	六味地黄丸	Six Ingredient Pill with Rehmannia
Liù Yī Sǎn	六一散	Six-to-One Powder
Lóng Dǎn Cǎo Cā Jì	龙胆草擦剂	Gentian Liniment
Lóng Dǎn Xiè Gān Tāng	龙胆泻肝汤	Gentian Decoction to Drain the Liver
Pí Fū Píng Ruǎn Gāo	皮肤平软膏	Skin Smoothing Ointment
Píng Wèi Sǎn	平胃散	Calm the Stomach Powder
Pí Shī Yī Hào Gāo	皮湿一号膏	Eczema Ointment No. 1
Pǔ Jì Xiāo Dú Yǐn	普济消毒饮	Universal Benefit Drink to Eliminate Toxin
Qīng Dài Sǎn	青黛散	Indigo Powder
Qīng Liáng Gāo	清凉膏	Clearing and Cooling Ointment
Qīng Rè Shèn Shī Tāng	清热渗湿汤	Clearing Heat and Draining Dampness Decoction
Qū Shī Sǎn	祛湿散	Damp-Removing Medicinal Powder
Rùn Jī Gāo	润肌膏	Flesh Moistening Ointment
Sān Huáng Xǐ Jì	三黄洗剂	Three Yellow Cleanser Formula
Sān Miào Wán	三妙丸	Three Marvel Pill
Sān Xīn Dǎo Chì Yǐn	三心导赤饮	Three-Pith Guide out the Red Powder
Shā Shēn Mài Mén Dōng Tāng	沙参麦门冬汤	Glehnia & Ophiopogon Combination
Shé Chuáng Zǐ Tāng	蛇床子汤	Cnidium Fruit Decoction
Shēn Líng Bái Zhú Sǎn	参苓白朮散	Ginseng, Poria, and Atractylodis Macrocephalae Powder
Shēng Má Tāng	升麻汤	Cimicifuga Decoction
Shēng Má Xiāo Dú Yǐn	升麻消毒饮	Cimicifuga Decoction to Eliminate Toxins
Shī Zhěn Sǎn	湿疹散	Eczema Powder
Sì Huáng Gāo	四黄膏	Four Yellow Cream
Sì Huáng Sǎn	四黄散	Four Yellow Powder
Sì Jūn Zǐ Tāng	四君子汤	Four Gentlemen Decoction
Sì Wù Tāng	四物汤	Four Substance Decoction
Sì Wù Xiāo Fēng Yǐn	四物消风饮	Eliminate Wind Drink with the Four Substances
Wèi Líng Tāng	胃苓汤	Calm the Stomach and Poria Decoction

Pīnyīn	Chinese	English
Wǔ Huáng Gāo	五黄膏	Five Huang Cream
Wǔ Líng Sǎn	五苓散	Five Ingredient Powder with Poria
Wǔ Wèi Xiāo Dú Yǐn	五味消毒饮	Five Ingredient Decoction to Eliminate Toxins
Xiāo Ér Huà Shī Tāng	小儿化湿汤	Children's Dampness Removing Decoction
Xiāo Fēng Dǎo Chì Tāng	消风导赤汤	Eliminate Wind and Guide Out the Red Decoction
Xiāo Fēng Sǎn	消风散	Eliminate Wind Powder
Xiāo Yáo Sǎn	逍遥散	Rambling Powder
Xiè Huáng Sǎn	泻黄散	Drain the Yellow Powder
Xīn Sān Miào Sǎn	新三妙散	New Three Marvels Powder
Xuè Fǔ Zhú Yū Tāng	血府逐瘀汤	Drive Out Stasis in the Mansion of Blood Decoction
Yǎng Xuè Dìng Fēng Tāng	养血定风汤	Nourishing Blood and Subduing Wind Decoction
Yǎng Xuè Rùn Fū Yǐn	养血润肤饮	Nourish the Blood and Moisten the Skin Drink
Yín Qiào Sǎn	银翘散	Honeysuckle and Forsythia Powder
Zào Shī Xǐ Gāo	燥湿洗膏	Damp-Heat Eliminating Ointment
Zēng Yè Tāng	增液汤	Increase the Fluids Decoction
Zhī Bǎi Dì Huáng Wán	知柏地黄丸	Anemarrhena, Phellodendron, and Rehmannia Pill
Zhǐ Yǎng Xǐ Jì	止痒洗剂	Anti-Itch Wash
Zǐ Sè Xiāo Zhǒng Fěn	紫色消肿粉	Purple Powder to Reduce Swelling
Zī Yīn Chú Shī Tāng	滋阴除湿汤	Yin-Enriching, Dampness-Eliminating Decoction

Appendix IV: Source Text Bibliography

Pīnyīn Title	Chinese Title	English Title	Author (English)	Author (Chinese)	Published
Chuāng Yáng Jīng Yàn Quán Shū	疮疡经验全书	Complete Manual of Experience in the Treatment of Sores	Dòu Hàn-Qīng	窦汉卿	Appeared in 1569, publishing year differs depending on the source
Dān Xī Xīn Fǎ	丹溪心法	Essential Teachings of [Zhū] Dān-Xī	Zhū Zhèn-Hēng, aka Zhū Dān-Xī	朱震亨 (朱丹溪)	1481
Dòng Tiān Ào Zhǐ	洞天奥旨	Collection of Secrets of External Medicine	Chén Shì-Duó	陈世铎	17th century–18th century
Huáng Dì Nèi Jīng	黄帝内经	The Yellow Emperor's Classic of Internal Medicine	Unknown	未知	Between the late Warring States period and the Hàn Dynasty
Jì Shēng Fāng	济生方	Formulas to Aid the Living	Yán Yòng-Hé	严用和	1253
Jīn Guì Yào Lüè	金匮要略	Essentials from the Golden Cabinet	Zhāng Jī	张机	ca. 220
Liú Juān Zǐ Guǐ Yí Fāng	刘涓子鬼遗方	Liú Juān-Zǐ's Ghost-Bequeathed Formulas	Liú Juān-Zǐ	刘涓子	499
Nèi Kē Zhāi Yào	内科摘要	Summary of Internal Medicine	Xuē Jǐ	薛己	1529

Pīnyīn Title	Chinese Title	English Title	Author (English)	Author (Chinese)	Published
Pǔ Jì Fāng	普济方	Prescriptions for Universal Relief	Zhū Sù et al.	朱橚等編	1406
Rú Mén Shì Qīn	儒门事亲	Confucians' Duties to Their Parents	Zhāng Cóng-Zhèng	张从正	1228
Shèng Jì Zǒng Lù	圣济总录	Comprehensive Recording of Divine Assistance	Goverment, Imperial Court of the Sòng Dynasty	宋代政府	1111–1117
Tài Píng Huì Mín Hé Jì Jú Fāng	太平惠民和剂局方	Formulary of the Pharmacy Service for Benefiting the People in the Taiping Era	Imperial Medical Bureau	太医局	1107–1110
Wài Kē Dà Chéng	外科大成	Great Compendium of External Medicine	Qí Kūn	祁坤	1665
Wài Kē Jīng Yì	外科精义	Quintessence of External Medicine	Qí Dé-Zhī	齐德之	1335
Wài Kē Xīn Fǎ Yào Jué	外科心法要诀	Essential Teachings on External Medicine	Wú Qiān	吴谦	1742
Wài Kē Zhēn Quán	外科真诠	Personal Experience in Wài Kē	Zōu Yuè	邹岳	1838
Wài Kē Zhèng Zhì Quán Shū	外科证治全书	Complete Treatise of Patterns and Treatments in External Medicine	Xǔ Kè-Chāng	许克昌	1831
Wài Kē Zhèng Zōng	外科正宗	Orthodox Lineage of External Medicine	Chén Shí-Gōng	陈实功	1617
Wēn Bìng Tiáo Biàn	温病条辨	Systematic Differentiation of Warm Pathogen Diseases	Wú Jū-Tōng (Wú Táng)	吴鞠通 (吴瑭)	1798

Pīnyīn Title	Chinese Title	English Title	Author (English)	Author (Chinese)	Published
Wǔ Shí Èr Bìng Fāng	五十二病方	Prescriptions for Fifty-Two Diseases	Unknown	未知	1065–771 BC
Xiān Shòu Lǐ Shāng Xù Duàn Mì Fāng	仙授理伤续断秘方	Secret Formulas to Manage Trauma and Reconnect Fractures Received from an Immortal	Lìn Dào-Rén	蔺道人	846
Xiǎo Ér Yào Zhèng Zhí Jué	小儿药证直诀	Craft of Medicinal Treatment for Childhood Disease Patterns	Qián Yǐ	钱乙	1119
Yáng Kē Huì Cuì	疡科会粹	A Gathering of External Sores	Sūn Zhèn-Yuán	孙震元	1802
Yáng Kē Xīn Dé Jí	疡科心得集	Collected Experience on Treating External Sores	Gāo Bǐng-Jūn	高秉钧	1805
Yī Fāng Jí Jiě	医方集解	Medical Formulas Collected and Analyzed	Wāng Áng	汪昂	1682
Yī Fāng Kǎo	医方考	Investigations of Medical Formulas	Wú Kūn	吴昆	1584
Yī Zōng Jīn Jiàn	医宗金鉴	The Golden Mirror of Medical Tradition	Wú Qiān et al.	吴谦等	1742
Yòu Yòu Jí Chéng	幼幼集成	Complete Work on Children's Diseases	Chén Fù-Zhèng	陈复正	1750
Zhāng Zhì-Lǐ Pí Fū Bìng Yī Àn Xuǎn Cuì	张志礼皮肤病医案选萃	A Collection of Zhang Zhili's Medical Experience in Dermatology	Zhāng Zhì-Lǐ	张志礼	2000
Zhào Bǐng-Nán Lín Chuáng Jīng Yàn Jí	赵炳南临床经验集	Zhào Bǐng-Nán's Clinical Experience Set	Zhào Bǐng-Nán	赵炳南	1975

Pīnyīn Title	Chinese Title	English Title	Author (English)	Author (Chinese)	Published
Zhōng Huá Rén Mín Gòng Hé Guó Wèi Shēng Bù Yào Pǐn Biāo Zhǔn Zhōng Yào Chéng Fāng Zhì Jì Dì Wǔ Cè	中华人民共和国卫生部药品标准中药成方制剂第五册	Drug Standards for Traditional Chinese Medicine Prescriptions Volume V	Pharmacopoeia Committee of the Ministry of Health of the People's Republic of China	中华人民共和国卫生部药典委员会	Appeared in 1992, publishing year differs depending on the source
Zhōng Yī Bìng Zhèng Zhěn Duàn Liáo Xiào Biāo Zhǔn	中医病证诊断疗效标准	Criteria for Diagnosis and Treatment of TCM Syndromes	State Administration of Traditional Chinese Medicine	国家中医药管理局	1994
Zhōng Yī Pí Fū Bìng Xué Jiǎn Biān	中医皮肤病学简编	Compendium of TCM Dermatology	Chéng Yùn-Qián	程运乾	1979
Zhǒu Hòu Bèi Jí Fāng	肘后备急方	Emergency Formulas to Keep Up One's Sleeve	Gě Hóng	葛洪	ca. 363
Zhū Bìng Yuán Hóu Lùn	诸病源侯论	General Treatise on the Etiology and Symptomology of Diseases	Cháo Yuán-Fāng	巢元方	610
Zhū Rén-Kāng Lín Chuáng Jīng Yàn Jí	朱仁康临床经验集	A Collection of Zhū Rén-Kāng's Clinical Experiences	Zhū Rén-Kāng	朱仁康	1979
		Complete External Therapies of Chinese Drugs	Xú Xiàng-Cái	徐象才	1998

Subject Index

Herb Index

Formula Index